Concepts of Epidemiology

Concepts
of Epidemiology
Integrating the ideas, theories, principles, and methods of epidemiology

THIRD EDITION

Raj S. Bhopal, CBE, MD, DSc (hon), MPH, BSc (hon), MBChB, FFPH, FRCP(E)

Alexander Bruce and John Usher Professor of Public Health, University of Edinburgh, and Honorary Consultant in Public Health, NHS Lothian Board, UK

formerly

Professor and Head of the Department of Epidemiology and Public Health, University of Newcastle Upon Tyne, UK

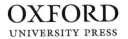
OXFORD
UNIVERSITY PRESS

OXFORD

UNIVERSITY PRESS

Great Clarendon Street, Oxford, OX2 6DP,
United Kingdom

Oxford University Press is a department of the University of Oxford.
It furthers the University's objective of excellence in research, scholarship,
and education by publishing worldwide. Oxford is a registered trade mark of
Oxford University Press in the UK and in certain other countries

First Edition published in 2002
Second Edition published in 2008
Third Edition published in 2016

Impression: 1

Published in the United States of America by Oxford University Press
198 Madison Avenue, New York, NY 10016, United States of America

British Library Cataloguing in Publication Data

Data available

Library of Congress Control Number: 2016945263

ISBN 978–0–19–873968–5

Printed in Great Britain by
Clays Ltd, St Ives plc

Dedication to the Third Edition

I dedicate this third edition to my wife Roma, my sons Sunil, Vijay, Anand, and Rajan, my daughter-in-law Hannah, and my grandson Leo, for their love, which enriches my life.

Dedication to the Second Edition

I dedicate this second edition to my brothers Sohan, Kalwant (deceased 1989), Jaswant, Surinder and Mhinder, and my sisters Harbans, Sheila, and Baljinder for their love, support, example, and direction.

Dedication to the First Edition

I dedicate this book to my mother Bhagwanti Kaur Bhopal[†] for impressing on me (and my siblings) the importance of education, and encouraging us to make up for her own lack of schooling and formal education; and to my father Jhanda Singh Bhopal[†] for setting an example of how to work hard, shoulder responsibility, and strive for self-improvement.

[†](deceased 2010)

Foreword

Foreword to the Third edition

A concept is a general idea or understanding, usually of something abstract rather than concrete. Raj Bhopal's *Concepts of Epidemiology* conveys the general ideas and understanding of epidemiology supremely well, perhaps better than any other monograph on the discipline of epidemiology. It has the added virtues of being clearly and concisely written, and provides comprehensive cover of all essential aspects. I thought the first edition was the best book of its kind that I had ever read. The second edition was even better; and now this third edition clarifies the ideas and enhances understanding even better than ever. It is a book that ought to be bedside reading for all epidemiologists everywhere.

John M. Last
Emeritus Professor of Epidemiology
University of Ottawa

Foreword to the second edition

The exciting, innovative features of Raj Bhopal's book are the emphasis throughout on a conceptual approach and the systematic focus on underlying concepts and fundamental principles. This approach leads students of epidemiology, the intended readers of the book, to a logical understanding of the methods and procedures used in epidemiological research and practice. That was why I endorsed the first edition with unqualified enthusiasm.

The second edition is a thorough revision of the first. There is extensive rewriting and updating throughout the text, which remains crystal clear, easy to read, and easy to understand. The details are specified in the Preface. Students of epidemiology who use this book to enter upon their study of epidemiology have every reason to be grateful to Raj Bhopal for making their task easier and more pleasurable than it might otherwise be.

I am happy to endorse this new edition with the same unqualified enthusiasm with which I greeted the first edition.

John M. Last
Emeritus Professor of Epidemiology
University of Ottawa

Foreword to the first edition

When I was learning epidemiology in the late 1950s, I was inspired by the first edition of Jerry Morris's now—classic little monograph, *Uses of Epidemiology*, but there were hardly any comprehensive current textbooks to guide me. The few available books were either unreadable, unhelpful, or failed to orient my thoughts along the directions my ideas were taking. How times have changed! Now there are so many good books that it is difficult for the uninitiated to select the most suitable one to meet their needs. In 1997, Raj Bhopal reviewed 25 textbooks of epidemiology, discussing their approach to the subject, and their strengths and weaknesses, in a critical commentary that is helpful to teachers and learners alike. Now, from the University of Edinburgh (where I spent five happy years in the 1960s), Raj Bhopal, who holds the Usher chair of public health, has written his own introductory textbook for graduate students who are embarking upon the detailed study of epidemiology.

This is an excellent introduction. Raj Bhopal's approach is conceptual—he describes and explains the underlying concepts and methods of epidemiology with clarity and with apt examples, and simple, elegant illustrations. Frequently throughout the text he asks penetrating questions that will test the limits of his readers' intellectual capacity—an admirable feature that other authors could copy with benefit to themselves and their readers. All the essentials are here: the person-population dyad, variation, error, bias, confounding, causality, the spectrum of disease, the 'iceberg' concept, risk and its relationship to disease frequency, study design, the ethical framework within which we practise epidemiology and conduct research, the relationship of epidemiology to other scholarly pursuits, and finally, some thoughts about the way the discipline has evolved and is likely to continue to evolve in the lifetime of those now entering upon careers in this field.

If I may speak directly to students starting the study of epidemiology: you can be grateful that there is a book like this to guide you along the fascinating pathway that leads to epidemiological enlightenment and understanding. This book will enable you to comprehend the connections between individual and population health, the natural history of disease, the methods of epidemiology, the interventions that work and don't work, and the role of epidemiology as the fundamental public health science. This is a book for you to buy, to read, to study, and to enjoy.

John M. Last
Emeritus Professor of Epidemiology
University of Ottawa

Preface

Preface (incorporating that for the first and second editions)

After the first edition in 2002 and given the durability of concepts and methods I thought I could rest up, perhaps for ever! Instead, numerous changes and additions were required for a second edition only six years later. I was amazed to find so much new to do for the third edition only seven years on.

A concept is a complex idea, or a cluster of interrelated ideas. A concept lies behind the word or phrase we use to describe something. This book aims to explain and illustrate the ideas underlying the language, principles, techniques, and core methods in epidemiology.

I explain the key concepts underpinning the science of epidemiology and its applications to research, policy-making, health-service planning, and health promotion. I emphasize theory, ideas, and epidemiological axioms to counter the criticism that epidemiology is an atheoretical discipline.

There are 10 chapters. Many introductory courses are designed around 10–15 or so sessions. I envisage that the core of this book could be grasped in 10 days of committed study, preferably in the context of a taught course, but also independently. I have written the book with the special needs in mind of students who are studying independently or online. Appendix 1 provides some ideas for teachers on potential curriculae for taught courses for undergraduate and postgraduate students and in continuing education.

The learning objectives introducing each chapter are expressed mostly in terms of the reader acquiring understanding. I believe that understanding is the highest form of learning, from which may flow durable knowledge, changes of attitude, and the achievement of skills. Understanding often comes from solving problems and answering questions (i.e. active learning). I have incorporated numerous challenging exercises, some of them requiring basic mathematical concepts and calculations. Mostly, these are embedded in the text but some conclude each chapter.

This book is deliberately thorough in its discussions, and not simply brief and descriptive, and this is to help readers to achieve a deeper understanding and to help bridge the world of theory to that of practice.

The book places emphasis on integrating the ideas of epidemiology. The interdependence of epidemiological studies and their essential unity is a particularly important theme.

In the first edition I stated that this book differs in many ways from alternatives, for example:

- The concepts of epidemiology are discussed in detail, and in an integrated way.
- The concepts are dominant whereas in other books the methods dominate.
- The epidemiological idea of population is explicitly the foundation of the whole book. In most other books, the population idea is implicit, and in some it is neglected.
- The practical applications of each concept are considered, and illustrated with examples drawn from contemporary research and public health practice, including health-care policy and planning. The idea is that the reader will acquire the depth of knowledge to use the concepts and not merely be aware of them.

- The work is rooted in the basic ideas of the science of epidemiology, which are wholly applicable worldwide.
- The emphasis is on gaining understanding, and not on calculations, except where this is essential to understanding.
- Most of the exercises require reflection not calculation.

I think this analysis is still correct.

Second Edition

In preparation for the second edition, I looked to criticisms and comments of book reviewers, previous students, and co-teachers. Surprisingly, the book earned much praise and little criticism. Nonetheless, I made many changes, some of them in response to specific feedback, including:

- simpler writing, particularly to meet the needs of students whose main language is not English, and those without a medical/clinical background;
- several new questions, answers, problems, and exercises, including 20 questions in Chapter 9 to develop students' understanding of study design;
- a brief introduction in Chapter 1 to incidence, prevalence, and study design;
- a set of questions with model answers so students can test themselves at the end of each chapter;
- a brief introduction to genetic epidemiology;
- extra concepts including correlation/regression, regression to the mean, and regression dilution bias, effect modification and interaction, receiver operating curves, the counterfactual approach, and birth cohort analysis in relation to cross-sectional and secular trends;
- an introduction to the purposes and principles of reviews, systematic reviews, and meta-analysis;
- a clearer exposition of epidemiology's relation to statistics, based on the principles underpinning epidemiological analysis of data;
- expansion in many directions including on epidemiological variables and data privacy.

Third Edition

My focus remains on the ideas, strategies, methods, and applications of the discipline. What added value might readers expect in this revision? In addition to more rigorously edited and updated and yet expanded text, with further simplification of language, readers will find:

- The use of exemplars, highlighted in panels, to illustrate the concepts and methods under consideration in every chapter
- Much more emphasis on causality, and an introduction to the language and approaches of causal graphs
- Introduction to the language (including an expanded glossary) and approaches of the directed acyclic graph (DAG), translating the technical terms into more familiar epidemiological words and phrases (with an exemplar)
- More and deeper consideration of the qualities of epidemiological variables
- Expansion of previously introductory material on how new genetic technologies are changing epidemiology, with special emphasis on the Mendelian randomization study (with an exemplar)
- Fuller consideration of the technical, ethical, conceptual, and practical epidemiological issues arising from computerized linkage of records (with exemplars)

- A clearer explanation of the way one moves from data to information and intelligence through systematic analysis and interpretation
- A clearer exposition of difficult ideas including non-differential misclassification, effect modification, and its statistical equivalent of interaction
- An expansion of the study design chapter
- In line with trends in epidemiology, a clearer distinction between proportions and rates, including adoption of distinctive terminology when appropriate
- Consideration of the potential implications for extremely large influence on tens of millions, if not hundreds of millions, of people

The old favourites in previous editions are still there; for example, thought exercises embedded in the text, numerical calculations, historical references (also see Appendix 2 for further reading and useful websites), and the links between epidemiology and both clinical and public health practice. Readers acquainted with the first edition will recognize the style, and hopefully they will agree it has matured and improved, and not just grown fatter over time.

I meet readers of *Concepts of Epidemiology* in all corners of the globe and I am heartened by their remarks. They tell me that this book explains complex issues simply. I have worked to ensure this third edition will make difficult ideas even easier. Let me know whether you agree (email me at raj.bhopal@ed.ac.uk).

Happy reading!

Raj Bhopal
December 2015

Acknowledgements

Acknowledgements for the Third Edition

I will never forget my debts to those who have helped me to write this book, and they are recorded in the Acknowledgements for the first and second editions (abridged). This page, as a result, is short. First, I thank my secretary Anne Houghton whose help in a myriad of tasks made this revision possible. The motive to take on the task came from OUP's commissioning editor and much help was given by Caroline Smith and James Cox.

Dr Debbie Lawlor has given me many insights into the topic of interaction. Dr Snorri Rafnsson, Dr Markus Steiner and Dr Colin Fischbacher's (co-teachers) have helped in my new writings, the latter two especially on causality and DAGs. Professor Harry Campbell checked the new writings on Mendelian randomization. I am solely responsible for any errors or misinterpretations.

I thank my students, colleagues, and fellow writers across the world. I am indebted to the University of Edinburgh for providing the challenging yet stable academic environment required for this kind of endeavour. Permissions for reproducing others' work are recorded separately, but I also express my gratitude here. I thank John Last for his generous foreword.

Finally, I have dedicated this edition to my immediate family, which is the least they deserve.

Acknowledgements for the Second Edition (abridged)

OUP has proven itself a most supportive publisher with many highly professional colleagues— I thank especially Helen Liepman, Georgia Pinteau, Rosemary Bailey, and Claire Caruana for their feedback, encouragement, and help over the years that has spurred me to prepare this edition.

Professor John Last's support has been constant and reflected in his splendid second Foreword for me. Dr Colin Fischbacher's comments on all the new sections were invaluable for he has a keen and critical eye. My postdoctoral colleague Dr Charles Agyemang gave prompt, enthusiastic, and able feedback on the new material. Professor Harry Campbell offered expert guidance on my introduction to genetics. Professor Richard Heller provided excellent material on population impact numbers, so if my distillation has impurities, this is my responsibility. Dr Sarah Wild helped me think about the section on interaction.

My family is now used to me and my scribbles. I thank my children Sunil, Vijay, Anand, and Rajan for the joy and fulfilment they give me. Without the tolerance and love of my wife, Roma, I would not have had the peace of mind, focus, and drive to pursue my academic passions. In trying to thank her I am, for once, lost for words!

February 2008

Acknowledgements for the First Edition (abridged)

My foremost debt is to the innumerable people who have taught me, whether in the classroom, seminar, and conference, or by their writings. One absorbs ideas and facts from others and over time synthesizes them with one's own thoughts and experiences. Eventually, it is impossible to distinguish one's own ideas from those of others. If my readers recognize their own ideas, and think they are incompletely acknowledged, then please accept my thanks and let me know.

Marcus Steiner, an MSc (Epidemiology) student and graduate at Edinburgh University, was my postgraduate reader-critic and helper. His advice and help, particularly with the technical preparation and development of the figures, was immensely useful.

Dr Sonja Hunt stimulated me to think about Figure 10.1. Dr Colin Fischbacher helped me proofread the manuscript and made several thoughtful observations. Professor John Last enthusiastically agreed to write the Foreword.

Others who provided academic advice on one or more specific chapters include: Professor Carl Shy, Dr David Chappel, Dr Eileen Kaner, and four anonymous referees who commented on the book proposal and chapter outlines.

I thank Dr Mike Lavender for permission to use extracts from our joint unpublished paper on the role of epidemiology in priority setting, and co-authors on various publications that I have drawn upon (these are referenced). I have drawn heavily on my publications to prepare Chapter 10 and Acknowledgements, details of which are given below.

Helen Liepman, Commissioning Editor at Oxford University Press, deserves thanks for her enthusiasm, expert support, and patience.

I conceived this book while in my post as Professor of Epidemiology and Public Health at the University of Newcastle upon Tyne, England. The embryonic and fetal growth stages of the idea were nourished during my sabbatical at the Department of Epidemiology of the School of Public Health at the University of North Carolina at Chapel Hill, and on my return to Newcastle. The birthplace of the book, however, was in Edinburgh University.

Secretarial support was provided chiefly by Lorna Hutchison, Carole Frazer (both Newcastle University), Betsy Seagroves (University of North Carolina), Janet Logan, and Hazel King (both Edinburgh University).

I offer grateful thanks to my wife Roma for encouraging me to finish the project, for accepting the sleep disruption caused by early morning shuffling as I slipped out of bed and into the study, and for my lack of enthusiasm for late night revelries. I have four sons, Sunil, Vijay, Anand, and Rajan, and I ask their forgiveness for sometimes being too busy and distracted to give them and their passions the attention they deserved.

R.S.B.
2001

Contents

Abbreviations

AIDS	Acquired Immune Deficiency Syndrome
AR	Attributable risk
AUC	Area under the curve
BCG	Bacillus Calmette–Guérin
BMI	Body mass index
BMJ	British Medical Journal
BSE	Bovine spongiform encephalopathy
CDC	Centers for Disease Control and Prevention
CHD	Coronary heart disease
CHI	Community Health Index
CI	Confidence intervals
CJD	Creutzfeldt-Jakob disease
CVD	Cardiovascular disease
DAG	Directed acyclic graph
DALY	Disability-adjusted life years
DNA	Deoxyribonucleic acid
ECG	Electrocardiogram
ECT	Electroconvulsive therapy
ERSPC	European Randomized Study of Screening for Prostate Cancer
EQUATOR	Enhancing the QUAlity and Transparency Of health Research
GBD	Global Burden of Disease
GIS	Geographical information systems
GNP	Gross National Product
GRACE	Global Registry of Acute Coronary Events
GWAS	Genome-wide association study
HALY	Health-adjusted life year
HDL	High-density lipoprotein
HEA	Health Education Authority
HIV	Human Immunodeficiency Virus
ICD	International Classification of Diseases
ICMJE	International Committee of Medical Journal Editors
IEA	International Epidemiological Association
LDL	Low-density lipoprotein
LVH	Left ventricular hypertrophy
MI	Myocardial infarction
MINAP	Myocardial Ischaemia National Audit Project
MMR	Measles, mumps, and rubella
NEPP	Number of events prevented in a population
NHANES	National Health and Nutrition Examination Surveys
NHS	National Health Service
NIH	National Institutes for Health
NNT	Number needed to treat
NNP	Number needed to prevent
NICE	National Institute for Clinical and Public Health Excellence
OR	Odds ratio
PAHO	Pan American Health Organization
PAR	Population-attributable risk
PI	Physical inactivity
PM	Proportional mortality
PMR	Proportional morbidity or mortality ratio
PODOSA	Prevention of diabetes and obesity in South Asians
PPOD	Population pattern of disease
PSA	Prostate specific antigen
PYLL	Potential years of life lost
QALY	Quality-adjusted life years
RCT	Randomized controlled trial
RNA	Ribonucleic acid
ROC	Receiver operating characteristic
RR	Relative risk
SEP	Socio-economic position
SHELS	Scottish Health and Ethnicity Linkage Study
SIDS	Sudden infant death syndrome
SMR	Standardized mortality ratio
SNP	Single nucleotide polymorphism
TB	Tuberculosis

UNESCO	United Nations Educational, Scientific and Cultural Organization	UV	Ultraviolet
UK	United Kingdom	WCEC	World Council on Epidemiology and Causation
USA	United States of America	WHO	World Health Organization
US	United States (of America)	YOLL	Years of life lost

Glossary of selected terms

The glossary focuses on clinical terminology, and terminology relating to directed acyclic graphs (introduced in the third edition), and excludes many terms and concepts considered in the main text, which can be accessed via the index.

Acute An adjective commonly applied to diseases that have a short time course.

Adenocarcinoma A cancer of mucosal cells.

Aetiology/aetiological Causation/about causation.

AIDS Acquired immune deficiency syndrome, the serious multisystem disease resulting from infection by the human immunodeficiency virus (HIV).

Allele *see* **Gene.**

Ancestor In DAG (see entry) terminology all preceding factors in the causal line that are linked to the exposure under study.

Anorexia Impaired appetite for food which can lead to serious illness; when caused by psychological factors it is called anorexia nervosa.

Angina *see* **Rose angina.**

Arrhythmia An abnormal rhythm—usually applied to the heart.

Association A link, connection, or relationship, between risk factors, between diseases, and most usually between risk factors and diseases.

Asthma A respiratory disease characterized by difficulty in breathing caused by narrowing of the airways (which is reversible).

Atherosclerosis/atherosclerotic The process of deposition of lipids and other materials in the walls of arteries leads to their narrowing and to inflammation. Such an artery is atherosclerotic (also known as arteriosclerosis/arteriosclerotic).

Atrial fibrillation An irregular heart beat resulting from very rapid and irregular contractions of the atrium (one of the chambers of the heart).

Attenuation Reduction of the measured effect of a cause in epidemiology. In microbiology it means that the virulence of microbes is reduced through processes that attenuate the effects (e.g. in the production of vaccines).

Autopsy *see* **Necropsy.**

Autosomal A genetic disorder relating to any chromosome except the sex (X and Y) chromosomes.

Backdoor path A non-causal path arising from an association with a third factor between a putative cause and outcome. In epidemiology, this is the effect of the confounding variable. In a DAG the arrow for this path points to the exposure.

Blocked/Blocking A causal path that is closed off as a result of the third factor (confounder).

Blood pressure Usually refers to the pressure in the systemic arteries (not veins and pulmonary arteries), as measured by sphygmomanometer (see below).

Brucellosis An infection caused by Brucella microorganisms, characterized by recurrent fevers.

Capture–recapture method A technique whereby two or more incomplete data sets are used to estimate the true size of the population of interest. Usually in epidemiology, the method is applied to populations that are hard to count (e.g. the homeless).

Cancer *see* **Neoplasm**.

Carcinogen(ic) A substance that increases the risk of developing a cancer (an adjective describing such a substance).

Case A person with the disease or problem under investigation.

Caseous An adjective applied to cheese-like lesions produced in response to inflammation (e.g. in tuberculosis).

Cataract An opacity in the lens of the eye.

Causal diagram A general term for a variety of approaches to showing the relationships between variables in graphic form. Within epidemiology these diagrams set out the relationship between exposure variables and outcomes, in relation to other variables such as confounders. One formal causal diagram is the directed acyclic graph (DAG).

Causal graph *see* **Causal diagram** (synonym).

Causation The term is commonly used in epidemiology, public health, and medicine as an alternative to aetiology.

Cause Something which has an effect; in the case of epidemiology this effect being (primarily) a change in the frequency of risk factors or adverse health outcomes in populations.

Causality The relationship between causes and effects.

CAD or coronary artery disease *see* **Coronary heart disease**.

Cholesterol A lipid (fatty substance) that is essential to many bodily functions that is transported in the blood via lipoproteins. Cholesterol and other lipids carried by low/very low-density lipoproteins (LDL/VLDL) are a risk factor for cardiovascular diseases, while those carried by high-density lipoproteins (HDL) may be protective.

Child In DAG terminology—the immediate descendant of the variable.

Chromosome *see* **Gene**.

Chronic An adjective commonly applied to diseases that have a long-lasting time course, and usually applied to non-toxic and non-infectious diseases.

Chronic bronchitis A lung disease characterized by production of excess sputum, wheezing, shortness of breath, and eventual respiratory failure.

Circadian A rhythm with a cycle lasting about 24 hours, corresponding to each day.

Collapsibility The situation where measure of association remains unchanged despite omission of variables from the model and where stratified and un-stratified results are the same. Collapsibility is not the same as confounding but a more general concept including both confounding and M-bias.

Collider A term used in DAGs for a variable where both the exposure and the outcome have an arrow (path) leading to it. In other words, the exposure and outcome, together, are the causes (parents) of the collider.

Competing causes (or competing risks) A concept where alternative causes of disease, or more usually causes of death, are in competition with each other; for example, in African Caribbean populations one explanation of the comparatively low CHD rates is that the atherosclerotic process kills people from stroke. If stroke were to be controlled, it may be that CHD would become more common.

Collider stratification bias *see* **M-bias.**

Community medicine *see* **Public health.**

Conditioning bias *see* **M-bias.**

Confidence interval The interval, with a given probability (e.g. 95%), within which is contained the population value of a summary measure such as a mean from a sample.

Confounding The distortion of the measure of an association between two variables by other (confounding) factors that influence both the variables under study.

Contagion/contagious The infectious diseases that may be transmitted from person-to-person.

Congenital A health problem present at birth.

Cooling tower A term that describes a structure, sometimes including evaporative condensers, designed to extract heat from a liquid—usually water—before its recirculation.

Coronary heart disease/coronary artery disease A group of diseases resulting from reduced blood supply to the heart, most often caused by narrowing or blockage of the coronary arteries that provide the blood supply to the heart.

Correlation analysis The extent that variables are associated with each other. The word is usually applied to continuous variables. The association can be measured by a statistical technique giving the correlation coefficient which varies from –1 (inverse correlation) to +1 (positive correlation).

Cot death A synonym for the sudden infant death syndrome, which is unexplained death in infancy.

Crohn's disease A disorder usually of the lower part of the small intestine, characterized by inflammation.

Cutaneous Associated with the skin.

D-connected/connection A path that is open.

D-separation or D-separated A path that is closed, either through confounding or M-bias or both. So it consolidates the ways in which a causal path con be blocked.

DAG Acronym for directed acyclic graph; *see* **Causal diagram** and **Directed acyclic graph.**

Deep vein thrombosis Clotting of blood in the deep veins usually of the calves, thigh, and pelvis. The clots may lead to a pulmonary embolus.

Degenerative An adjective applied to disease thought to be resulting from deterioration of tissues over time (i.e. with age).

Demographic transition The change in the age structure of the population after death rates and fertility rates decline, with a comparatively older population being the result.

Demography The scientific study of population, particularly the factors that determine its size and shape, including birth and death.

Depression A serious clinical illness with a characteristic set of symptoms and behaviours that, in its most severe form, may lead to suicide.

Descendants The variables arising from a postulated effect (in DAG terminology).

Developmental origins of disease *see* **Fetal origins of disease hypothesis.**

Diabetes mellitus A disease characterized by high levels of glucose in the blood caused by either lack or ineffectiveness of the hormone insulin.

Diethylstilboestrol A medication containing the hormone oestrogen.

Differential diagnosis A preliminary list of the most likely diseases in a patient, to be confirmed by further investigation.

Directed acyclic graph (DAG) A formal mathematical method for producing a postulated causal diagram. The diagram shows one-way relationships, hence it is called acyclic, and the direction of relationships is shown by arrows.

Disease A bodily dysfunction, usually one that can be described by a diagnostic label. (For simplicity, this book concentrates on discussing diseases and uses this word loosely when other words describing other health problems would be more specific, e.g. death, disability, illness, sickness, etc.)

Distribution The frequency with which each value (or category) of a variable occurs in the study population. The distribution of many variables takes on a characteristic shape. *Also see* **Normal distribution**.

Dizygotic Usually refers to non-identical twins who have shared the womb, but result from two fertilized eggs (*see* **Monozygotic**).

Down's syndrome A congenital genetic disorder, leading to mental retardation and a characteristic face, caused by the presence of three chromosomes instead of two at the site of the twenty-first chromosome.

Edge The line that is the basis of the arrow in a DAG.

Effect modifier A factor that alters the causal impact of another factor, the classical example being that smoking cigarettes greatly modifies (increases) the risk of lung cancer after exposure to asbestos and vice versa.

Elective In health care, a procedure done at a time chosen for its convenience, as opposed to being dictated by an emergency (e.g. elective surgery).

Electrocardiogram (ECG) A recording of the electrical activity of the heart made by an instrument called an electrocardiograph.

Emphysema When applied to the lungs (pulmonary emphysema) a condition caused by destruction of lung tissue with gaseous distension.

Endogenous selection *see* **M-bias**.

Environment A broad concept in epidemiology, sometimes meaning everything except genetic and biological factors, and sometimes more qualified and narrow (e.g. physical environment).

Epidemiological transition The change in disease patterns that accompanies the demographic transition, with both transitions usually following economic, educational, or social improvements.

Epidemiology See text, but in short, the study of the pattern of diseases and their causes in populations.

Epilepsy A disease of the brain characterized by temporary, involuntary, altered states of consciousness, including fits (convulsions).

Equity/inequity An equality that is required by our rules on fairness and justice. An inequality that is unfair or unjust is called an inequity. Inequity is a subset of inequality, as not all inequalities are unfair.

Estimability *see* **Identification**.

Ethnicity The group you belong to, or are perceived to belong to, or a mix of both, as a result of cultural factors such as dress, religion, diet, name, ancestry, and physical appearance (e.g. skin colour).

Exchangeability A concept indicating that two groups are the same in terms of their probability of an event (e.g. on outcome). In other words, the groups are alike.

Exogeneity An econometrics term meaning absence of confounding.

Exposure A general term to indicate contact with the postulated causal factors (or agents of disease) under study and used in a way similar to risk factor.

External validity *see* **Generalizability** and **Validity**.

Fetal origins of disease hypothesis The phrase encapsulating the idea that early life circumstances, particularly in utero, have an important and lasting effect in determining health and disease in later life.

Gaussian *see* **Normal distribution**.

Gene The discrete basic unit (made of DNA or deoxyribonucleic acid) of the chromosome, which itself consists of numerous genes and other DNA material. Genes carry information coding for specific functions (e.g. making proteins). There are two copies of each gene, one on each of the pair of chromosomes. The two copies of the gene at a particular location on the pair of chromosomes are called alleles. There are 23 pairs of chromosomes in each cell in human beings (46 in total), and the number of genes is estimated as 20–25 000 (until recently the estimate was 50–100 000).

Generalization and generalizability Drawing principles or conclusions that go beyond the data at hand and, often in epidemiology, the population studied. In sciences, epidemiology being no exception, generalizability is a much coveted property.

Genetic drift Genetic evolution, characteristically observable in small populations, arising from random variations in gene frequency.

Gestational diabetes High levels of blood glucose in association with pregnancy (*see* **Diabetes mellitus**).

Gonorrhoea Sexually transmitted infection caused by the bacterium *Neisseria gonorrhoeae*.

HDL *see* **Cholesterol**.

Heaf test A skin test similar to the Mantoux test (see below).

Health A desired ideal, which includes being alive and free of disease, disability, and infirmity, characterized by well-being and efficient functioning in society.

Helicobacter pylori A bacterium that lives in the human stomach, and in some circumstances causes gastritis, ulcers, and stomach cancer.

Herd immunity The resistance of an entire community to spread of infection arising from immunity to the infection in a high proportion of the population thereby preventing easy spread of disease.

Herpes Infection with the herpes simplex virus, characterized by small blisters, usually in and around the mouth (type I virus) and on and around the genitals (type II virus).

Histology The examination of tissues microscopically.

Human papillomavirus (HPV) A viral microorganism that causes, among other problems, cervical cancer.

Hypersensitivity reaction An abnormally powerful reaction by the immune system to exposure to some substances (allergens) such as peanuts, fur, or pollen.

Hypertension A condition of having blood pressure above an arbitrarily defined level (presently 140/90). Hypertension is associated with many adverse outcomes, particularly atherosclerotic diseases.

Hypertrophy Unnatural enlargement of the tissues or structures.

Hypothesis A proposition that is amenable to test by scientific methods. In sciences, including medicine, public health and epidemiology a hypothesis is an evolved, advanced written statement that offers an explanation for a natural phenomenon as a prelude to empirical research. (*See also* **Theory** and **Null hypothesis**.)

Illness The state of being unwell, usually due to disease.

Impaired glucose tolerance An abnormality of glucose metabolism detected after glucose measurements following a fast and the ingestion of a standard glucose load. It predicts a higher risk of CHD and of diabetes.

Inequity *see* **Equity**.

Instrumental variable A variable that is not directly, but indirectly, related to the exposure of interest (e.g. a gene variant that codes for a higher level of cholesterol). Such instrumental variables are usually not related directly either to confounding variables or to outcomes, but this assumption should be tested.

Intermediate variable A variable that lies on the postulated causal pathway between the exposure under study and the outcome.

Kaposi's sarcoma A cancer of cells (called reticuloendothelial cells) that is characterized by brown/purple patches on the skin.

LDL/VLDL *see* **Cholesterol**.

Latent variable An unobserved variable.

Lead time The extra time gained by earlier than usual detection of disease, as in screening.

Legionnaires' disease A pneumonia usually caused by the bacterium *Legionella pneumophila* (so-called because of the major outbreak among the US Legionnaires attending a convention in Philadelphia in 1976).

Leprosy A multisystem infection caused by the bacterium *Mycobacterium leprae*.

Leukaemia A group of cancers of blood cells, with various types (e.g. chronic myeloid leukaemia, acute leukaemia, etc.).

Life-grid approach A technique of data collection where the information of interest, say, smoking habits, is linked to key life events (e.g. date of marriage, change of job, etc.).

Logistic regression *see* **Multiple regression**.

Lyme disease An infection caused by the microorganism *Borrelia burgdorferi*, characterized by skin rash and arthritis.

Lymph, and lymph glands or nodes The fluid from the spaces between cells drains into the lymphatic system, a network of tubes. The lymph glands/nodes are organs connecting into the lymphatic system, and are important in the immune system.

M-bias A term that denotes collider bias. The M relates to the shape of the association shown in the relevant DAG.

Mantoux test A skin test to assess the level of immune response to tuberculosis, using a protein derived from the tubercle bacillus.

Mean A statistical measure of the average, where the values for all the members of a group are added up, and the total is divided by the number of members.

Median A statistical measure of the average; the value that divides a group into two equal parts, those below and those above the median.

Mediation analysis Analysis that examines the relationship between the exposure-mediator, and mediator-outcome, taking into account confounders for these relations.

Melanoma A skin cancer of the pigment producing cells of the skin or eye.

Meningitis/meningococcal meningitis An inflammation of the lining around the brain (meninges) as, for example, caused by infection by the meningococcus bacterium.

Miasma An impurity in air thought (wrongly) to be capable of causing diseases; the impurity arising from a number of sources including decaying matter and from cases of disease.

Microorganism A term to refer to unicellular organisms including viruses, bacteria, protozoa, and algae.

Mm Hg Pressure recorded as millimetres of mercury (Hg) because traditionally mercury was used in the sphygmomanometer.

Mode A statistical measure of the average; the most commonly occurring value.

Moderator The moderator variable is a variable that subgroups the exposure (independent) variable (e.g. young versus old people). The effects may differ. So, it is a variable that may lead to effect modification (i.e. a statistical interaction).

Monozygotic Refers to identical twins born from one fertilized egg. Twin studies are important in epidemiology to help judge the relative importance of environment and genes.

Multiple (logistic) regression In regression analysis a mathematical model is constructed to describe the relation between one variable X (say, height), and another Y (say weight). The method then predicts Y, knowing X (the independent variable). Multiple regression permits the simultaneous assessment of the relation between several variables (X1, X2, etc.) and Y. The multiple logistic regression model is a variant where the predicted variable (Y) is the probability of an event and hence is of particular interest in epidemiology.

Mutagen A substance such as radiation that damages the structure of DNA (or RNA) through mutations (i.e. permanent alterations) in the chemical structure of DNA. A single nucleotide polymorphism (SNP) is an example of the outcome of mutation at the gene level, where the nucleotide structure is altered.

Myocardial infarction The death of heart muscle from insufficient blood supply to the heart, usually caused by blockage of the coronary arteries (*see* **Atherosclerosis** and **Coronary heart disease**).

Natural history of disease The course of disease from inception to resolution (or death) with no medical interference.

Necropsy An autopsy, that is, an examination of the dead body by a pathologist usually to find the cause of death or to find evidence in the case of crime. This is a very important way of judging the accuracy of death statistics.

Neoplasm/neoplastic A new and inappropriately regulated growth, usually applied to a cancer/ an adjective usually used to describe something that is cancerous.

Node The variable in the DAG terminology.

Normal distribution A statistical distribution that describes many biological variables well. The mean, median, and mode values are identical, the distribution is symmetrical around this value, and one standard deviation above and below the mean includes about 68 per cent, and two standard deviations about 95 per cent, of the population.

Null hypothesis A statistical, not biological, hypothesis stated in a way that implies that there is no difference between comparisons, other than that which could occur by chance alone.

Osteoporosis Loss of bone density caused by loss of calcium and phosphorous from bone.

P-value *see* **Significance test**.

Parasuicide A suicide attempt that does not lead to death.

Participant The word that is replacing study subject, as in study participant.

Pathogen An organism (usually reserved for microorganisms) that causes disease.

Pathogenesis The mechanisms and processes by which disease occurs.

Pathology The study of the processes leading to, during, and following disease. Pathology is a vital partner to epidemiology.

Pellagra A nutritional deficiency disease caused by lack of the vitamin niacin (B3), with problems including dermatitis, diarrhoea, and neurological disorders.

Person-to-person spread Direct transmission of disease, usually infections, usually resulting from close proximity of persons.

Phenylketonuria A genetic disorder in which the amino acid phenylalanine cannot be metabolized properly, leading to mental deficiency.

Placebo An inactive substance or procedure used as a therapeutic intervention for psychological effect; and commonly used in the control group in a trial.

Population A complex concept with multitude meanings in epidemiology, but crucially, the group of people in whom the problem under study occurs, and in whom the results of the research are to be applied.

Post-mortem *see* **Necropsy** Also used more loosely to mean an investigation after some problem has arisen.

Potential outcome (framework) The outcome under hypothetical circumstances, which can be used as an alternative to counterfactual logic.

Probability The chance that an event will occur expressed between the values of 0 (no chance) and 1 (100% chance). The cumulative incidence rate is the main epidemiological measure of probability.

Prognosis Forecast of the outcome of a disease or other health problem with appropriate management (cf. natural history, which is without such management).

Propensity analysis/score A method for calculating the probability of being exposed or having an outcome given a set of characteristics (variables). The score instead of individual variables can be used for adjusting for differences between groups.

Proportional mortality (or morbidity) ratio (PMR) A summary measure of the proportion of deaths/disease due to a specific cause in the study population compared to either all causes or another cause.

Prostate A gland at the base of the male bladder.

Psychosis/Psychotic A term used for some serious mental health problems (e.g. schizophrenia). A person with such a disorder would be psychotic.

Public health (medicine) An activity to which many contribute, most usually defined as the science and art of prolonging life, preventing disease, and promoting health through the organized efforts of society. Public health medicine is one of the many names given to the specialty of medical doctors who focus on public health.

Pulmonary Associated with the lungs.

Pulmonary embolus A blood clot lodged in the arterial structure of the lungs.

Race The social group you belong to, or are perceived (or assigned) by others as belonging to, based on a limited set of physical characteristics, particularly skin colour, hair, and facial features. Race has been seriously discredited as a useful scientific construct and is being super-seded by ethnicity.

Regression *see* **Multiple regression.**

Reverse causality The possibility that the causal relationship is in the opposite direction to that postulated, for example, we think of lack of physical activity as causing a higher risk of heart disease but perhaps heart disease causes a disinclination to exercise.

Risk factor A factor associated with an increased probability of an adverse outcome, and poten-tially but not necessarily a causal factor.

Rose angina Angina is the characteristic chest pain arising from a shortage of oxygen to the heart muscle. Rose angina is the measure of whether chest pain is angina using the Rose angina questionnaire.

Rubella syndrome A complex set of congenital malformations caused by infection of the mother by German measles (rubella) and transmitted to the fetus.

Sampling The approach to selection of people to participate in studies. In epidemiology, the sam-pling methods are chosen to minimize selection biases, given other restraints.

Sarcoidosis A disease of unknown cause, where the histology resembles tuberculosis. Most com-monly it affects the lungs, liver, eyes, and skin.

Scurvy A disease caused by vitamin C deficiency, characterized by symptoms/signs including bruising and bleeding readily.

Senile dementia Brain disease of unknown cause characterized by loss of intellect, which is usu-ally irreversible and caused by degenerative processes associated with old age.

Sexually transmitted diseases (STDs) The group of diseases mainly transmitted during sexual behaviour (e.g. syphilis). Some STDs may be transmitted in other ways too (e.g. AIDS).

Sickle cell disease/anaemia A genetic disorder, whereby haemoglobin, the oxygen-carrying molecule in red blood cells, crystallizes when oxygen in the cell is low and distorts the blood cell into a sickle shape.

Sickness The state of being unwell or dysfunctional, usually because of disease.

Significance/significant Commonly, misleading shorthand for the phrase statistical signifi-cance, or statistically significant, as given by the P-value (*see* **Significance test**). Significance and significant, alone, should be reserved to mean importance.

Significance test Shorthand for tests of statistical significance whereby the P-value indicates the probability that the observed difference could have been obtained by chance alone. The evalu-ation of data using these tests has been severely criticized in epidemiology.

Single nucleotide polymorphism (SNP) *see* **Mutagen/mutation.**

Smallpox A severe viral disease, now extinct, characterized by skin blistering.

Sphygmomanometer A device for measuring arterial blood pressure using an inflatable cuff (usually applied to the upper arm). The cuff is inflated until blood flow stops, then deflated until blood flow begins (systolic blood pressure) and then occurs freely (diastolic blood pressure).

Standard deviation A measure of variation around the mean, measured as the square root of the variance (see below).

Standardized mortality (or morbidity) ratio (SMR) A comparative, summary measure of the rate of death/disease in a population adjusted for one or more confounding factors (usually age or sex or both) using the indirect method. The ratio is of deaths observed/deaths expected if the rates in the standard population had applied in the study population.

Statistical significance *see* **Significance** and **Significance test**.

Stratified sample The people selected for (or participating in) a study where the list of those to be sampled is organized by subgroups (e.g. men and women, or age groups). Then random samples are chosen within each subgroup.

Streptococcus/cocci One of a number of species of bacteria, some of which cause serious human diseases.

Subject A person who is studied, that is, a member of the population under study (*see* **Participant**).

Suicide Purposive action that leads to one's own death.

Target population The population about which inferences or generalizations are to be made or interventions designed for.

Theory A system of ideas offered to explain and connect observed factors or conjectures. A statement of general principles or laws underlying a subject. Theories are built on hypotheses and supporting data. They summarize the state-of-the-art.

Trisomy 21 *see* **Down's syndrome**.

Tuberculosis A multisystem infection caused by the bacterium *Mycobacterium tuberculosis*.

Validity The degree to which an observation or measurement can be shown to be true and accurate.

Variables Measure that vary and so are important in epidemiology. Variables can be in exposures (risk factors), intermediate or mediating factors, confounders, colliders, and outcomes.

Variance A measure of the variation in a set of observations. Each value is subtracted from the mean value and squared (always a positive number), and the total is divided by the degrees of freedom (often the number of observations minus 1).

Vertices Synonym for node.

Zoonoses Diseases transmitted from animals to humans.

Brief information on people mentioned in the text

Aristotle Greek philosopher, scientist, and general scholar living 384–322 BC.

Berkson (Joseph) 1899–1982, The Berkson's bias, explained in the text, was first described by this American statistician.

Bradford Hill (Austin) 1897–1991, Statistician renowned for his work on smoking and cancer, and clinical trials, and for guidance on causal interpretation of data.

Crick (Francis) 1916–2004, One of three scientists receiving the Nobel Prize for discovering the structure of DNA in 1953.

Davey Smith (George) 1959–, Epidemiologist, working primarily in life-course epidemiology and inequalities in health.

Durkheim (Emile) 1858–1917, French social theorist and eminent sociologist.

Einstein (Albert) 1879–1955, Physicist, most famous for the theory of relativity.

Evans (Alfred) 1917–1996, Epidemiologist who developed ways of assessing causality, based on the Henle–Koch postulates.

Galton (Francis) 1822–1911, British scientist who made numerous contributions including to biology (genetics) and statistics. Founder of eugenics, the science of good breeding, that was widely abused by governments across the world, including the United States and subsequently Nazi Germany.

Goldberger (Joseph)   1874–1927, American public health doctor and epidemiologist famed for his work demonstrating the nutritional basis of pellagra.

Gregg (Norman)   1892–1966, Australian ophthalmologist famed for his hypothesis that rubella (German measles) in the mother could lead to congenital abnormalities in the fetus (Rubella syndrome).

Henle (Jacob)   1805–1885, German pathologist who provided three of the four (Henle–Koch) postulates that underpin analysis of whether a microbe causes disease.

Hippocrates   (460–377 BC approximately) Influential teacher and leader of a school of medical thought that continues to be influential, and not only in relation to the Hippocratic Oath.

Hume (David)   1711–1776, Scottish philosopher and historian.

Jenner (Edward)   1749–1823 British medical practitioner who tested a hypothesis that exposure to cowpox protects against smallpox. This laid the scientific foundation for the eradication of smallpox and immunization.

Koch (Robert)   1843–1910, German bacteriologist who established the bacterial cause of many infectious diseases, including anthrax (1876), tuberculosis (1882), conjunctivitis (1883), and cholera (1884).

Kuhn (Thomas)   1922–1996, Science philosopher, who is renowned for his work on the nature of scientific revolutions.

Lind (James)   1716–1794, British naval physician who did a controlled trial (one of the first on record) of treatments for scurvy, finding that oranges and lemons were curative.

Mendel (Gregor)   1822–1884, Published in 1866 his research on the laws of heredity based on his observations and experiments on garden peas. This was the beginning of the science of genetics.

Pearl (Judea)   1936–, Professor of computer science and statistics who has played a key role in articulating causal thinking using DAGs and structural equation modelling.

Popper (Karl)   1902–1994, Philosopher, who contributed to science by, for example, promoting the key idea of falsifying rather than proving hypotheses.

Ramanujan (Srinivasan)   1887–1920, Mathematician, renowned for his intuition that led him to enunciate complex formulae that are still being proved.

Rothman (Kenneth)   1945 to 19–, Epidemiologist, known for conceptual and technical advances, and for his text *Modern Epidemiology*.

Skrabanek (Petr)   1940–1994, Epidemiologist renowned for his capacity for critical appraisal.

Snow (John)   1813–1858, Pioneer in both epidemiology and anaesthetics. His investigations of cholera were pivotal in the development of epidemiology.

Tesh (Sylvia)   1937–, Public health scholar and author of a wide-ranging and controversial book on public health called *Hidden Arguments*.

Watson (James)   1928–, American scientist who in 1953 co-discovered the structure of DNA, winning the Nobel Prize in 1962 (*see also* **Crick**).

Chapter 1

What is epidemiology? The nature, scope, variables, principal measures, and designs of a biological, clinical, social, and ecological science

Objectives

After reading this chapter you should understand:

+ that the prime focus of epidemiology is on the pattern of death, disease, disability, and ill health (disease for short) in populations;

+ that epidemiology combines elements of clinical, biological, social, and ecological sciences;

+ that epidemiology is mostly dependent on clinical practice and the clinical sciences to make a diagnosis, which is essential to most epidemiological work;

+ that the central goal of epidemiology as a science is to understand the causes of variation in diseases in different populations, and use this knowledge to improve the health of populations and individuals;

+ that the central goal of epidemiology as a practical discipline is the prevention and control of disease in populations, guiding health and health-care policy, and planning and improving health care for individuals;

+ the nature of variables in epidemiology;

+ that useful epidemiological variables should assist the purposes of epidemiology;

+ the definitions of core measures of disease frequency and main study designs in epidemiology;

+ that both research and practice in epidemiology are based on theories, although these may not be explicit.

1.1 The individual and the population

Humans cherish the fact that they are unique, not only in their physique but also in their character, personality, and behaviour. The health of an individual is also unique, and only the facts of birth and death are universally shared. Some people who smoke develop lung cancer and other smokers do not. Some people drink alcohol and become aggressive, while others become passive. These outcomes are not predictable on an individual level. Such individual level prediction remains an elusive goal of health sciences. It is self-evident, however, that the characteristics of individuals play a part in causing their diseases. According to Hippocrates, writing more than 2000 years ago, medicine should consider the health of the inhabitants of a place, for example, 'are they heavy drinkers and eaters and consequently unable to stand fatigue or, being fond of work and exercise, eat wisely but drink sparely?' Hippocrates also wrote about the role of the environment on disease, particularly the seasons, the winds, and water (see Chadwick and Mann, 1950).

It is less intuitive than with individuals, but population groups have distinctive patterns of disease. For example, the commonest cancers in the United Kingdom are those of the lung while the commonest in China are those of the liver; tuberculosis is rare in Norway but common in Pakistan; and blood disorders such as sickle cell disease are common in the equatorial region but rare in the northern and southern latitudes. Before reading on, reflect on why this is so, and consider the role of individual behaviour, social interaction, genetic factors, and the natural environment.

These distinctive patterns are a result of the varying exposure of population groups to the causes of disease. If different populations were exposed equally to the causes, they would have much the same patterns of disease, although some variation would remain due to genetic differences, which are small between populations.

The pattern of disease is dependent on the characteristics of individuals comprising the population and the individuals' interaction with each other and their environment. For example, sexually transmitted diseases arise only when having more than one sexual partner is common in society. If a non-diseased person had multiple sexual partners in a society where a single sexual partner was the norm for others, this would not raise his/her own risk of sexually transmitted disease (or that of others in the society). Herd immunity is the name for protection given to people who are not immunized, by the immunization of others. A population's pattern of disease arises from its intrinsic social characteristics. If society changed, the individual's risk of disease would also change, even when the individual does not—as reflected in the examples of sexually transmitted disease and immunization. Patterns of diseases in populations, therefore, result from the characteristics of individuals, their societies, and their environment (as discussed in detail in Chapter 2). The science and practice of epidemiology seeks to describe, understand, and utilize these population patterns to improve health.

1.2 Defining epidemiology and a statement of its central idea

The identity of the person who coined the term *epidemiology* is unknown, but it is derived from the Greek words meaning *study upon populations* (*epi* = upon, *demos* = people, *ology* = study). This derivation does not convey what is studied or the nature of that study, and is effectively the same as demography, which is the study of the characteristics of populations, such as size, growth, density, distribution, and vital statistics. Epidemiology is concerned primarily with disease, and how disease detracts from health. Most epidemiologists are interested in health but study it indirectly through disease, partly because of the difficulty of measuring health directly. Epidemiologists tend to use the word *disease* broadly to include a range of health problems, for example, accidents and being unwell even though, strictly, these are not diseases. I have taken this approach too. Epidemiologists are embroiled in studying the consequence of diseases, such as disability and death, especially premature death. A more descriptive word for the discipline would be *epidemiopathology* (*pathos* is the Greek word for suffering and disease), but it is too clumsy to recommend.

The word *epidemic* was used by Hippocrates, but his writings were mainly compilations of the case histories of affected people and not a study of the causes, nor the pattern of epidemic in the population. The early applications of epidemiology were in the study of infectious disease epidemics, environmental hazards, and social and nutritional problems. Most epidemiology is on human populations, but veterinary epidemiology is also important, both in its own right and in the study of the interaction between humans and animals, causing the diseases known as the *zoonoses*.

Porta's (2014) dictionary gives a long definition of epidemiology that includes 'The study of the distribution and determinants of health-related states or events in specified populations, and the application of this study to control of health problems'. The definition includes the study of the populations of animals and plants (for the first time).

Based on what it has done in the last 150 years, epidemiology will be defined here as the science and practice that describes and explains disease patterns in populations. It uses this knowledge to prevent and control disease, and improve health. The central idea of epidemiology is that patterns of ill health and disease in populations may be analysed systematically to understand their causes and to improve health. The strategy of epidemiology is to seek differences and similarities ('compare and contrast') in the disease patterns of different populations to gain new knowledge. Nearly all of the examples in textbooks and in collections of landmark epidemiological papers are based on this. The valid measurement of disease frequency, factors that may influence disease (and are therefore potential explanations for the observed patterns), and the consequences of disease is crucial (Chapters 3, 4, 7, and 8). Measurement, however, is a means to an end. Excellence in measurement will not, in itself, yield excellence in epidemiology. The quality of epidemiology must be judged by its contributions to its goals. The same applies to the design of epidemiological studies (Chapter 9).

1.3 Directions in epidemiology and its uses

A great expansion in the scope of epidemiology is underway. This book contains many references to the history of epidemiology, including historical landmark studies, for example, in section 10.14. You may wish to look at them as part of your introduction to the subject. The ideas that have proven themselves in the study of disease are used increasingly to study health and health care. Epidemiology is useful in the laboratory, both in contributing to ideas to help understand biological processes, and in pragmatic ways such as defining ranges for the normal values of biological measures. Normal values are usually derived by either demonstrating the distribution of the values in healthy populations or, much better, by demonstrating the health problems associated with particular values, which are, therefore, abnormal.

Epidemiology plays a central role in the practice of clinical medicine, and though its uses have been insufficiently demonstrated, its potential for the professions allied to medicine, such as nursing and physiotherapy, is promising. Epidemiology underpins the movement known as 'evidence-based medicine'. Epidemiology is important to animal health and there is a move to unite the human and animal health agendas (known as 'one health').

The standard definitions of epidemiology, such as the science of the distribution and determinants of disease, or the occurrence of disease in populations, do not capture the essence of applied epidemiology in health-care settings, though they do describe well the tradition of the science. Morris's (1964) classic book, *The Uses of Epidemiology*, fully recognized the huge contribution of epidemiology to health care, opening the chapter on community diagnosis with the words, 'Epidemiology provides "intelligence" for the health services' (1964, 2nd edition). Modern epidemiology is more than just a science: it is a craft, vocation, and profession—in this sense, it is a partner of public health and clinical care, not just a science of these disciplines. Currently, epidemiology is seen as useful in:

◆ yielding understanding of what causes or sustains disease in populations (humans, animals, and now also plants);

◆ measuring the burden of disease in populations;

◆ assessing the effectiveness of interventions;

- preventing and controlling disease in populations (public health);
- guiding health and health-care policy and planning (management);
- assisting in the management of disease in individuals (clinical epidemiology).

1.4 **Epidemiology as a science, practice, and craft**

Nearly all definitions of epidemiology describe it as a science, and there are regular claims for it to be the underlying science of public health (Chapter 10). Some critics have claimed epidemiology is not a science at all, but rather a toolkit of methods for other sciences and professions to use. An understanding of whether epidemiology is a science is important in an era when the label 'science' is vital to the credibility of both research and professional practice. Try the exercise in Box 1.1 before reading on.

Science is about knowledge, for the word is derived from the Latin *scientia*, meaning knowledge, and the French *scíre*, to know. Dictionary definitions of science tend to be complex, for example:

1. the observation, identification, description, experimental investigation, and theoretical explanation of phenomena;

2. such activities restricted to a class of natural phenomena;

3. any branch of knowledge based on systematic observations of facts and seeking to formulate general explanatory laws and hypotheses that could be verified empirically.

Clearly, not all systematic study is science; for example, literature, art, philosophy, and religion are not sciences, though they may be rigorous and systematic, and even emulate the methods and measurement techniques of science. A painter who systematically observes and measures what pigments mixed together produce the most realistic sky in a landscape painting does not, obviously, become a scientist. The content of the work is the central matter. Science is the systematic study of natural phenomena. Furthermore, science is not just about the methods and techniques, which can be applied in many non-scientific circumstances (e.g. political polling), but the mode of thought. The scientific mode of thought pursues new knowledge based on theory and hypotheses tested by direct, research-based observation. Scientists are engaged in extending or consolidating the knowledge base, sometimes through deliberate repetition of research. Science is a creative endeavour that relies as much on questioning, imagination, and exploration as art, but the difference is that science tests out its ideas by seeking empirical evidence rooted in the natural world.

The idea to be tested in scientific research is often stated as a question. The question may be expressed in a way that lends itself to systematic testing. If so, it is called a hypothesis. Now reflect on the importance of the testable question, as emphasized in Box 1.2.

Box 1.1 The nature of science in relation to epidemiology

- What are the characteristics of a science?
- Name some disciplines that are sciences and some that are not.
- Compare the disciplines that are sciences to those that are not.
- Is public health a science? Is medicine a science?
- Is epidemiology a science?
- Is epidemiology a practice?

Box 1.2 The question as the basis of science

'That is the essence of science: ask an impertinent question, and you are on the way to a pertinent answer.'

Jacob Bronowski (1908–74), British scientist, author of *The Ascent of Man* (1973)

The idea, the question, the testable hypothesis, the research test, and the interpretation of the research data to advance understanding of natural phenomena, when put together, comprise science. Epidemiology studies the nature of diseases and their causes and consequences by using systematic methods of measurement to test ideas, set out as questions and hypotheses—hence it is a bioscience, serving medicine and public health, just as medical sciences such as pathology and microbiology do. Epidemiology has historically been particularly relevant to medicine rather than laboratory science, but the increasing collaboration between geneticists and epidemiologists is changing the balance.

Epidemiology is, however, concerned with disease and health risks in populations. Human populations live in societies, where behaviour and attitudes are shaped by interaction among people. People create the conventions and laws of a society and these influence health. Epidemiology studies disease within a sociocultural context, and is therefore not only a bioscience, but also a social science.

Populations exist in a physical environment, which is dominant in determining their health. The study of life in relation to the environment is *ecology* (the word being derived from the Greek for *house*), so epidemiology is, in addition, the science of the ecology of disease.

The science of epidemiology, therefore, combines elements of biology, social sciences, and ecology: a biosocial–environmental science focusing on disease in populations. By its nature, epidemiology is multidisciplinary. The closest partners of the epidemiologist are the statistician, the clinician, the biological and the social scientist for reasons that will become apparent.

Epidemiological science is easily applied. Understanding the causes of diseases, more than any other information, transforms the practice of clinical care and public health. For example, the epidemiological work showing that smokers have a much higher risk of a multiplicity of diseases than non-smokers has transformed health care, public health, and health politics. Epidemiological data has value for creating health policy, whether for the nation, or for patients, for example, those with cancer or risk of cancer.

While many epidemiologists are simultaneously engaged in both research and practice, some only apply available knowledge. Their applied work is not science, although it draws upon science. In this regard, epidemiology is no different to, for example, medicine, nursing, geology, and chemistry, where there are scientists and practitioners, and often the two roles are combined. Scientific research and practice in epidemiology are symbiotic, but not identical, activities. Recent criticisms of epidemiology may partly arise from a failure to separate the roles of epidemiology as a science, and as a craft or practice (see Chapter 10). Analogously, there are criticisms of physics for discoveries that have underpinned poor energy policy (e.g. disasters in nuclear energy power plants, and the use of the nuclear bomb), and criticisms of biology for the unethical and erroneous interpretation of data on human intelligence (e.g. the Immigration Bill of 1924 in the United States of America kept Jews from migrating to America on the basis of their supposedly low intelligence). Criticisms of the research need to be separated from those of its application.

The practice of epidemiology operates somewhat differently from the science of epidemiology. The research questions, the value of various methods, and data analysis, presentation, and interpretation may differ; something that needs to be appreciated. These differences and their implications will be emphasized throughout this book.

Finally, sometimes epidemiology is criticized as being observational. That is a curious criticism. It is true that experiments are done comparatively rarely in epidemiology, but when these are possible and necessary, they are done. Nearly all sciences are primarily observational, for example, astronomy, geology, biology, and even physics. Being mostly, but not wholly, observational is a strength, not a weakness.

1.5 **The nature of epidemiological variables**

The word *variable* is in common use in research disciplines including epidemiology, but its meaning is seldom defined. Most people have used the word variable. Before reading on, ask yourself—what is it?

A variable is anything that varies and hence has different values. Clearly, this applies to most phenomena, but only a few are chosen for epidemiological study. Variation in populations' disease patterns is the foundation of epidemiology, but in epidemiology the word *variable* is not usually applied to diseases, which may sometimes be referred to as *outcome variables* or, more commonly and simply, *outcomes*. It is usually applied to factors that help to describe and understand disease pattern, which are called *exposure variables* or *risk factors* (see Chapter 7). There are also *confounding* (Chapter 4), *mediator* and *moderator* (Chapter 5), and *instrumental variables* (Chapter 9). Unless otherwise stated, *variable* in this book refers to an exposure variable or risk factor. A brief definition of some kinds of variables can be found in Table 1.1.

A variable does not have intrinsic qualities, and so logically can be all of the aforementioned types in different contexts. So, cigarette smoking (usually exposure), diabetes mellitus (usually an outcome), endothelial dysfunction (usually a mediator), age (usually a confounder), and sex/gender (usually a moderator) can be used differently depending on the question under investigation. We will return to these ideas, especially in Chapter 5 in relation to causal graphs, but try the exercise in Box 1.3 before reading on.

In question 1 cigarette smoking is assigned, by the investigator, the role of exposure (potentially causal) variable. In question 2 smoking is the outcome variable, and as is usually the case, we would wish to reduce this. In question 3, we have assigned the role of confounding factor

Table 1.1 Some types of variable in epidemiology

Type of variable	Description
Exposure or risk factor (often simply variable)	The variable that we are interested in studying as a potential associated (risk) factor or cause of an outcome
Mediator	The variable that we think is important in the pathway, or mechanism, that leads from the exposure to the outcome (see Chapter 5)
Outcome	The variable (usually undesirable) that we are wanting to understand better, so we can (usually) reduce it in the population
Moderator	The variable that we believe may alter the effect of an exposure (see Chapter 5)
Confounder	The variable that we are not presently interested in studying for the relationship between the exposure and outcome, but we need to include because it is associated with both the exposure and outcome (see Chapter 4)

Box 1.3 Cigarette smoking and types of variable

Reflect on cigarette smoking as a variable in the five questions below, and indicate which of the five roles of variables it is playing in this context.

1. Does smoking cigarettes increase the risk of cancer?

2. Does parenting style influence the risk of taking up cigarette smoking in the teenage years?

3. Might the higher risk of coronary heart disease in South Asian men of Pakistani origin in Scotland be a result of more cigarette smoking compared to White Scottish men?

4. Is the effect of asbestosis in increasing lung cancer affected by smoking cigarettes?

5. Is the higher risk of hospitalization for respiratory disorder in children from poorer than richer households a result of their greater exposure to second-hand cigarette smoke?

to cigarette smoking. It might be an explanation for higher risk in Pakistani men (the role of cigarettes as a cause of coronary heart disease is well known). In question 4 we assign the role of moderating (or modifying) factor to cigarette smoking. In question 5 we have assigned cigarette smoke as a mediating variable. The roles are assigned, and investigators interpret the data in the light of these. This process requires knowledge of the subject under investigation and needs to be resolved prior to data analyses (see Chapters 4, 5, and 9).

As this discussion shows, epidemiological variables are of many types and with different qualities. These qualities include the numerical values they can have, as follows (see also Chapter 9 for further information):

♦ Categorical variables are those where the individual is put into two or more categories, or groups. Sex is an example, that is, male or female. Another is dead or alive. These are called binary variables. Categories may be in some order, for example. social class, where there is an expectation that as we move through the classes, say from 1 to 5, there is a step change, for instance, in access to resources, or likelihood of smoking. Categorical variables are of great importance in epidemiology as risk factors (exposures), confounding factors, moderators, mediators, and outcomes. The categories are usually assigned numbers for data analysis, for example, alive = 1, dead = 2. (Categorical variables are also called qualitative data, but this risks confusion with qualitative research.)

♦ Numerical or quantitative variables are those where there is no prior grouping, and the values rise from zero onwards, with no imposed upper limit. The variables can be whole numbers, for example, the number of episodes of asthma a person had over the last year, or the number of times a person took exercise in the last month. Such variables can also be continuous, for example, age (measurable in seconds, days, years, etc.) or amount of alcohol consumed (litres, millilitres, etc.). Continuous measures are often converted to whole numbers such as age in years, or alcohol consumption to the nearest unit. It is also common and practical, but often not advisable, to convert quantitative variables into categorical ones as this will reduce precision, for example, age into young/middle-aged/old or into 5-year or 10-year groupings.

Quantitative variables are commonly risk factors, mediators, and confounding factors, but less commonly outcome variables in epidemiology, simply because death, disease, and illnesses are the outcomes of greatest interest and these are categorical variables. States that are intermediate between health and disease are often measured quantitatively, for example, blood pressure, or weight in relation to height, otherwise known as body mass index (BMI). These are usually called

Box 1.4 The epidemiological exposure variable (risk factor)

♦ What characteristics should an exposure variable have to make it important and useful in epidemiology?

♦ How do the purposes and uses of epidemiology help to assess the potential value of an exposure variable?

intermediate traits. Driven by the needs of clinical practice, these are often converted to categories, for example, mild or severe hypertension, or normal, overweight, and obese.

Epidemiological variables aid the description, analysis, and interpretation of disease patterns. Analysis of disease by age, sex, economic status, social class, occupation, country of residence, country of birth, region of residence, and racial or ethnic classification are powerful ways of showing and interpreting variations in diseases and health states.

Many variables used in epidemiology are markers for complex underlying phenomena, which cannot be measured easily, if at all. For example, social class is an indirect indicator of various differences between populations in factors such as occupation, income, education, and styles of consumption. It is important, therefore, that we can disentangle and study separately the component influences of such epidemiological variables. Before reading on, do the exercise in Box 1.4.

A good epidemiological exposure variable should:

♦ have a potential causal impact on health status in individuals and populations;

♦ be measurable accurately;

♦ differentiate populations in terms of patterns of disease or other health outcomes;

♦ differentiate populations in some underlying characteristic relevant to health, for example, income, childhood circumstance, hormonal status, genetic inheritance, or behaviour relevant to health;

♦ achieve one or more of the following:

  • generate testable causal hypotheses

  • help to develop health policy

  • help to plan and deliver health care

  • help to prevent and control disease.

These characteristics, which align with the purposes of epidemiology, can help to assess and choose from a multiplicity of exposure variables (risk factors). In Chapter 10, and other parts of the book, these characteristics will be used to illustrate the strengths and weaknesses of epidemiological variables, particularly in the context of the controversies around race and ethnicity (see section 10.10.3).

Table 1.2 summarizes the concepts here in the context of age, the most influential and important of all epidemiological exposure variables. Before reading on, however, try the exercise in Box 1.5.

In most populations, age is accurately measured by asking people. Alternatively, age can be obtained from birth registration data. In some populations, mainly in developing countries, where registration at birth is not operative or effective, age may not be known accurately (as is the case for this author—I was born in India and do not have a birth certificate). In some societies, for social reasons, there is a tendency to exaggerate age on self-report, while in others to understate it. In the context of developing countries, this can be an important limitation. In developed countries, it may be relevant to studies of migrants and ethnic minority groups.

Table 1.2 Age as an epidemiological exposure variable

Characteristics of a good epidemiological variable	Characteristics in relation to age
Impact on health in individuals and population	Age is a powerful influence on health
Be accurately measurable	In most populations age is measurable to the day, but in some it has to be guessed and may deliberately be reported wrongly
Differentiate populations in their experience of disease or health	Huge differences by age are seen for virtually every disease, health problem, and for factors which cause health problems
Differentiate populations in some underlying characteristic relevant to health, e.g. income, childhood circumstance, hormonal status, genetic inheritance, or behaviour relevant to health	Differences in disease patterns in different age groups reflect a mix of biological changes, varying exposure to environmental risk factors and may reflect population changes in genetic factors, particularly in populations where migration has been high
Generate testable causal hypotheses	While generation of hypotheses is easy, they are hard to test because there are so many underlying differences between populations of different ages
Help in developing health policy	Age differences in disease patterns profoundly affect health policy decisions
Help to plan and deliver health care	Knowing the age structure of a population is critical to good decision-making in health care as it influences the kind of problems seen
Help to prevent and control disease	By understanding the age at which diseases start, preventive and control programmes can be targeted at appropriate age groups

Biological changes related to ageing have a profound influence on susceptibility to many diseases. For example, disorders of growth and development occur in the young; degenerative diseases such as osteoporosis or senile dementia mostly in the old. Therefore, age is associated with and influences health of populations.

Age is superb at showing variations in most diseases (see Table 8.19, Chapter 8). Variations by age seldom yield easy explanation, for their causes are a complex mix of social, environmental, and biological factors. Causal hypotheses about age and disease are not easily tested.

Box 1.5 Thinking about age as an epidemiological exposure variable

◆ Is age easily and accurately measured?

◆ Is age good at showing population differences in disease experience?

◆ What underlying differences between people does age reflect?

◆ How can these differences be used to advance understanding of disease causation, improve health policy or health-care planning, or prevent and control disease?

Generally, the more complex the variable, the harder it is to explain the underlying reason for the associated variation in disease experience. This is why it is imperative to understand the underlying concept behind the variable, as with causal studies, additional data will be needed and these will be dependent on such understanding. The epidemiological concept of ageing is a mix of biological and environmental components. As the body grows older its biology changes, but at the same time absorbs a barrage of environmental insults. The combined effects lead to differences in disease patterns in different age groups and in different generations (see section 9.8 on cohort effect). Furthermore, the social circumstances, and particularly social support networks, of people change at different ages and these also affect health. Age differentiates populations in characteristics relevant to health; for example, the likelihood of exposure to hepatitis B virus, unfiltered cigarettes, and poverty and obesity in childhood depend on a person's age. The differences in disease experience at different ages are profoundly important to clinical care, preventing and controlling disease, making sound health policy, and for effective health-care planning. In practice, given its complexity, age is usually treated like a confounding rather than exposure variable (see Chapter 4), which is sometimes a missed opportunity for causal thinking.

The epidemiological concept of sex is also, in practice, a mix of biological and social factors. Epidemiological studies do not tend to collect data on sex (biological construct), although there is a good case for that. They tend to collect self-reported or observed sex and interpret this as biological sex (rather than gender). Try the exercise in Box 1.6 before reading on.

To begin to understand the sex variation in the occurrence of coronary heart disease, or any other outcome, the investigator needs to know what differences there are between men and women in the population studied. Table 1.3 categorizes some of these differences as biological, coexisting disease (or comorbidity), behavioural, social, occupational, economic, and health care. There are complex differences between men and women, so using this variation to explain the different patterns of heart disease is immensely difficult. To ascribe differences solely to genetic factors would be a serious, though tempting, error. By contrast, differences between men and women in the risk of breast cancer are likely to be biological and for cervical cancer are, of course, wholly biological because men do not have a cervix. The depth of the analysis will, therefore, be disease and context specific. Differences in health care between men and women (and indeed between other population groups) as explanations for disease variations arouse great controversy, because inequitable health care is unethical and unjust.

Scientific understanding of the reasons for the variation by sex is extremely helpful in designing preventive interventions, but in its absence, the variations can be used to set priorities and target resources.

Box 1.6 Categorizing the differences between sexes in relation to diseases

List the differences between women and men which could explain their different patterns of disease. (You may wish to focus your thinking using coronary heart disease, which is more common in men than women.) Can you put these differences into categories?

Table 1.3 Categorizing and analysing the factors which may underlie an epidemiological variable: examples of differences in coronary heart disease

Category of underlying difference	Example of possible specific differences by sex	Implications for science of epidemiology
Biological	Hormonal, e.g. oestrogen levels	Collect biological data
Coexisting diseases	Women are less prone to the other diseases which raise the risk of heart disease, e.g. diabetes	Collect clinical data
Behavioural	Women eat more fruits, vegetables, and salads than men, and generally smoke less	Collect data on behaviours relating to health
Social	Women spend more time with friends and family	Collect psychosocial data as potential explanations
Occupational	The pattern of working, including likelihood of employment, the hours worked, and the type of occupation is substantially different	Collect data on employment histories
Economic	Women earn less money than men	Collect data on differences and their effect on lifestyles and stress levels
Health care	Women with heart disease are treated differently than men by health-care professionals	Collect data on level and timing of interventions and quality of care

For the science of epidemiology, which is mainly concerned with the advance of causal knowledge, variables that highlight variations between and within populations in diseases of unknown aetiology are *potentially* of great value. If disease variation has not previously been demonstrated, it is of particular value. The repetitious demonstration of variations is, however, seldom of scientific value, although it may be important for getting a problem acknowledged and thus, policy implemented.

For example, huge variations between countries in the incidence of cancer have been demonstrated, and these conclusively demonstrate that population variation in cancer is largely determined by environmental factors. New observations on such variations would be of scientific value only if they refuted, rather than confirmed this interpretation. A great deal of effort is presently underway to show racial and ethnic variations in cancer. These mainly reconfirm the insights from international studies. Their additional value in aetiological research needs to be questioned. In his analysis of epidemiology as a science, Skrabanek (1994) argued that epidemiologists must advance understanding of the causes of the associations between epidemiological variables and diseases. He cited a review of 35 case–control studies of coffee drinking and bladder cancer, which failed to provide important information on whether coffee causes bladder cancer. He likened such research to repetitively punching a pillow: a dimple forms and refills, while the totality of the blows is no more than the first. He called this 'black box' epidemiology, and another epidemiologist, Kuller (1999), has criticized a similar phenomenon that he called circular epidemiology. As public health advocates know well, policy and service action are driven by local and up-to-date data. This kind of demand is one explanation for circular epidemiology. It is, nonetheless, poor science.

1.6 **Definition and diagnosis of disease: an illustration of the interdependence of clinical medicine and epidemiology**

Investigating the causes of health problems is the essence of the science of epidemiology. Taking steps to prevent and control the problem, including providing the appropriate health services, is the essence of public health policy and health-care planning. The craft of epidemiology lies in presenting the scientific evidence in ways that help lead to effective public health and clinical action. Epidemiology cannot work properly until some basic clinical and pathological issues have been resolved, for example, on the definition of the disease. The science of epidemiology, therefore, functions in close partnership with clinical medicine and medical sciences, particularly pathology. Read Box 1.7 and try the questions before reading on.

Sickness X (Box 1.7) illustrates why epidemiology requires clinical collaboration. As the cause is unknown, the disease must be defined on the clinical picture or non-specific laboratory tests. If a definition cannot be agreed or is inaccurate, cases cannot be diagnosed accurately and epidemiology is paralysed, or led to error.

The first question in epidemiology is the nature and validity of the definition of the disease or other health problem under investigation. Clinicians need to study cases and agree on a definition, which will permit the classification of sick people into one of two groups: probably suffering from the disease, or probably not. Diagnoses are statements of probability, and their accuracy will depend on the clarity of their definition. Epidemiologists need to help to achieve this clarity. A definition of sickness X that accepted only patients with a rash as being cases would miss those without a rash. To accept cases of disease without a rash, however, means that more people suffering from other disorders will be wrongly diagnosed with sickness X.

Pragmatic choices need to be made. For scientific investigation, a definition which includes people with a high probability of disease is likely to be better than one which includes many people without disease. For public health, a strict definition may be inadequate, for it can underestimate the size of the problem and miss the people most likely to benefit: those with early symptoms and few signs. A possible definition would be that a case of sickness X is, for the purpose of epidemiological research and public health surveillance:

♦ an illness diagnosed by a physician;

♦ one of a cluster or outbreak of cases;

♦ one that occurs in an ill person who has at least two out of these three problems:

  • gastrointestinal disturbance

  • skin rash

  • mental disturbance

♦ one with no other clear diagnosis.

Using this pragmatic definition, physicians can be asked to inform researchers of the occurrence of cases, which can be counted and studied. The effect of error in the definition on the estimated frequency of the disease may be huge, for example, solitary cases are excluded here. The comparison of different populations is likely to be misleading, as will be discussed in Chapter 3, but a pragmatic definition is still essential.

Consider, for comparison, the definition used by Fraser and colleagues (1977) in their investigation of the 1976 Legionnaires' disease outbreak in Philadelphia: a case had 'a fever of at least 102 degrees and a cough, or a fever allied to chest X-ray evidence of pneumonia, plus some association

Box 1.7 A puzzle for medicine and a challenge for epidemiology: sickness X

A sickness of unknown type, which appears as an outbreak, sometimes affecting whole communities, is spreading across a large part of continental Europe. Years later it will emerge in the United States of America. It will be shown to be present in many countries, though it may remain unrecognized in normal medical practice, for it can occur as solitary cases or in small numbers, and not outbreaks. Sick people have a wide range of symptoms and signs on examination. Their many symptoms include simply feeling unwell, with loss of appetite and abdominal pain, disturbances of the gastrointestinal tract including diarrhoea, a skin rash on parts of the body exposed to the sun, and mental disturbances.

Sickness leads to progressive physical and mental deterioration. People who contract the sickness are likely to die, with the mortality rate being as high as 60 per cent in some outbreaks. If a sufferer recovers, the sickness can recur.

The sickness clusters in families, and it affects poor people living in rural areas more than any other group. Growing corn is common in areas where the disease occurs. The system of sharecropping is common where the disease is common, that is, the landowner decides what is to be farmed. The tenants do the work, and then the crop and resulting profits are shared. The problem is greatest in spring, though the early symptoms occur in winter. The sickness is common in prisoners and patients in asylums, however, it does not affect staff in these institutions.

Physicians cannot agree on the cause of the sickness and the many 'cures' tried by physicians give variable and unpromising results.

Questions

◆ Can you form a definition of this sickness X?

◆ If not, how would physicians make a diagnosis? How could the number of cases of the sickness be counted for epidemiological purposes? How would the epidemiologist find cases for study?

◆ If you can define sickness, how would you do it? What would be the components of your definition?

Hint: Imagine you are asking local doctors to let you know when they see a person they think has sickness X. What would you say to them?

---

with the Legion convention'. The definition was designed to separate those who were probably linked to the outbreak from those who probably were not. Later, when the importance of the Bellevue Stratford Hotel in Philadelphia as the source of disease exposure became clearer, the definition was revised to include only people who were American Legion conventioneers, or who had entered the Bellevue Stratford Hotel after 1 July 1976. The change in definition caused confusion in the minds of the public and the media, and changed the numbers of cases involved and dead. Similarly, a change in the definition of AIDS and in myocardial infarction (heart attack) some years ago led to changes in the numbers of cases. Changes in case definition are common, reflecting the fact that diagnosis is often pragmatic, and is influenced by advancing knowledge and new techniques.

Box 1.8 The nature and possible causes of sickness X

- ◆ What thoughts come into your mind about the nature of the sickness?
- ◆ What kind of sickness/disease is it? Is it, for example, genetic, congenital (present at birth), degenerative (wear and tear of age), cancer, injury, infection, toxic, nutritional, or immune disorder?
- ◆ What kind of sickness/disease is it not?
- ◆ What sort of factors could cause a sickness such as this? Think of these factors at the level of individual, family, community, and national society.

Even at this stage, some possibilities in the causation of sickness X can be ruled out using general clinical and pathological principles about the nature of disease. Try the exercise in Box 1.8 before looking at Table 1.4.

Table 1.4 summarizes some reasoning on the nature of sickness X. This disease is not a chromosomal or gene defect, congenital, an immune disorder, a result of injury, a degeneration of age, or a result of uncontrolled cell division (cancer). It may be a result of infection, exposure to toxins, or a deficiency of some essential substance. This analysis is based on epidemiological reasoning and draws upon other relevant sciences. Population studies may be used by the clinician in managing the individual patient, for example, the clinician may utilize knowledge of an ongoing outbreak to help reach a diagnosis and to decide whether the patient needs hospitalization (or isolation), or can be managed in the community. At the time of writing (2015), the world is responding to the Ebola virus epidemic. Clinicians are basing their management of people travelling from West Africa and who are unwell on the epidemiological knowledge of which countries are affected. Therapeutic ideas may be sparked off by understanding of causation and then tested on populations of patients. The results derived from populations will then be applied to individuals. Clinical practice, public health, and epidemiology are intertwined.

Table 1.4 Types of disease and some preliminary reasoning on causes of sickness/disease X

Type of disease	Reasoning for and against sickness X being this kind of disease
Genetic	Genetic diseases do not vary in their frequency over short periods of time, and do not selectively avoid certain populations, e.g. staff in institutions
Congenital	Congenital problems are present at birth, are usually diagnosed in the young, and are usually permanent
Degenerative	As for genetic. They do not tend to affect the young
Cancers	As for genetic. They do not exhibit marked seasonal variation
Injuries	The cause of injuries is usually apparent
Infections	The picture fits, though the reason for some populations being immune is unclear
Toxins	The picture fits but the nature of the toxin is obscure
Nutritional deficiency	The picture fits but the nature of the deficiency is obscure
Immune disorders	These do not present as epidemics

1.7 **The basic tools of epidemiology: two measures of disease frequency and five study designs**

The toolbox of epidemiology is powerful, growing, and changing—and it needs to be applied with great care. As with any tool wrongly applied, it can be damaging, and even dangerous. The tools are best used with a proper understanding of the purposes, theories, principles, and pitfalls of epidemiology. It is for this reason that the main tools are discussed later on in this book—Chapters 7–9. Some readers may, nonetheless, wish to read about the tools in advance of the more general material in Chapters 2–6. Others may find the brief introduction given in this section sufficient for the present.

The fraction (or ratio) of the number of outcomes of interest (usually diseases or similar problems) in relation to the population under study provides the core measurement tool. The most important of these measures are incidence rates and prevalence proportions, and from these building blocks, a multiplicity of specific disease measures arise.

Table 1.5 outlines these two measures, which are discussed in Chapter 7. The study types that are mostly used in epidemiology can be seen in Table 1.6. As we will see in Chapter 9, there is much conceptual and methodological overlap between these study designs. Moreover, each study design is capable of generating many different kinds of measure.

Exemplar 1.1, which can be found at the end of this chapter, also illustrates some of the conceptual and methodological issues discussed so far.

1.8 **Conclusions and seeking epidemiology's theoretical foundations**

A theory is a statement that provides an explanation or coherent account of a group of ideas, facts, or observed phenomena, such as the theory of evolution. Epidemiology has been criticized as an atheoretical discipline, comprising a mixed bag of tools, useful for solving particular problems but neither adding up to a science, nor providing a theoretical basis to the study of health and disease. Epidemiology, however, both draws upon and contributes to theories of health and disease. It may be that epidemiologists spend little time reflecting on the theories underpinning their work, but the same criticism would probably apply to other sciences. In most disciplines, theories are at the core of thinking and practice. Priscilla Alderson (1998) has argued that it is not possible to think

Table 1.5 Introduction to incidence rates and prevalence proportions

Measure	Key features	Type of study	Formulae*
Incidence	Count of new cases over a period of time in a population of known size defined by characteristics (age, sex, etc.), and place and time boundaries	Disease register supplying data (case series or population case series) Cohort Trial	New cases ÷ population at risk or New cases ÷ time spent by the study population at risk
Prevalence	Count of cases (new and old) at a point in time in a population of known size defined by characteristics (age, sex, etc.) and place	Cross-sectional Disease register (case series or population case series)	All cases ÷ population at risk

*The fractions arising are multiplied to create a whole number, e.g. by 100, or 100 000.

Table 1.6 Epidemiological designs and applications: an overview

Study design	Essential idea	Some research purposes
1. Case series and population case series (synonym, register studies)	Count cases (numerator) and relate to population data (denominator) to produce rates and analyse patterns	Study signs and symptoms, and create disease definitions Surveillance of mortality/morbidity rates Seek associations Generate/test hypotheses Source of cases or foundation for other studies
2. Cross-sectional	Study health and disease states in a population at a defined place and time Measure burden of disease and its causes	Measure prevalence (very rarely incidence) of disease and related factors Seek associations between disease and related factors Generate/test hypotheses Repeat studies (on different samples) to measure change and evaluate interventions Repeat study on same sample to create a cohort study
3. Case–control	Look for differences and similarities between a series of cases and a control group	Seek associations Generate/test hypotheses Assess strength of association
4. Cohort	Follow-up populations, relating information on risk factor patterns and health states at baseline, to the outcomes of interest	Study natural history of disease Measure incidence of disease Link disease outcomes to possible disease causes, i.e. seek associations Generate/test hypotheses
5. Trial	Intervene with some measure designed to improve health, then follow-up people to see the effect*	Test understanding of causes Study how to influence natural history of disease Evaluate the effects (side effects and benefits) and costs of interventions

*Measures designed to worsen health or to make no difference would be ethically unacceptable though this has been common from a historical viewpoint. This may currently be done (with ethical or regulatory approval) on animals.

about health care without theory, even though it may be implicit rather than explicit. Before reading on, do the exercise in Box 1.9.

The main epidemiological theories and principles that have guided this chapter include:

◆ Disease in populations is more than the sum of disease in individuals (described in depth in Chapter 2).

◆ Populations differ in their disease experience and this is because of variation in disease susceptibility or exposure to the causes.

◆ Knowledge about health and disease in human populations can be applied to individuals and vice versa.

Principles arising:

◆ Disease variations can be described, and their causes explored, by assessing whether exposure variables are associated with disease patterns.

◆ Health policies and plans and clinical care can be enriched by understanding disease patterns in populations.

Box 1.9 Spotting theories and principles underlying epidemiology

Can you discern any theories which have guided this chapter so far? What general principles follow from these theories?

Methods and techniques in epidemiology are designed to achieve the potential inherent in these theories and principles. In turn, new methods and techniques lead to new or refined theoretical understanding. Epidemiology's contribution to the theory of health and disease will be a recurrent theme throughout the book, and will be summarized and expanded upon in Chapter 10 (section 10.1).

In this third edition, I am introducing more material on causal diagrams as a means of strengthening the theoretical basis of epidemiology. I recommend that these diagrams should be introduced routinely into data analysis plans for research projects and into the introduction section of reports and scientific papers. Furthermore, these diagrams should be used to convey how theoretical thinking has altered as a result of empirical research. This step will alter the way we analyse and interpret data, for reasons I will explain in Chapter 5.

As Nancy Krieger (2011) has demonstrated, it is important that epidemiology is a theory-based, and not merely a methods-orientated, discipline.

Exemplar 1.1: Dawber, T.R., Kannel, W.B., and Lyell, L.P. (1963) An approach to longitudinal studies in a community: The Framingham Study. *Annals of the New York Academy of Sciences*, Volume 107, pp. 539–56

Background

By the middle of the twentieth century, coronary heart disease (also known as ischaemic heart disease, or CHD) was becoming an important cause of death and disability. The view that it was a natural, degenerative disorder of ageing, which was still the case when I studied medicine in the 1970s, was giving way to a perception that the underlying causes could be understood to impede the further rise of the epidemic. (The situation is now the same for the dementias of old age.) The Framingham Study was pivotal in transforming our understanding. In this paper, the investigators explain the underpinning reasoning and exemplify many of the key points covered in this chapter.

My summary of the paper

Introduction

While epidemiology has been successful in understanding the causes and prevention of infectious and nutritional diseases, it has not yet demonstrated its value in chronic diseases. Epidemiology works through demonstrating associations between possible causal factors and diseases, and proof of causality is seldom provided.

Laboratory, animal, or clinical research is often needed for demonstrating cause and effect, unless field trials can also be done. There are ways of judging whether an association is likely to be causal. One advantage of a prospective study is that the suspected causal factors are present prior to disease onset.

The Framingham Study

The study started in 1948 in the town of Framingham, in the state of Massachusetts, United States of America. The authors explain the factors contributing as to why this town was suitable including stability of its population, allowing long-term follow-up and community support. It studied adults with the aim of measuring the incidence of CHD and how host and environmental factors influence this. The authors point to their good fortune that the factors they selected were shown to be associated with CHD. They also emphasized the importance of clear research questions and various objectives focused on this one outcome. The hypotheses were generated by a consultation process including a committee of cardiologists. Prior information, including from case/control comparisons, was used.

The age group 30–59 was selected for reasons which included population stability and that the number of cases of CHD in those younger would be low. The sample required was estimated at 6500, of whom 5000 would be disease-free at onset.

A random sample was obtained of the 10 000 people in the age group, but it was supplemented by volunteers. Men and women were studied. The authors estimated there would be about 1500 cases over 20 years.

The variables studied and case definition

The outcome was CHD assessed as a binary variable from death certificates, medical reports, hospitalization and other records, follow-up clinic examinations, etc. After the study began, new laboratory tests (cardiac enzymes) were introduced and were incorporated into the definition of the outcome, clinical CHD. This outcome included:

myocardial infarction based on electrocardiogram (ECG) (and later, enzymes);

angina pectoris based on chest discomfort;

coronary insufficiency based on symptoms and ECG;

sudden death;

death apparently due to CHD with no specific diagnosis.

Records were reviewed by the medical staff. Two independent observers were needed to agree the diagnosis.

The exposure variables included age, sex, family history, lipid levels, blood pressure, smoking, and physical activity.

Analysis

Machine processing of data was required (NB: this is before the era of the desktop computer). The period of observation was assumed to be uniform for each subject (the measure of incidence would hence be a cumulative incidence). The risk of developing CHD was examined in subgroups defined by the level of the risk factor. The authors emphasize how difficult and time-consuming the analysis was and they admit some mistakes were made in the process, for example, grouping of data rather than coding the actual measurements.

Example results

a) *Cholesterol*

In men 30–59 years at study entry, the risk of developing 'heart attack' (authors' quotation marks) over 10 years was calculated as a ratio with the whole population given a risk value of 100. For those with serum cholesterol levels below 200 mg/dL (5.18 mmol/l) the risk was 50 (half that of the whole population) and for those with cholesterol level of 260 mg/dL (6.73 mmol/l) or more it was 186. This was nearly a fourfold difference.

b) *High blood pressure, an ECG abnormality not due to CHD and high cholesterol combined*

In the group with none of these three abnormalities the risk was 53, and in those with all three it was 435. This was more than an eightfold difference.

These results were interpreted as identifying highly susceptible individuals.

Authors' conclusions

Community-based studies of this kind are difficult and methods need to be developed. Through knowledge of the epidemiology of chronic disease, methods of control and prevention may be developed.

Concluding remarks

The Framingham Study is one of a few that established epidemiology as a dominant force in chronic disease control. More than 1200 papers have been published from the original study and its extensions. The study has transformed the field of causal factors in cardiovascular disease from being somewhat mysterious to well understood. This paper provides unusually deep insights into the way the investigators thought through the methods and even the mistakes they made. It explains, not just describes, the epidemiological approach. Several of the risk factors that were studied in this study are now widely accepted as causal.

Summary

Populations, as with individuals, have unique patterns of disease. Populations' disease patterns derive from differences in the type of individuals they comprise, in the mode of interaction of individuals, and in the environment. The science of epidemiology—which straddles biology, clinical medicine, social sciences, and ecology—seeks to describe, understand, and utilize these patterns to improve population health. As a science, epidemiology's central paradigm is that analysis of population patterns of disease, particularly by linking these to exposure variables (risk factors), provides understanding of the causes of disease. Epidemiology is useful in other ways too, including preventing and controlling disease in populations, and guiding health and health-care policy and planning. Causal understanding is not always essential in these latter applications. Epidemiology can also help clinicians to manage the health care of individuals.

A useful epidemiological exposure variable reflects the purposes of epidemiology, and is: measurable accurately; differentiates populations in their experience of disease or health; and generates testable aetiological hypotheses, and/or helps in developing health policy and health-care plans, and/or to prevent and control disease. For advancing causal knowledge, variables that highlight the differences between and within population subgroups in diseases of unknown aetiology are *potentially* of great value. The more complex the concept captured by the variable, the harder it is to understand the reasons for the associated variation in disease experience. For health policy and planning, variables that show variations in diseases for which effective interventions are available are particularly valuable.

Understanding the epidemiology of a disease demands clinical collaboration. Clinicians need to agree on a definition that will permit screening or diagnosis. The first question for the epidemiologist, in any investigation, is the nature, validity, and usefulness of the definition of the disease or other problem under investigation. Then follow questions on which populations are to be studied, and the methods for making accurate measurement of the frequency and pattern of disease, as well as the postulated risk factors and other relevant variables. In turn, epidemiological knowledge is used by clinicians to help make diagnoses in individuals, to prescribe effective treatments, and to offer patients information on the natural history and prognosis of their diseases.

Epidemiology has evolved a large toolbox. At its core lies the measurement of the prevalence and incidence of risk factors and outcomes. These measurements are generated by study types (designs) that serve the various purposes of epidemiology. Of the many kinds of available study, the most important are case series (register studies), cross-sectional, case–control, cohort, and intervention (trials) studies. One of the most important of these studies is summarized in Exemplar 1.1. Epidemiology is both founded on, and contributes to, theories of health and disease, though these are too seldom made explicit.

Sample questions

Give yourself 10 minutes for each question.

Question 1 The phrase 'outcome variable' is often used in epidemiology. Explain the meaning of this phrase, and indicate how it differs from exposure variable.

Answer The outcome variable usually refers to the disease, illness, death, or preceding processes leading to these; for example, hypertension, or obesity/overweight. The outcome variable is the variable that the study is trying to understand or explain the causes of. The potential explanations are usually referred to as exposure variables, or even more commonly, risk factors. There is an overlap in these two types of variable because sometimes epidemiologists study the effect of one disease (now exposure variable) on another (outcome variable), and sometimes of one exposure on another (now outcome variable).

Question 2 Define epidemiology and briefly outline its principal strategies.

Answer Epidemiology is the study of the patterns of health, and disease, in populations. It focuses on describing and understanding these patterns, thereby shedding light on the causes of ill health and disease. Its central strategy is to compare and contrast populations over time and between places, and using differences and similarities in risk factors and disease outcomes to aid understanding. Epidemiology uses several designs to gather data and frameworks for causal reasoning to interpret it.

Question 3 In what respects is epidemiology a science? In what respects is it not a science?

Answer Epidemiology is a science, in that it studies a natural phenomenon—the causes of health and disease in populations—using systematic approaches to developing hypotheses, implementing methods, and interpreting data. It uses and develops theories of health and disease. It is a science with elements of biological, social, and ecological sciences.

Epidemiology also measures the burden and distribution of disease for applied purposes, for example, health-care planning and setting public health priorities. In this context, epidemiology is not about the study of causes or exploring hypotheses and theories—but is rather a practice or craft, rather than a science.

References

Alderson, P. (1998) The importance of theories in health care. *British Medical Journal*, **317**, 1007–10.

Bronowski, J. (1974) *Ascent of Man*, Chapter 4. London, UK: BBC.

Chadwick, J. and Mann, W.N. (1950) *The Medical Works of Hippocrates*. Oxford, UK: Blackwell Scientific Publications.

Dawber, T., Kannel, W., and Lyell, L. (1963) An approach to longitudinal studies in a community: the Framingham Study. *Annals New York Academy of Sciences*, **107**, 539–56. (Reprinted in Buck *et al.* 1988, pp. 619–30).

Fraser, D.W., Tsai, T.R., Orenstein, W., *et al.* (1977) Legionnaires' disease: description of an epidemic of pneumonia. *New England Journal of Medicine*, **297**, 1189–97.

Krieger, N. (2011) *Epidemiology and the People's Health. Theory and Context*. New York, NY: Oxford University Press.

Kuller, L.H. (1999) Invited commentary: circular epidemiology. *American Journal of Epidemiology*, **150**, 897–902.

Morris, J.N. (1964) *Uses of Epidemiology*, 2nd edn. Baltimore, MD: The Williams and Wilkins Company.

Porta, M. (2014) *A Dictionary of Epidemiology*, 6th edn. New York, NY: Oxford University Press.

Skrabanek, P. (1994) The emptiness of the black box. *Epidemiology*, **5**, 553–55.

Chapter 2

The epidemiological concept of population

Objectives

On completion of this chapter you should understand:

♦ the meaning and applications of the idea that epidemiology is a population science;

♦ the profound influence of the characteristics of a population on its disease patterns;

♦ the potential and limitations of epidemiology in the absence of demographic population size and structure data;

♦ the expansion of possibilities in epidemiology which occurs when demographic population data are available;

♦ the impact of change in the size and characteristics of the population on health.

2.1 The individual, the group, and the population

Epidemiology is a population science. It is primarily concerned with understanding the distribution and causes of disease through comparing the pattern of disease in populations over time, between places and in different types of people, as symbolized in Figure 2.1.

Populations, of course, comprise unique individuals. Humans, however, are social beings who thrive in families, groups, and communities, and it is extremely rare for people to live in isolation. (Solitary confinement is one of the severest penalties in society.) The family is the basic social unit, but nearly all humans live in much larger populations. The study of human groups is the keystone of epidemiology. No epidemiological study can be done on one person, but other medical sciences such as pharmacology, pathology, and physiology may study one person, or even parts of a person.

To compare and contrast health status and disease patterns you need groups. While epidemiology may be based on very large groups— sometimes millions of people, but nearly always hundreds or thousands—it can be also done on very small groups. The classic experiment of Lind in 1747 was on 12 persons, divided into six pairs of two, with each pair receiving a different intervention to try to prevent scurvy (Lind 1753—see Exemplar 10.1). A definitive study of adenocarcinoma of the vagina by Herbst and colleagues (1971) was based on eight cases and 32 people without disease as controls (see also section 5.6.3).

Epidemiology aggregates the health experiences of individuals as groups and tries to generalize the findings to the population from which these groups have come, and beyond this to other populations. These aggregate health experiences are analysed in terms of the questions summarized in Box 2.1 to seek patterns over time, between places and between subpopulations with different characteristics. This is known as the epidemiological triad of time, place, and person. Time, place, and person can be thought of as very broad exposure variables. The strategy of epidemiology, as

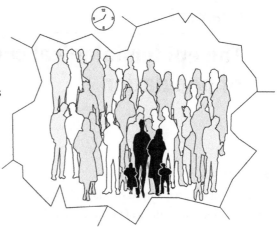

- Populations comprise individuals, families, groups and communities
- Epidemiology seeks variations in disease patterns over time, between subgroups and between places
- Understanding such variation yields knowledge on causation and prevention of disease

Fig. 2.1 The individual and population: the triad of time, place, and person.

we saw in Chapter 1, is to discover the causes of these patterns, and ultimately the causes of disease. (A theme developed in later chapters, particularly Chapter 5.)

Answer the questions in Box 2.2 on disease X (described in Chapter 1, Box 1.7), before reading the answers in Table 2.1.

As the analysis in Table 2.1 shows, epidemiological thinking can help us to progress understanding of the causes of disease in populations, and also to forecast the probability (risk) of disease and its outcome in individuals. For example, we can reassure staff in institutions where disease X is present that their chance of developing disease is low. In studies to pinpoint the cause of the disease, we will be looking for associations with particular types of environmental exposure.

Epidemiological conclusions are directly applicable to the groups studied, but only indirectly to individuals, and then only to those who are reasonably typical of the population studied. For example, for populations, the causal link between smoking and lung cancer is solid and can be accurately quantified. Indeed, it is usually possible to extrapolate causal associations of this kind beyond the study population, and even globally. For an individual the causal link may not apply, for there may be environmental or genetic reasons why that person is not susceptible to the carcinogenic effect of tobacco. The risk of disease outcomes for individuals, especially well ones, can seldom be estimated accurately. The exception to this include extremely sick people—for example, those in deep coma.

This contrasts with some other fields of life. For example, school examination grades can be predicted fairly accurately for an individual from previous examination achievements. Individuals

Box 2.1 The triad of epidemiological questions—time, place, and person

- How does the pattern of this disease vary over time in this population? (Time)
- How does the place in which the population lives affect the disease pattern? (Place)
- How do the personal characteristics of the people in the population affect the disease pattern? (Person)

Box 2.2 Exercise: application of the triad of time, place, and person to disease X

Apply the questions in Box 2.1 to disease X. (See Chapter 1, Box 1.7)

- ◆ Now, does this information help you to understand, or at least develop ideas on, the causes of the disease?
- ◆ How might you use this information to begin more detailed scientific investigation?
- ◆ How does the information help to plan for the control or prevention of disease?

can also assess the risk of being struck by a car while crossing the road, based on their own experiences. The difference is that most diseases are rare so few individuals get them; many diseases only occur once; and you either have the disease or you do not. By contrast, school grades are estimated many times and crossing the road is a daily event. Predicting the individual's risk of developing the common cold over, say, a five-year period is more feasible than predicting whether an individual will develop, say, stroke or lung cancer.

The knowledge gained by epidemiological studies still benefits individuals. Surprisingly, information gained from groups may sometimes be more helpful to individuals than information from the individuals themselves. Physicians from the time of Hippocrates have devoted much effort to

Table 2.1 The epidemiological triad of questions applied to disease X (Box 1.7) and its contribution to causal understanding

The epidemiological triad of questions	The questions applied to sickness X
How does the pattern of disease vary over time? (Time)	The sickness is a new, emergent problem
	It sometimes occurs as outbreaks
	It is seasonal
	It follows times of economic hardship
How does the place in which the population lives affect the disease pattern? (Place)	It is worst in people living in low-lying areas It affects people in institutions more, but only the inmates, not staff
How do the personal characteristics of the people in the population affect the disease pattern? (Person)	Living in poverty and sharecropping increase risk Being related to a person with the disease increases the risk It affects all ages, and both men and women

Moving from triad to causes

With the great variation in disease over time, between places, and by personal characteristics the evidence points to an environmental rather than a genetic cause. The various associations, e.g. emergence in the spring, the link to poverty, the effect on those living in institutions, etc. permit hypotheses to be developed and tested. Also they point to populations for study, e.g. those living in institutions and farmers practising sharecropping. At this stage, no specific control or preventive actions are compelling but the disease seems to be preventable. In Chapter 1 (Table 1.4 and associated text) we favoured toxic, infectious, and nutritional hypotheses. These can be tested using a mix of the epidemiological designs outlined in Chapter 1 and discussed in Chapter 9. See section 2.4 for the story of the cause of sickness.

Box 2.3 Thought exercise on prognosis (prediction of progression of illness)

- ◆ How would you assess the prognosis for a patient with a terminal illness who asks, 'how long have I got to live?'
- ◆ How would you advise a parent of a 5-year-old son with asthma who asks, 'will my child have asthma for the rest of his life?'

prognosis, the prediction of outcome once a disease has occurred, which is essential to both the practice and the science of medicine. A great deal of attention has been paid to symptoms, signs, and tests which indicate the prognosis of an individual, but prognosis remains an erroneous business. Before reading on, reflect on the questions in Box 2.3.

Even in the dying person, the outcome is difficult to predict accurately. In a study in Chicago hospices of the terminally ill, experienced physicians overestimated survival by a factor of 5.3. This is not simply an issue of over-optimism, but one of complexity. There are too many factors at play. The likelihood of an individual child with asthma continuing to have it in adulthood cannot be predicted from the signs, symptoms, or characteristics of the individual. Prognosis can, however, be expressed as a probability derived from population studies. This probability only informs the individual what happens on average, although the physician may use the individual's data to try to refine the prediction. Imperfect and unsatisfactory as this extrapolation from the population to the individual is, the approach has been widely adopted within medicine as the best available, pending the development of accurate measures of prognosis based on the characteristics of individuals (this is a massive challenge for future clinical research which will, hopefully, be greatly assisted by advances in genetics). The potential and progress of personalized medicine is a hot topic in both scientific journals and the mass media. To date, the experience does not instil optimism. Epidemiology will remain the dominant means of prediction of risk and prognosis for the foreseeable future, at least in conditions that are chronic, and not recurrent. In essence, epidemiology has become a substitute for the experience of the clinician and has superseded the clinician's case series.

Where a disease occurs repeatedly in the same person, individual-based prediction becomes possible, and is likely to be superior to epidemiological predictions. For example, the experience of a child who has an asthma attack once or twice a week, mostly at nights, can be used to predict the occurrence, timing, and outcome of the next attack. By contrast the risk of occurrence and outcome of meningococcal meningitis, which is rare, is only predictable from population studies.

Information about the demographic and socio-economic characteristics of a population tells us about the health of individuals within that population. For example, knowing that a population is rich predicts a pattern of death for most individuals that is dominated by heart disease, stroke, and cancer—and not by infections and nutritional deficiency disorders. These generalizations are possible as population characteristics influence individuals' risk of disease, as discussed next.

2.2 Harnessing variety in individual and group-level disease and risk factor patterns

Epidemiology is interested in understanding the factors that shape population patterns of disease as in disease X in Box 1.7. These factors are usually complex interactions between individuals,

---

Box 2.4 Heterogeneity (dissimilarity) and homogeneity (similarity) of exposure to potential causes of disease in epidemiology

- How would epidemiology study the link between tobacco and lung cancer in a society where every adult smoked 20 cigarettes per day?

- How would one investigate epidemiologically the effect, in the long term, of the gas nitrogen on human health? What about oxygen?

- Neutrinos are cosmic particles which penetrate deep into the Earth. There are billions going through us every second. How would we investigate, epidemiologically, their impact on health?

---

their physical environment, and their society. To understand the pattern, therefore, needs understanding of the circumstances in which the population lives.

Investigation of disease patterns should be, therefore, on populations characterized in terms of location, size, age and sex structure, and a wide range of data on the life and environmental circumstances of the people. The idea is to utilize the inherent variety of populations, and measure characteristics that are potential explanations for disease variation. In studying variation in chronic bronchitis, for example, we need to know whether the populations studied are exposed to air pollution, tobacco, poverty, or poor housing. This is the central message in the famous quotation from Hippocrates (Chapter 1), and in most definitions of epidemiology. As populations change over time, it is imperative that researchers state when they performed their fieldwork, but, amazingly, this information is commonly missing in publications. Do the exercise in Box 2.4 before reading on.

In a society where everyone smoked cigarettes, say 20 per day, epidemiology would be virtually powerless to assess the effect, for while lung cancer would be common, the exposure to the major cause would be uniform. The key strategy of comparing and contrasting the disease pattern in people with and without the postulated cause (exposure) is not possible here. The solution would be to persuade some of the population to decrease or stop smoking; in other words, to do an experiment. Experiments usually need to be justified by data supporting the hypothesis; in the circumstances described, this would be difficult.

While experimentation might be possible for tobacco, it could not be accomplished easily with respect to oxygen, nitrogen, and neutrinos, as experimentally stopping, or even substantially reducing, exposure to these substances would not be feasible except for short periods of time. The effects of such gases and particles on long-term human health are not open to rigorous epidemiological study. Nonetheless, useful information might come from experimental studies on animals or cell cultures.

Paradoxically, the variety that is so vital to epidemiology poses challenges in interpreting and applying research. While tobacco and alcohol, for example, are damaging to health in populations as a whole, there are people and groups for whom these substances are harmless and perhaps even beneficial in some respects. For example, tobacco use is linked to fewer problems with ulcerative colitis, and it suppresses the appetite and prevents weight gain. Alcohol in small amounts may reduce the risk of atherosclerotic heart disease. Whether, for a particular individual, tobacco or alcohol consumption is advisable or not is, surprisingly, beyond epidemiology, which only permits valid judgements at the population level. (This limitation does not, however, stop the use of epidemiology in this way.) The health damage caused by tobacco in populations unequivocally far outweighs the health benefits. The position concerning alcohol consumption is less clear, but the harm and damage at a population level, in most societies, is certainly more in balance than that for tobacco. Epidemiology aids policy development in these controversial areas.

Section 2.3 will discuss why the disease and risk factor patterns in populations are not merely the sum of the same measures as applied to individuals.

2.3 Disease patterns as an outcome of individuals living in changing social groups

Diseases are expressed biologically in individuals. It is tempting, therefore, to assume that the causes of diseases, and the solutions to their control and prevention, are also biological and lie at the individual level. Many diseases, however, are caused only by the interaction of individuals, and most are profoundly influenced by such interactions. In other words, the causes of disease are often social and biological. Individuals shape society, and in turn society exerts a powerful influence on individuals, including their attitudes, behaviour, and diseases.

Do the exercise in Box 2.5 before reading on.

Chapter 1 introduced the idea that disease patterns were influenced by the interaction of social, environmental, and individual level factors. This central concept applies to many diseases. Suicide is a clear-cut example. While suicide and parasuicide are linked to psychotic disorders, particularly depression, they are hugely influenced by convention. Durkheim, a French sociologist working in the nineteenth century, held that common values underlie social order, and that the loss of such values leads to social and individual instability, and suicide. Durkheim's studies (1951) showed huge variations in suicide, which he believed to be an attribute of the society, or social reality, which in turn determined the suicide-related behaviour of individuals. This principle, that society influences mortality, has now been demonstrated in wider circumstances, and most recently in the context of inequalities in health.

Mortality rates generally, and for some specific causes of death, are associated with increasing inequality of wealth in society. For a given level of wealth, societies that distribute the wealth more equally have higher life expectancy (and other health outcomes are better) than those that distribute wealth less equally. Economically unequal societies also have poorer mental and physical health than expected. Such societies show an excess of both overtly social problems such as murder and accidents, and other apparently biological problems such as cardiovascular diseases.

Box 2.5 Impact of social organization on disease patterns in populations

Imagine a world where humans lived an isolated lifestyle, avoiding others whenever possible, using technologies to communicate, and using physical barriers to reduce contact. Children would be raised by one parent, perhaps. Imagine that the physical and economic environment remained similar to that we experience now; that is, people lived in housing of similar quality and used similar cars, etc.

+ What would be the effect on disease patterns?
+ Which diseases would be more common and which less so?
+ What would be the influences on lifestyles?

The explanations for these observations are complex and controversial. The main hypothesis under examination is that unequal societies are less likely to invest in activities that improve health, and/or that they undermine social cohesion, and increase stress. There is some evidence that the adverse effects of income inequality are greatest in the poorer and middle-income groups and least in the wealthiest groups. In short, being poor is associated with poor health, and being poor in an economically unequal society adds a further burden on health. Many industrialized countries, including the United Kingdom and United States, have become both wealthier and more unequal in the last 30–40 years, so these observations have particular relevance to modern public health.

Society even has an impact on genetic diseases. Down's syndrome, a genetic disorder called trisomy 21, shows how social expectations and behaviours alter disease patterns. Societies that encourage birth at older ages have a higher rate of Down's syndrome than those that encourage childbirth in the young, because the genetic abnormality becomes more common as the mother ages. Prenatal screening is available for this disorder, and the choice of abortion of the affected fetus is possible. So, the number of people with Down's syndrome depends on age of the mother at conception, availability and uptake of screening, and the acceptability of abortion—all socially determined. The pattern of this genetic disease depends, therefore, on the way society is organized.

Individuals and their societies live in a physical environment, which is the prime determinant of health and illness in populations (an argument developed in Chapter 4 on causal thinking).

In the imaginary future world in Box 2.5, which is feasible, diseases that are transmitted from person-to-person would occur rarely. So, an isolated individual or small group would not develop diseases such as tuberculosis, leprosy, influenza, the common cold, measles, mumps, AIDS, Ebola, and sexually transmitted diseases. Some of the microorganisms causing these diseases are exclusively human pathogens (e.g. the leprosy bacillus, mumps virus, measles virus) so they would not survive, and would become extinct. If humans also isolated themselves from animals, the zoonoses (diseases transmitted from animals to humans), including Lyme disease and brucellosis, would not occur. The human–animal cycle necessary for the propagation of parasitic diseases would be broken. The effect would not just be on the highly contagious diseases. Ulcers associated with infection by the bacterium *Helicobacter pylori* would be less common. Cancers linked to microorganisms would not occur, or their incidence would be profoundly reduced. For example, cervical cancer, which is primarily caused by human papillomavirus transmitted sexually, and gastric cancer, often a consequence of *Helicobacter pylori* infection, would decline sharply.

The pattern of mental health problems would be profoundly different. The stresses of living in complex societies would be replaced by problems of isolation and loneliness.

The influence on cancer and heart disease would also be huge, mostly from changes in behaviours which are influenced by social and peer pressures; for example, smoking, alcohol drinking, physical activity, and the amount and content of diet. The pattern of behaviour would change hugely, causing massive but unpredictable alterations in the pattern of disease.

The thought exercise in Box 2.5 is not theoretical. For most of their history, humans have lived as small groups of 20–100 hunter-gatherers and not in large settled communities. There are still humans who are, effectively, isolated. Influenza and measles are deadly disorders in populations previously unexposed to them and, therefore, lacking in immunity. Smallpox, a scourge for any society, was near genocidal in isolated populations exposed to it. Over the last few hundred years, isolated human groups have been rapidly exposed to populations of strangers with devastating consequences for their health. The Tasmanian aborigines were made extinct by their interaction with European settlers and North American Indians were decimated by the new patterns of disease arising from both their interaction with Europeans, and later the new social expectations and roles imposed upon them. As a form of germ warfare, European settlers gave American Indians 'presents' of blankets that had been contaminated with material from smallpox patients. In more modern times, in 1857 the British colonized the Andaman Islands (east of India, west of Thailand) where the tribe Great Andamanese comprised 5000 people. In 1988, 28 were left. Measles and influenza took their toll. In March 2015, 50 members of the Great Andamanese were alive, but all from the Bo speaking tribe had died. The Jarawa tribe remains isolated on the Andaman Islands but is making contact with the outside world. In the first edition of this book, I wrote that the result is predictable. Since then, there have been measles outbreaks and continuing encroachment of territory despite an Indian Supreme Court injunction, largely ignored, that the main road into the Jarawa territory be closed. Tourism has become a major problem for the Jarawa tribe with the introduction of alcohol, drugs, and sexual exploitation threatening to destabilize this isolated tribe of 400 people.

The swift move to urbanization following the industrial revolution in the eighteenth century, still continuing in the industrialized nations and accelerating in the developing ones, has exposed billions of people to new environments, new disease agents, and different forms of human interaction. Migration and population mixing has a profound effect on the disease patterns of society. As a generalization, over some generations, the migrant population takes on the pattern of disease of the host country. The process of change is usually slow, but it can be fast and surprising. Emigrants from India to wealthy industrialized countries develop chronic diseases such as heart disease and diabetes at a level far higher than predictable from the rate of disease in India and from their pattern of causal factors. The explanations for this are under study. Migration also changes disease on a local scale. For example, the strongest explanation for the observed high rates of childhood leukaemia around nuclear power stations is based on the pattern of childhood infections. There was substantial population mixing because of the inward migration of workers into the relatively isolated communities hosting power stations. If the hypothesis is correct, local migration changing the pattern of childhood infection, and not radiation from power stations, is the fundamental cause of the excess of leukaemia in these areas (see Kinlen *et al.* 1995).

The twenty-first century may see a reversal, at least in wealthy industrialized countries, of population mixing. First, easier transport and new communications technology are offering people the chance of enjoying the benefits of the city while mostly living in isolation, either in the countryside or within fenced and guarded compounds in the city. Computer links at home, work that can be done solo, environmental concerns, and an increase in costs of office space in cities are likely to accelerate these trends. Secondly, with increasing inequality in income the wealthiest people have both the resources and incentives to isolate themselves geographically from their societies.

The population, then, has patterns of health and disease which are caused by the interactions of individuals living in a complex, organized society. Some diseases would not arise at all in isolated individuals and small groups. For nearly all diseases, the pattern would be greatly different if the social organization differed. Disease patterns are generated in, and by, populations so need to be described, explained, and predicted in populations. While all individuals must sicken and die, the nature of the population they live in has a profound effect on which sicknesses they develop, when they develop them, and at what age they are likely to die within the range determined by biological processes. The close link of epidemiology to public health, which is defined as the science and art of prolonging life, preventing disease and promoting health through the organized efforts of society, is clear in this context. This sets the stage for considering the late Geoffrey Rose's idea of the sick population.

2.4 **Sick populations and sick individuals**

Rose proposed a radical and still controversial vision in his book, *Strategy of Preventive Medicine* (Rose 1994). This controversy has not abated and its resolution is unlikely in the near future. His central proposition was that people with overt diseases and health problems—people with hypertension, alcohol problems, or obesity—are simply at one end of the spectrum, or distribution, in the population. They are not to be seen as deviant, but an integral part of the whole. To prevent such problems requires changes in the population, with a shifting of the whole distribution of risk factors. For example, in Rose's argument, prevention of alcoholism requires that the entire distribution of alcohol consumption shifts, so the average and total consumption declines. To quote Rose, 'the supposedly "normal" majority needs to accept responsibility for its deviant minority—however loth it may be to do so'. Leaving aside the slightly pejorative term 'deviant minority', we can see what the controversy is: it is hard to accept, for example, that my eating or drinking habits are responsible for someone else's obesity or alcoholism. However, the idea is aimed at society as a whole, and not on you or me, or anyone else.

Rose developed the idea of sick and healthy populations, distinct from sick or healthy individuals, by reflecting on questions arising from international studies of high blood pressure and cardiovascular disease, and the exercise that follows is based on that. Currently a systolic blood pressure of 140 mmHg or more is considered a matter of concern and one of 160 mmHg would cause some alarm. Here, consider a value of 140 mm as indicative of hypertension. Before reading on, reflect carefully, but broadly, on Figure 2.2 using the questions in Box 2.6. Figure 2.2 is a graph showing the systolic blood pressure on the x-axis and the percentage of the population with that level of pressure in each of two populations on the y-axis.

Figure 2.2 shows that the shape of the two distributions of blood pressure is broadly similar, and of the shape that is described as a normal (or Gaussian) distribution as shown in Figure 2.3 (normal distributions are symmetric; the mean, median and mode values are the same; and 68% of the population lies within one standard deviation of the mean value, and 95% within two standard deviations—see glossary). The distribution of blood pressure in London civil servants is far to the right of that of Kenyan nomads. One simple indication of the impact of this on the amount of disease is the percentage of the population with hypertension. Based on the cut-off of 140 mmHg,

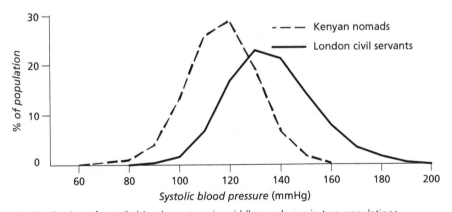

Fig. 2.2 Distribution of systolic blood pressures in middle-aged men in two populations.

Box 2.6 Reflection on the distribution of blood pressure values in Kenyan nomads and London civil servants

Examine Figure 2.2 and reflect on these questions:

◆ In what ways, broadly, do the shapes of the distributions differ (if at all) in the two populations?

◆ Roughly, what percentage of Kenyans and London civil servants have hypertension, that is, systolic blood pressure of 140 mmHg or above?

◆ Is there any suggestion from Figure 2.2 that the cause of high blood pressure in an individual Kenyan nomad and a London civil servant is likely to differ?

◆ What are the causes of the different distribution of blood pressure, in general terms, in the two populations?

◆ Are the causes of high blood pressure in the population, reflected in the distribution, different from those in the individual?

---

a large percentage of civil servants have hypertension (about 40%) and a small percentage of nomads do (about 10%). Based on a cut-off of 160 mmHg substantial numbers of civil servants have hypertension (about 15%), while such values are rare in nomads. Rose and Day (1990) showed that the population mean (average) predicts the number of people with the health problem. For systolic blood pressure, their data predicted a 10 per cent increase in the percentage of the population with hypertension for every 10 mmHg increase in mean systolic blood pressure.

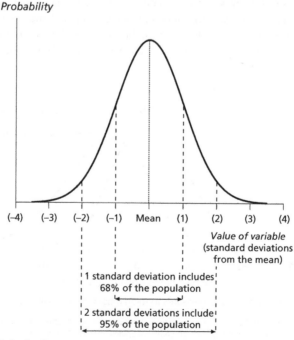

Fig. 2.3 The normal distribution.

The cause of high blood pressure in individuals is usually not pinpointed and is named essential hypertension. (In medicine, the prefix 'essential' really means 'we don't know the cause'.) In about 10 per cent of cases a specific cause (such as a kidney problem) is found. While Figure 2.2 does not inform us about the causes of hypertension in individuals, the similarity in the shape of the distribution, and the range of difference between the two extremes, suggest similarities in the forces that shape the distribution. Rose surmises that the specific causes of hypertension in nomads may be the same genetic, environmental, and behavioural factors as those operating on civil servants. Certainly, renal failure will cause hypertension in a Kenyan and a Londoner alike.

The stark difference is in the location on the x-axis, as opposed to the shape, of the blood pressure distributions. Explaining this is a typical epidemiological challenge. It is likely that the nomads are closer to the normal pattern for humans and that the Londoners' distribution has shifted rightwards. The question of what causes this difference between populations is a different one from what causes hypertension in an individual. We can speculate that the causes of the rightward shift are dietary factors (including high fat, high salt, high calories), obesity, insufficient exercise, stress, and the relationships between these and genetic factors. Such factors are largely generated in society and are acting on the population. For example, Londoners have created a society where a sedentary lifestyle is an option, which is not possible for nomads. The question of causes, therefore, needs to be studied in relation to the population and not just individuals. The causes of sickness in the population—for example, London civil servants who comprise a group with an abnormal blood pressure distribution—are conceptually different from the causes of sickness in the individual, and need to be studied differently too. Rose emphasizes that information on the population distribution of the risk factors and outcome (as in Fig. 2.2), and the shape of the risk factor–disease outcome relationship (see dose–response, Chapter 5) is vital to the population approach in preventive medicine.

Similar analysis could be done for many other health problems such as alcoholism, obesity, and diabetes. Before reading on, reflect on alcohol and alcoholic liver disease. While the cause of alcoholic liver cirrhosis is alcohol (by circularity of argument in the definition), its incidence varies hugely between populations and indeed within subgroups of the population. What is the cause of this population variation? Plainly, there are differences in populations in the consumption of alcohol. Why are there such differences?

The individual may be an alcoholic as a response to anxiety, depression, unemployment, role models in the family, or genetic variants promoting addictive behaviours, or simply a fondness for alcoholic beverages that led to addiction. Populations, however, have high and low consumption for different reasons including stigma, religion, tradition, customs of hospitality, availability, laws, policies, income, and taxes.

Understanding the causes of such phenomena in the population is the primary responsibility of population scientists, and in regard to health and disease, of epidemiologists.

Rose referred to the causes of population variations as the causes of the causes. These are also known as distal causes, with the immediate causes being proximal. The major cause of lung cancer is tobacco. What causes people to take up smoking even when they are knowledgeable about its harm? Why does the amount of smoking vary so much between populations? The causes of the causes, reflected in these questions, tend to be social and environmental, not biological.

The idea that the causes of diseases in individuals differ from causes in populations, leads to a radically different strategy for disease control based on both the causes, and the causes of the causes. The goal becomes changing the distribution of risk factors in populations as opposed to individuals. Figure 2.4 illustrates the strategic difference between the so-called high-risk and population-based approaches. A distribution of alcohol consumption is shown in part (a), with the level at which health risk increases (say risk of alcoholic liver damage). Part (b) of the figure

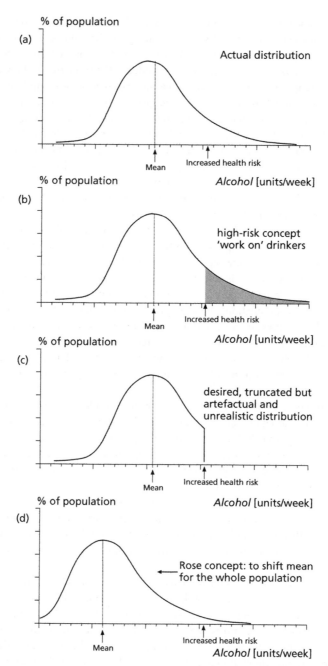

Fig. 2.4 The actual, high-risk, truncated, and shifted distributions: example of alcohol.

shades the high-risk group. The high-risk approach concentrates on this group. If the strategy is successful, the end result would be as shown in (c), a highly artificial result that has never been seen. The population approach accepts that a distribution like (c) is not feasible. To achieve a similar result in terms of reducing risk, we could shift the entire distribution leftwards. Such shifts require social action whereby the average levels of consumption are based on reducing the harm,

Box 2.7 Sickness X: individual and population perspective

- ◆ Was sickness X (Box 1.7) a disease of sick individuals or of sick populations?
- ◆ What might have been the causes of the causes in sickness X?

not merely in individuals, but the population as a whole. We have to apply the idea carefully and thoughtfully. For example, if the entire BMI distribution were shifted leftwards, some thin people would become dangerously underweight. This matter is discussed again in section 2.8. Do the exercise in Box 2.7 on whether sickness X is a disease of individuals or of populations, before reading the material in Box 2.8. (You may wish to re-read the material in Box 1.7.)

Isolated cases of sickness X did occur, usually in the mentally ill, or in people with addictions such as alcohol. More usually it occurred in outbreak or epidemic form in whole communities. Knowledge of the specific 'causal' agent did not achieve control of the disease at the population level, although it did cure the individual once treated.

Sickness X is pellagra, a disease caused by deficiency of a vitamin now called niacin (vitamin B3). The investigation of the causes of pellagra by Joseph Goldberger starting in 1914 is a compelling, classic tale (Roe, 1973). At that time an infectious cause was favoured, but Goldberger's traditional review of the scientific literature in 1914 led him, rapidly, to favour a nutritional cause, even though in 1914 a USA government commission had concluded otherwise. Goldberger (and a colleague, Edgar Sydenstricker) pursued the investigation for over more than 20 years with a mix of epidemiological designs (including a cohort study and trial), and in addition to laboratory-based animal research. The biology of the disease is now clear. However, to say the cause of pellagra is niacin deficiency, or even a nutritional deficiency, is a simplification, particularly as it does not provide a course of action for controlling the disease in the population. The characteristics of the disease in a population context, some of which are identified in Box 2.8, give clues to the wider causes of the cause (niacin deficiency): poverty; loss of freedom of populations and individuals to

Box 2.8 Some observations on disease X as a sickness of populations

Sickness X

- ◆ Never occurred in humans free to choose their own way of life
- ◆ Occurred after populations were thrown into poverty
- ◆ Did not decline even after its specific cause was well understood in biological terms
- ◆ Continued to occur, in hundreds of thousands of people every year, in some extremely rich countries that would not accept that the cause had been discovered even though other countries virtually eliminated the problem by acting upon available knowledge
- ◆ Declined when a war led to a change in the mode of life in the United States
- ◆ Declined when economic disaster led to a marked change in the mode of living and working in rural areas
- ◆ Was virtually defeated by government action

choose their diet; and eating too narrow a range of foods. The causes of the disease are, therefore, nutritional deficiency of niacin, lack of milk and meat in the diet, lack of variation of foods in the diet, poverty, farming practices inappropriate to the needs of the population, and loss of the freedom to farm according to one's own judgement.

The effective actions to bring the disease under control have included: treatment of diseased individuals with niacin; free distribution to healthy populations or at risk populations of yeast, which is rich in niacin to supplement niacin intake; increasing the range of foods offered to captive populations; phasing out the type of farming called sharecropping; flour enrichment; reduced unemployment; military service; and food rationing. In the United States, flour enrichment started in 1941 and this action virtually wiped out pellagra. Pellagra outbreaks continue to occur, but are now rare. A pellagra outbreak with 908 cases between July 1999 and February 2000 occurred in Kuito, Angola, mostly in war refugees.

Exemplar 2.1 summarizes Rose's ideas with five commentaries examining their current relevance.

2.5 Individual and population-level epidemiological variables

Information collected carefully and precisely at the individual level may not portray the true state of the population's health. Equally, information on a population or the environment may not have meaning in relation to health at an individual level. Before reading on, reflect on the questions in Box 2.9.

Individual attributes such as age, age at death, blood pressure, and serum cholesterol can usually be aggregated and meaningfully used to describe an aspect of a population's health. To provide a meaningful picture the data must be from either the whole population or a characteristic (representative) sample. If this is not the case the description of the population's health status may be grossly inaccurate, even though the individual measures are accurate.

Imagine a study of the mean value of cholesterol in a population aged 18–64 where the methods ensured accurate measurement. If the investigators call for volunteers to participate, the population data may be erroneous because the people studied are untypical. For example, people who have cardiovascular problems, or poor diet, may come forward for testing while those who are fit, active, and disease-free may not perceive a need for this. The result will be an erroneously high mean level of cholesterol. For this reason, epidemiology is generally based on studies of the entire population of interest and, when this is too large, on representative samples (e.g. by random sampling, stratified sampling, etc.). The investigator exerts control of who is studied. As representativeness is often a key requirement in epidemiology, particularly for measuring the burden of disease and risk factors, small studies on representative samples may be of greater value than large ones on unrepresentative samples. (In causal research, representativeness is hard to achieve and as it is less important here, investigators may not, and even should not, strive to achieve it.). Typically, the response rate in population studies would be 60–70 per cent of those invited, sometimes repeatedly, to participate. Participation is usually least in young poor men living in the inner city.

Box 2.9 Individual and population measures

Under what circumstances might individual measures be meaningfully applied to populations and vice versa? Reflect on such measures as age (individual), sex (individual), blood pressure (individual), household size (not individual), population density (area), and gross national product (national).

Box 2.10 Some individual measures which, conceptually, have no meaningful epidemiological interpretation when aggregated into populations

- Fingerprint patterns
- Personality
- Eye colour
- Loneliness

Even with excellent measurements and best practice in sample selection, therefore, the end result may be inaccurate as a population measure.

The population needs to be described by both the frequency distribution of the health status measure, as in depicted in Figures 2.2 and 2.3, and summaries such as the mean and standard deviation (see Chapter 9 for further guidance on analysis of data). The population distribution of most biological measures follows a normal or Gaussian distribution as shown in Figure 2.3. The mean, median and mode value is then the same (or, in practice, similar). One standard deviation includes about 68 per cent of the population, and two standard deviations include 95 per cent of the population. This observation underlies many statistical tests. In epidemiological studies, the population distribution must be examined to assess whether it follows the normal distribution. If it does, the mean and standard deviation provide an accurate picture of the distribution, for instance, like Figure 2.3. If not, the distribution should be shown because summary statistics do not allow the reader to envision it accurately. The measures made on representative samples of individuals usually provide meaningful information on the whole population.

Sometimes individual measures have no value when aggregated. Box 2.10 lists fingerprint patterns and personality as examples of measures that are meaningful and useful at an individual level, but not in aggregate. Societies do not have a personality or a fingerprint pattern and summarizing such individual data into group data is purposeless quantification.

Measures of the population or the environment also may be meaningless when applied to the individual. Epidemiological findings based on such variables may be applicable only at the population level. Some population and environment level variables of this kind are listed in Table 2.2. It is a paradox that some data collected from individuals (e.g. the number of people who live in the household), when used in aggregate (e.g. as population density of an area), cease to be meaningful

Table 2.2 Some population and environmental variables, which conceptually have no direct and meaningful individual interpretation

Population variables	Environmental variables
Population density	Air quality
Income and wealth inequality index	Road traffic density
% of population unemployed	Ambient temperature
Indexes of socio-economic deprivation	Hardness of the water
Gross national product	Land use

at the individual level. While social variables are usually measured in individuals, environmental variables are usually not so measured.

Contemporary challenges in epidemiology include the accurate measurement of environmental exposures in individuals, and the measurement of social characteristics in aggregate. Social characteristics including cohesion in society, teamwork, and the state of economic transition, are likely to have profound effects on health and yet be incompletely captured and described through the usual individualized approaches to measurement. Section 2.6 examines the interdependence of demography and epidemiology.

2.6 Epidemiology and demography: interdependent population sciences

Demography is the study of population structure, including the impact of birth, death, fertility, marriage, migration, and other social factors.

There is an obvious overlap in epidemiology and demography. Epidemiology is hugely dependent on demography and is difficult when demographic data are not available or are wrong. To understand the importance of demography in epidemiology, try the exercise in Box 2.11 before reading on.

It is hard to imagine a place without demographic data, for in modern times we are bombarded with population statistics. A census of population or a register of citizens is fundamental to modern life. The United States census has taken place every 10 years since 1790 and the United Kingdom one since 1801. Indeed, our first epidemiological, public health action in a society without a population count would probably be to undertake a survey of population size (census) or setting up a population register. Accurate population counts are hardest to obtain in fast-changing societies and in places where people do not live in built homes on land they own or rent. Nomadic and refugee populations are such examples.

Even in the industrialized world, there may be a lack of reliable population size data in the inner city, in economically deprived areas, in holiday towns where there is a flux of population, holiday theme parks (although these may operate turnstile counts), war zones, refugee camps, or at major public gatherings such as pop festivals. Some industrialized countries, for example, The Netherlands, do not have a census but rely on compulsory registration of population to get demographic data. In most developing countries, census data are usually available but may not be reliable, particularly for small localities, or between censuses.

Lebanon is an advanced middle-income country in the Middle East. It is unusual in not having had a census since 1932. The reason is political. Population size and structure is, nonetheless, estimated in various ways. With the recent civil war (1975–1990), the continuing border

---

Box 2.11 The importance of demography to epidemiology

- ◆ Imagine a country or region where there were no demographic data, so the number of people and the age and sex composition of the population were unknown
- ◆ Imagine also that an epidemic (say of pneumonia or food poisoning) is suspected
- ◆ You are asked to develop a plan to prevent and control the epidemic in the area
- ◆ You are also asked to advise on the future needs for medical personnel in the area
- ◆ How would you do this and what obstacles can you foresee?

- Count of cases possible
- Limited health-care planning possible on case count
- Trends in case counts useful if population is stable in size and structure
- Changes in case count cannot be interpreted easily if population is changing in size and structure

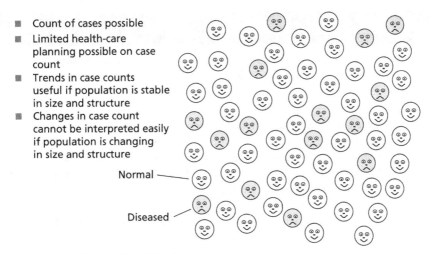

Normal

Diseased

Fig. 2.5 Potential and limits of undefined populations.

battles and the large number of refugees and soldiers, an accurate population count is not possible. Furthermore, registration of deaths takes place at the locality of family origin as registered in the last census and not at the place of residence or death. A medical diagnosis is not a requirement for a death certificate but death registration is, though its completeness is unclear. Without such basic information, describing disease patterns on a national scale and monitoring trends is difficult. The circumstances of a refugee camp, though extreme, illustrate the principles well.

Imagine that the epidemic referred to in Box 2.11 occurs in a refugee camp, where the population size is variable and where there has been a large intake in recent days (the camp population is represented in Figure 2.5 with each circle being a person and cases of sickness/disease are shaded). An outbreak of pneumonia is suspected. What can the epidemiologist do? This scenario illustrates the key principles that apply in large populations but that are often glossed over.

The epidemiologist can count the cases, and note the date of disease onset, date of diagnosis, and the age and sex of the patients. This information is useful to assess need for care and monitor population health. For example, if there are 20 cases who become sick today perhaps we can assume there will be a similar number tomorrow. So, facilities can be organized and supplies ordered. What if the number of cases per day declines or rises? The daily trend can be described and used to make a prediction and the facilities and supply order adjusted. Using information on the age, sex, or other characteristics of cases, appropriate refinements can be made to the plan of needs. So, if 90 per cent of the cases are children, the need for antibiotics can be adjusted, because they need small doses and possibly different drugs. This is a useful and practical application of epidemiology. The daily counts can be used to assess whether the problem is being brought under control or worsening. Nonetheless, the information is sorely limited.

Without a knowledge of population size and composition, we cannot estimate the number of cases that are to be expected in normal circumstances, so we cannot say whether there are more than expected, and hence whether an epidemic is underway or being controlled. Changes in daily numbers may simply be reflecting changes in population size. We cannot assess whether the disease is affecting some groups, such as men more than women, or whether it is commoner in some parts of the camp than others. The number of cases over time gives some, but not definitive, insight into whether the disease is controlled or not, for a rise may occur if the population is increasing, even in the face of successful control. Only if the population size is stable can change

Box 2.12 Developing a population profile

Imagine that accurate information on the age and sex composition of the refugee camp inhabitants is to be collected. How will this be done?

in the number of cases reflect change in disease incidence. Epidemiological investigations into the reasons why outbreaks (here pneumonia) occur usually focus on comparing cases with controls. This work is impeded by lack of information about the population of potential cases and potential controls, as will be discussed in Chapter 9 on study design. In these circumstances, a rational, epidemiologically based, disease control strategy is hard to design, implement, and monitor. Try the exercise in Box 2.12 before reading on.

The first step in an accurate count of population, a local census, is to set boundaries (Fig. 2.6). Where does the camp begin and end? The second step is to define a time for the census. The count is likely to differ by time of year, day of week, and probably time of day. The third step is to define who is to be included. It is likely that some people are visitors, others are helpers, some are staff, and some refugees will move in and out of the camp. The fourth step is to decide what information is to be collected and how. Once these decisions are made, the number, age, and sex of the inhabitants can be ascertained. Now that we have done a census, the case numbers can be expressed as a proportion of the population from which they arose. The number of cases per unit of population can be calculated either overall or separately by the characteristics of the people in the camp (e.g. by age, sex, type of resident, etc.). Chapters 7 and 8 consider the epidemiological approach to collecting and analysing such data.

If there is a change in the number of cases over time, there are two main explanations: either the number or type of people has changed, or the rate of disease has changed. Since the population

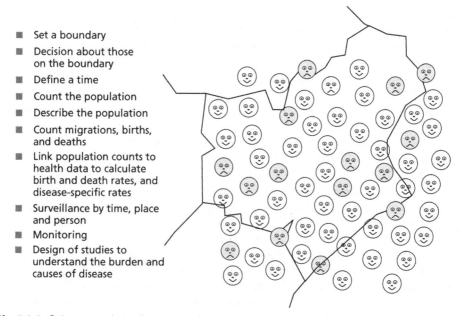

- Set a boundary
- Decision about those on the boundary
- Define a time
- Count the population
- Describe the population
- Count migrations, births, and deaths
- Link population counts to health data to calculate birth and death rates, and disease-specific rates
- Surveillance by time, place and person
- Monitoring
- Design of studies to understand the burden and causes of disease

Fig. 2.6 Defining a population by setting a boundary.

Box 2.13 A public health and epidemiological framework for solving the problem of the camp epidemic

Imagine yourself as the health officer of this camp, responsible for controlling the epidemic.

◆ Which questions do you need to answer to bring to bear a rational control strategy and to declare the problem under control?

◆ Which epidemiological data do you need, in general terms, to answer the questions?

◆ How does the census help you?

is unlikely to remain stable for long in a refugee camp, the number of cases will change due to population size fluctuations. The obvious answer is to re-count the population regularly, perhaps weekly, but this will be impractical in a camp and in most real-life circumstances. In practice, the occasional census needs to be supplemented by keeping track of population changes, which requires recording deaths, births, and migration. These 'vital' statistics permit the census data to be updated routinely.

The collection of vital statistics is, in practice, incomplete and error prone, so population counts become out of date, particularly in small geographical areas, and the census needs to be repeated. In the setting of a camp this need may arise monthly. Most nations repeat the census every 5–10 years or so. Cities where population change is rapid generally need counts between census years. Reflect on the questions in the exercise in Box 2.13 before reading on.

The questions the health officer needs to ask and the answers are summarized in Table 2.3. These questions are generalizable to a multiplicity of epidemiological problems. The data will come from a variety of sources and study designs, although in the specific context of a refugee camp the epidemiology is likely to be fairly basic. With the population count by age and sex, basic but important epidemiological questions of whether the disease frequency has altered, and is altering in the face of control measures, can be answered (see part (a) of Table 2.3). For understanding of cause (part (b) of Table 2.3), the level of information needed is greater. For designing, implementing, and evaluating effective strategies for the prevention and control of disease, knowledge of the culture and politics of the refugee camp and the society it is in will need to be integrated with the epidemiology.

The work of demographers and statisticians who calculate disease rates clearly overlaps with that of epidemiologists, and yet it differs in one important goal: epidemiology needs to understand, explain and use, and not just describe, the patterns of disease. That means understanding enough about the population to generate and test causal hypotheses. The epidemiological population, as with a demographic one, is usually defined using geographical boundaries (Fig. 2.6). The epidemiological population may also be defined by the characteristics of the population such as age and sex, or consist of, say, people with diabetes, children attending a particular school, or the homeless. The epidemiological population also needs to be bounded by time limits. In addition to population size estimates, epidemiology needs an understanding of the social and environmental circumstances of the people under study.

The idea of generalization (applicability elsewhere) is crucial to many scholarly disciplines and sciences. Ideally, epidemiological conclusions should be applicable not just to the people actually studied, but also to others similar to them elsewhere. In practice, as human populations are highly variable in biological, environmental, and social ways, generalization is fraught with difficulty. Figure 2.1 has deliberately shown human figures, for it is too easy to forget people when using

Table 2.3 Answering public health and epidemiological questions using data and study methods

The public health and epidemiological questions	Data needs	Study design usually used (Chapter 9)
(a) Frequency and pattern		
How common is this problem?	Case numbers alone are often sufficient for rare diseases and when the population is stable, otherwise population counts are essential	Case series/Disease registers/Cross-sectional studies
		Cohort studies
Is the problem increasing, decreasing, or about the same?	Accurate numbers of cases and population counts are essential	Repeat above studies/analyses over time
Where does the problem occur most?	Case numbers and population counts by area are essential	Analyse data by place
Who is affected most?	Case numbers and population counts by population characteristics, such as age, sex, economic status, and ethnic group are essential	Analyse data by the characteristics of the person
(b) Understanding the cause		
What are the causes of the problem?	Detailed information on the population and its social and environmental context is essential	Case–control study
		Cohort study
	The data need to be collected to test hypotheses on causation	Trials
(c) Control		
What strategy is needed to prevent or control the problem?	Understanding of what has worked elsewhere, the causal chain of the disease and of the resources available, together with an understanding of the population in its social context	Literature review, preferably systematic
Are control measures working?	Case numbers and population data are usually essential for monitoring effectiveness of control measures, together with an understanding of other changes occurring in the population and environment	Evaluation using pragmatic designs, e.g. before and after analyses of disease
		Repeat cross-sectional studies
		Trials

This scenario, set in a refugee camp, illustrates the principles that are applied on a grand scale in studying the health of nations, continents, and the world.

symbols (of which numbers are the prime example), but for simplicity most figures in this book use ovals to represent human beings. A clear and detailed description of the population, in its environmental and social context, is essential to assess the potential for generalization. Unfortunately, it is common for investigators to ignore this cardinal rule, to fail to provide the contextual data needed for generalization, to generalize too readily, and to err. When generalization is not appropriate, epidemiological data can still be used for local assessment and improvement of the health state of the people actually studied.

2.7 **The dynamic nature of human population and the demographic and epidemiological transitions**

In natural communities, the size and composition of populations is constantly changing owing to deaths, births, and migrations. However, even when the population size remains fixed, the population is still changing. Tackle the exercise in Box 2.14 before reading on.

Obviously, even when the population is fixed the individuals are getting older so the average age increases, changing the pattern of disease. Furthermore, the lives of these people are changing, for example, new foods, technologies, treatments, social norms, laws, and policies. Even fixed populations are dynamic.

In the industrialized world, we have witnessed increasing lifespan from better socio-economic conditions, nutrition, environment, and health care. The average lifespan has increased by several decades in the last two hundred years or so (and continues to rise). Simultaneously, such societies typically have smaller families, in some countries far too small to replace those dying. This has led to societies where the population is, on average, ageing. This is labelled the demographic transition. The accompanying shift in the pattern of diseases is called the epidemiological transition.

Consider a place where the number of people is fixed and whenever an individual dies, or leaves, they are replaced. Imagine that the age, sex, and ethnic composition of the group stay much the same. A place of this kind might be a prison or a nursing home. Even then, the population's health patterns are not fixed, because human behaviours are evolving and their environments changing. The prison environment in the United Kingdom has changed by, for example, the introduction of television, alteration in diet, and the development of a drug-taking culture. The wider social trends in behaviour, including smoking, influence these enclosed populations. In short, for epidemiological purposes there is no fixed human population, only dynamic ones, always in transition. Epidemiology is studying the pattern of disease in changing populations. To emphasize a point made earlier, it is because of this change and evolution that researchers should be giving the time when the research was performed, and not when it was published.

While human populations are dynamic, the concept of a fixed population is, nonetheless, helpful in thinking about the measurement of disease occurrence. Cohort studies (discussed in Chapter 9) are an attempt to create a defined or 'closed' population, while studies on vital statistics are on natural living or 'open' populations. In closed populations, people who are dying and migrating are not replaced. In open populations, there are gains as well as losses, as people are born and migrate into, and die or emigrate from, the population. The change in size of the closed population can be predicted from the death and emigration rates. The prediction of an open population's size is more difficult and requires, in addition to the aforementioned, estimates of immigration and fertility patterns. If the number of people entering a population is balanced by the number exiting, the population is in a steady, but not unchanging, state.

Changes in the environment and behaviour lead to time-period influences on disease patterns. For example, 30–40-year-old women were less likely to be smokers in the decade 1920–1930 than

---

Box 2.14 **Implications of changes in populations for studying epidemiology**

Reflect on the dynamism in human populations and its implications for studying the pattern of disease. In what ways is the population changing even when the number of people is relatively constant?

30–40-year-old women in 1950–1960. In an examination of the relationship between age group and lung cancer, say in 2008, the investigator would need to consider both the direct effect of age-ing, and the time period effect (also see section 9.8) of changing exposures to the causes of lung cancer.

The combination of the demographic transition and the effects of wider influences on health (wealth, environment, behaviour, etc.), leads to a profound change in the pattern of disease, with decline in infections and the dominance of chronic diseases. This epidemiological transition is emerging rapidly in middle-income countries such as Mauritius, Chile, and urban India. For epi-demiology, these transitions are a boon, because they have led to greater variation in disease patterns and exposures to causes, and provide the fuel for the epidemiological engine. Mostly, however, they are good for the public. The chronic diseases, an ageing society, and population growth are signs of success in controlling premature death.

In relatively wealthy and stable countries, improvements in most indices of health have been dramatic. In the face of economic, political, and social disturbance, health gains can be rapidly reversed. The decline in life expectancy for men in Russia and other East European countries fol-lowing the fall of communism and the introduction of markets, and of men and women in much of Sub-Saharan Africa because of AIDS, are examples of the epidemiological transition in reverse.

2.8 Applications of the epidemiological concept of population

The epidemiological concept of population has a huge influence on every aspect of public health, population research, and health care, but it is often implicit. Health policy is nowadays nearly always based on the concept of population. Policy is usually directed either at the whole popula-tion or at subgroups identified by some important characteristic, such as geographical location (a nation, a city, or economically deprived area), the age group, sex or gender, or some other char-acteristic such as ethnic or racial group.

Traditionally, health-care systems have been designed for those who express their need by consulting a doctor or other healer. Increasingly, health-care systems are incorporating goals of improving health by using the concept of population. They are planning services based on the pattern of health problems in the population, taking into account the health of subgroups, and not just of users of the service. They are delivering modified services to subgroups of the popula-tion who differ in their needs, including those who will not attend normal services, for example, the homeless, those in rural areas, or those who speak a foreign language. By using knowledge of population trends in health status, they are anticipating the need for future services and planning something different.

Health promotion is based on the population idea. Indeed, the social sciences and psychology, which underpin health promotion theory, emphasize how peer influences dominate the actions of individuals.

The population concepts of epidemiology, particularly as interpreted by Rose, may yet lead to a radical shift in practice. The concepts shift attention away from individual-orientated pro-grammes to the population. The concept requires a radical idea: the targeting of interventions at people in the middle of the distribution (the average person) and not just at the extremes.

In the nineteenth century, epidemiology established its credentials in medicine and is now an essential part of clinical research and practice. Clinical practice based on the epidemiological concept of population is potentially transformed. The clinician is presented with new challenges, a means of increasing the impact of medical science (especially through earlier intervention), personal responsibility to the wider society, and acute ethical dilemmas. Clearly, the purpose of the health professions is greater than just the alleviation of the pain and illnesses of individuals. Their purpose includes the acquisition of knowledge (research) and organization of care for the benefit of people who access the service, the people who need the service but do not access it, and the generations to come.

For the individual clinician the people to be served are primarily those who consult, whether in the self-referral manner of the American health-care system, or by registration with the general practitioner and referral to specialist services as in the British NHS. Clinicians have or develop a list of people for whom they are responsible. For clinicians, collectively, the list comprises all the people in the society within which they live and work. This population philosophy provides the foundation for clinical epidemiology and evidence-based health care.

The example of type 2 diabetes care illustrates the need for and power of this approach. This is a chronic disabling disease with a prolonged progression (or natural history, which is discussed in Chapter 6), which may be diagnosed after the damaging effects have occurred. Many people with diabetes are diagnosed late. This poses a huge problem for clinicians managing diabetes. The traditional form of clinical care would involve awaiting the development of symptoms and problems severe enough to lead the person with diabetes to present for clinical care, for example, infections, fatigue, blindness, renal failure, or even coma. The population approach is to take advantage of epidemiological knowledge to promote early diagnosis of disease and the prevention of complications. Diabetes clinicians are among the early adopters of the population perspective and are increasingly assessing their effectiveness in terms of how well diabetes is detected, diagnosed, prevented, and controlled in the population and not just in individual patients.

This requires them to identify all people with diabetes and to have means of indirectly influencing them through other health-care providers. Practising population-based medicine requires diabeticians to study health and disease in the community setting, to understand the epidemiology of the disease and to have access to information on the impact of their work in the population setting. The key tool for achieving all this is a population register of patients with diabetes. In future, such registers may also include people with impaired glucose tolerance and impaired fasting glucose, which are precursors commonly of diabetes. The same principles apply to most areas of clinical practice.

Biomedical scientists can use and apply the population concepts of epidemiology too. First, they can use hypotheses generated by epidemiological observations in populations for their own studies, whether on cells, organs, animals, or individual human beings. Secondly, they can test out hypotheses based on their research by seeing whether disease patterns in the populations are in line with their predictions. Thirdly, they can ground their own work in a defined sample of the population and not rely on cells, organs, and other specimens from volunteers, or from selected patients.

2.9 **Conclusion**

The concept of population drives epidemiology and its applications in public health, medicine, and health research. Population thinking emphasizes that disease patterns are the outcome of the interaction between individuals and their environment. It emphasizes that research on the causes and control of disease needs to be based on these interactions and not on an analysis of individuals in isolation. These interactions are complex and there is no single way to portray them. Many different accounts and diagrams to illustrate these accounts exist. It is a high level challenge to develop a general theory that links all these multilevel influences. In Table 2.4, I have produced a hierarchy of influences.

Table 2.4 Influences on human population health: a hierarchy from the Universe to the genome

Level	Example
Outer space	Radiation and other cosmic particles of known (X-rays) and unknown (neutrinos) effects
Earth's atmosphere	Ozone, cloud cover, CO_2 and other gases influencing climate and penetrability of radiation, including UV light (skin cancers)
Physical and chemical environment on and near the earth's surfaces	Population density from housing location and quality, roads, and air pollution all influencing health, e.g. respiratory health
Social, economic, and political environment	Poverty as a cause of a multiplicity of health problems
Mobility of populations	Travel-related diseases, including epidemics
Cultures, especially those influencing health care and health-related behaviours	Taboos on smoking in women in most cultures of the world, especially Asian ones. Taboos on alcohol in Islamic cultures
Health and social care and other relevant systems, e.g. education	Availability or not of hospital health services at no direct, personal cost at the point of need
Workplaces	Working hours, shift work, protective systems
Social networks	Sense of community and support systems
Home environment/family	Nuclear or multigenerational families, living alone, single parenthood
Individual—phenotype	Stunting, blood pressure, weight, height
—genotype	DNA and gene alterations leading to personal and familial risks

I have started with outer space. We are constantly and ubiquitously bombarded by electromagnetic radiation from outer space. As most of these exposures do not vary in ways we can study (e.g. neutrinos), we cannot study their effects in epidemiology. Yet, we know some of this electromagnetic radiation is both harmful and helpful, for example, UV light which causes skin damage and helps make vitamin D, and X-ray and other radiation that leads to mutation in the DNA that both cause defects and lead to evolution in beneficial ways. The DNA is placed, in my hierarchy, at the bottom, illustrating the connections between these levels.

The population approach promises to enhance the impact and effectiveness of clinical endeavour by providing a broad scientific rationale to practice. The movement now known as evidence-based medicine is based on population-based research, but hopefully, better understanding at the individual level will also be used. The population concept underlies the discipline of health and health-care needs assessment. No modern policy document or health-care plan is complete without a population view, and health promotion and health education work also thrive within the population perspective. Clinical practice is embracing the idea. Medical science has always had the ambition of being generalizable to the whole population and is increasingly moving from the study of the individual and the organs, to studying large populations.

The underlying theories that support this chapter are that disease patterns in individuals and societies are profoundly influenced by the mode of interaction of individuals with each other, animals, other living things, and the wider inanimate environment; and that the pattern of disease in society is more than the sum of disease in individuals. The central principle that can be drawn from this chapter is that the causes of disease lie in populations and their societies as much as in individuals and their biology. Given this, it is fitting that the exemplar in this chapter (Exemplar 2.1) develops this point using five commentaries on one of Rose's classic articles.

Exemplar 2.1: Five perspectives on Reproduced with permission from Rose G. Sick individuals and sick populations. *International Journal of Epidemiology*, Volume 14, Issue 1, pp. 32-38, Copyright © 1985 International Epidemiological Association

In this chapter, I have introduced Rose's views on sick populations and I have emphasized that these remain controversial, and no less so than when they were published. In 2001, the journal that published his classic paper in 1985 reprinted it with five commentaries. In this exemplar, I extract some points made by Rose and summarize the views of the commentators before making some concluding remarks.

Rose's paper (pp. 427–32)

The question 'Why did this patient get this disease at this time?' (attributed to Roy Acheson) concerns both clinicians and epidemiologists.

The epidemiological approach assumes the causal factors are heterogeneous (they vary). The hardest causes to identify are those that are universally present. Using the example of Kenyan nomads and London civil servants (Fig. 2.2), he makes his core point that the causes in individual cases differ from the causes of population differences for disease incidence. He uses this to explain why factors that are important causes in populations (e.g. high salt levels), may not explain disease in individuals and why factors important in individuals (e.g. genetics), may not explain disease patterns in populations.

He then proposes that the individual causes approach leads to targeting high-risk individuals, while the causes in the populations approach leads to a population strategy. He outlines the advantages and disadvantages of each approach. One key problem is that because more people are at low or medium risk, most cases may arise in these groups rather than in those at high risk. He identifies that the population approach is radical, and that it also has drawbacks including that for most people the benefits will be small. He articulates the prevention paradox, whereby a large benefit to the population may mean a small benefit to individuals. He calls for both approaches, but identifies the population-based strategy as the greater priority.

Commentary by Ebrahim and Lau (pp. 433–4)

The authors endorse the 'causes of causes' approach using the example of infant mortality. The cause of the causes is identified as poverty, while the proximate causes such as vitamin A and immunization are the generally favoured type of 'magic bullets' interventions. They also observe that notwithstanding the attraction of population strategies, the high-risk strategies are gaining support worldwide. Ebrahim and Lau call for solidarity among public health scientists, including epidemiologists, in advocating for this approach and in winning public support.

Commentary by James McCormick (pp. 434–5)

McCormick observes that little progress has been made on the population approach since Rose's paper was published. He identifies the need for causal evidence between risk factors and disease at the individual level and as a way of altering the risk factor. Population-level associations, he asserts, lead to ecological fallacy (see Chapter 9). While praising the paper, the author's view is that the population approach is an unreal aspiration.

Commentary by Schwartz and Diez-Roux (pp. 435–9)

The authors assert that one lesson from Rose's paper has been accepted, that is, more cases may arise from people at low risk than those at high risk. By contrast, that the causes of the causes differ from the causes had caused 'epidemiology wars'. These wars, they propose, arise from different ways of attributing causality. They offer the insight that proximal causes are easier to attribute but have less value than more distal ones, because they are also closer in time to the adverse outcome, leaving little opportunity for action. They also invoke Durkheim's idea of social facts (ways of acting in a society) and that we study disease in a particular fixed context (tacit causal field) that is then not influencing the outcome because it is not varying. To see these hidden causal effects, you have to move to places with different contexts and social facts. The causes of the causes, nonetheless, also need to affect the body and do so in complex ways. The authors end their analysis by extolling Rose's contribution for opening up new ways of thinking that deserve recognition.

Commentary by Weed (pp. 440–1)

Douglas L. Weed sees Rose's ideas as radical, lasting, and prescient. The study of the causes of the causes is study of the incidence of disease. Weed spotlights Rose's contention that if we can remove the causes of causes, then a focus on high-risk, susceptible individuals will not be needed. This approach should then be our primary focus. This responsibility lies with every-one, but also with the informed specialist, especially epidemiologists.

Commentary by Hunt and Emslie (pp. 442–6)

Kate Hunt and Carol Emslie find similarities between Rose's approach (causes of cases and causes of incidence) and social anthropology (causes of particular misfortune and causes of general misfortune). These authors then discuss the general public's (lay) understanding of the causes of coronary heart disease and conclude that this appreciates and incorporates the central point of the prevention paradox (i.e. that even if lifestyle advice works at the population levels there will be many exceptions, and many people may not reap the benefits). The authors found no parallels in lay epidemiology for Rose's observations on the fact that most cases may occur in people at low risk and on the inability to study the causal effects when there is no variability in the exposure. The authors point to the uncertainties in prediction highlighted in epidemiology, emphasized by Rose, and echoed in lay accounts and the certainties of simpli-fied health education messages. They want the public to be exposed to Rose's ideas.

Concluding remarks

The ideas introduced in this chapter and in this exemplar panel are as controversial, perhaps more so, than when they were published. Their importance to epidemiology as a science of causation of population health is evident. They will concern epidemiology, both as a science and as a practice, for decades. There is, however, a huge amount of work to be done, both conceptual and empirical. For example, conceptually what refinements do we need when we want to change distributions where the harms occur on both sides (i.e. high and low levels of the factor, e.g. weight, blood pressure, and possibly even alcohol use). Empirically, we need to develop and evaluate population-level interventions, and compare their effectiveness and costs with high-risk interventions.

Summary

Epidemiology is a population science in several senses. Firstly, it studies populations' disease patterns, which are hugely influenced by the interaction of individuals living in communities. Secondly, it depends heavily upon demographic population data to achieve its goals. Thirdly, its findings are drawn from, and applied to, groups (or populations) of people. Conclusions and recommendations from epidemiological data may be applied to individuals with caution (in a probabilistic way), and with open acknowledgement of individual variation. For epidemiology to work as a science, there needs to be variation within and between populations in the exposure and outcome variables of interests.

Epidemiology without demographic data is limited in its scope, for then disease patterns can only be studied in populations that are stable in size and composition. Even then, interpretation of comparisons between population groups is possible only when there are stark differences. Epidemiological studies do not work well, and are hard to interpret, without an understanding of the composition of the population under study. Serious errors in interpretation of data may arise from the use of erroneous demographic statistics. With demographic data, epidemiology examines disease over time, between places, and among population subgroups.

One critical yet still controversial concept, led by Geoffrey Rose, is that the causes of disease in individuals are not synonymous with the causes of disease in populations. This has implications for epidemiology and its application to public health.

Populations are dynamic, changing in age structure, ethnic composition, and behaviours. Epidemiology needs to work within the context of demographic and epidemiological transitions as societies change. Change occurs whether we are studying fixed or open populations.

One prime purpose of epidemiology is applying findings in health promotion, health care, and health policy to improve the health of populations. The focus on population in epidemiology distinguishes it from clinical research and the other medical sciences, which primarily study the individual, the organ, and the cell.

Sample questions

Question 1 Why is the population size and structure, as measured at census (or held in a population register), so important in epidemiology?

Answer A census of population, providing data on age, sex, and the social and economic structure of the population, is fundamental to modern epidemiology. Without such base information calculating disease rates, describing and interpreting disease patterns on a national scale, and monitoring trends, is extremely difficult.

Without knowledge of population size and structure, we cannot estimate the number of cases that are to be expected in normal circumstances, so we cannot say with confidence whether there are more than expected, and hence whether an epidemic is underway. We cannot assess whether the disease is affecting some groups, for example, men more than women, or whether it is commoner in some places than others. In these circumstances a rational, epidemiologically based disease control strategy is hard to design, implement, and monitor.

Question 2 Geoffrey Rose wrote that the causes of disease in populations may not be the same as the causes of disease in individuals. What did he mean?

Answer Rose meant that the causes of diseases in populations are often above and beyond the individual and relate to the way society is organized and the state of our environment. For example, the causes of asthma in populations relate to the way our housing is built, the state of the economy, the amount of allergens people are exposed to, the chemicals used, family size and structures, the hygiene of the environment, etc. By contrast, causal explanation at the individual level usually retains a focus on genetics, immune systems, and allergens. This is another and broader perspective on considering the wider determinants of disease in individuals. In Rose's vision it is not enough to consider disease causation at an individual level as, often, the solution does not lie there.

Question 3 Epidemiology is said to be a population science. Explain the meaning of this description in relation to either smoking or lung cancer.

Answer Epidemiology studies the pattern of disease (lung cancer) and its potential causes (smoking) in populations, comparing subgroups of the population to assess the difference in patterns of disease in those who do and do not smoke. It tracks changes in populations in time, by place, and by the characteristics of groups. It uses this knowledge to understand what causes such patterns and to implement interventions to reduce the level of the risk factor and ultimately the adverse outcomes.

References

Durkheim, E. (1951) *Suicide: A Study in Sociology*, translated by Spalding, J.A. and Simpson, G. Edited and with an introduction by Simpson. Glencoe, IL: Free Press. (First published 1897.)

Ebrahim, S. and Lau, E. (2001) Commentary: Sick populations and sick individuals. *International Journal of Epidemiology*, **30**, 433–4.

Herbst, A., Ulfelder, H., and Poskanzer, D. (1971) Adenocarcinoma of the vagina: Association of maternal stilbestrol therapy with tumour appearance in young women. *New England Journal of Medicine*, **284**, 878–81.

Hunt, K. and Emslie, C. (2001) Commentary: the prevention paradox in lay epidemiology--Rose revisited. *International Journal of Epidemiology*, **30**, 442–6.

Kinlen, L.J., Dickson, M., and Stiller, C.A. (1995) Childhood leukaemia and non-Hodgkin's lymphoma near large rural construction sites, with a comparison with Sellafield nuclear site. *British Medical Journal*, **310**, 763–8.

Lind, J. (1753) *A Treatise of the Scurvy in Three Parts, containing an inquiry into the nature, causes, and cure of the scurvy*. Excerpted from James Lind, *A Treatise of the Scurvy in Three Parts, Containing an enquiry into the nature, causes and cure of that disease*, together with a critical and chronological view of what has been published on the subject. Sands, Murray and Cochran, Edinburgh, and reprinted in Buck, C., Llopis, A., Najera, E., and Terris M. (1988) *The Challenge of Epidemiology*. Issues and selected readings, pp. 20–3. Washington DC, WA: Pan American Health Organization.

McCormick, J. (2001) Commentary: reflections on sick individuals and sick populations. *International Journal of Epidemiology* **30**, 434–5.

Roe, D. (1973) *A Plague of Corn: The Social History of Pellagra*. Ithaca: Cornell University Press.

Rose, G. (1985) Sick individuals and sick populations. *International Journal of Epidemiology*, **14**, 32–8.

Rose, G. (1994) *The Strategy of Preventive Medicine*. New York, NY: Oxford University Press.

Rose, G. and Day, S. (1990) The population mean predicts the number of deviant individuals. *British Medical Journal*, **301**, 1031–4.

Schwartz, S., and Diez-Roux, A.V. (2001) Commentary: causes of incidence and causes of cases—a Durkheimian perspective on Rose. *International Journal of Epidemiology*, **30**, 435–9.

Weed, D.L. (2001) Commentary: a radical future for public health. *International Journal of Epidemiology*, **30**, 440–1.

Chapter 3

Variation in disease by time, place, and person: Background and a framework for analysis of genetic and environmental effects

Objectives

On completion of this chapter you should understand:

◆ that virtually all diseases vary in their frequency over time, across geographical areas, and between populations and subgroups of populations;

◆ that disease variations can be partially or wholly artefacts of errors or changes in data collection systems;

◆ that variations must be analysed systematically to check that they are real and not artefacts;

◆ some basic genetics underpinning genetic epidemiology;

◆ that the potential role of genes in causing population level variations in disease is limited;

◆ that most real variations are caused by environmental and social change over the short term, with a genetic contribution in the long term;

◆ that variations, which are nature's experiments, provide a potentially powerful means of understanding the causal pathways of disease;

◆ that study of clusters and outbreaks, that is, abrupt changes in disease frequency, may yield both causal knowledge, and information to control the public health problem;

◆ that variations help to develop and target health policy and health care;

◆ that variations in risk factors and health outcomes generate observations of associations, which in turn spark causal hypotheses.

3.1 Introduction to variation in disease by time, place, and person

Health outcomes, including most diseases, vary in their population frequency over time, between places, and between populations. (We seldom understand why.) This simple but profoundly important observation, virtually without exception, is one of the axioms of epidemiology. Medicine and public health often take credit for bringing about a decline in disease when it is actually due to natural causes, but they rarely take the blame for rising disease rates. Diseases which have undergone massive natural change in incidence within the last 100 years include peptic ulcer, stroke, gastric cancer, AIDS, and infections including tuberculosis. Studying and understanding these variations is a challenge, but a rewarding one.

This chapter emphasizes a systematic framework of analysis of disease variations, particularly to ensure that observations of variation are real, and not just products of data errors and artefacts. The framework applies to all measures of disease frequency. For reasons discussed in Chapter 7 (sections 7.2 and 7.3, Table 7.2), for causal investigations, the soundest measure is the incidence rate, based on new cases. The likelihood of an artefact causing disease variations is greater with prevalence measures of existing disease than with incidence rates. For simplicity, we will focus on incidence in this chapter.

3.2 Reasons for analysing disease variations: environment and genetics

Consider the questions in Box 3.1 before reading further.

There are five principal reasons for investigating a change in disease frequency:

1. To help control an abrupt rise in disease incidence, especially when this comprises a cluster or outbreak of an infectious or environmental disease.

2. For understanding the factors which changed the disease frequency, and hence gaining insight into the causes of disease.

3. To use the time trend in disease, and its causes, to develop health policy and health-care plans.

4. To predict the future course of the disease.

5. To reduce, if not eradicate, the disease.

The investigation of a decline in disease frequency is, for understanding causes, as worthy of investigation as an increase. In practice, a rise in disease incidence is perceived by society as a problem, while a decline is not, and so given lesser priority.

The key strategy in epidemiology is to seek and quantify disease variations, and then develop and test hypotheses to understand their causes. The key question is—why does the disease vary over time, between places, and between populations? In the first instance, as discussed in more detail in Chapter 5, causes are distinguished as genetic and environmental, the latter broadly meaning everything that is not genetic.

Before reading on, do the exercise in Box 3.2.

Variation in disease occurs over time and between places in populations because the risk characteristics of the people or of their environment alter, often unequally. As such changes are not geographically uniform, this generates different patterns of disease in different places. In addition, even within apparently homogeneous populations the disease experience of subgroups usually varies too because of differences in their characteristics, including genetic inheritance, behaviour, and local environment. Even if the social and physical environment were constant, however, some changes in population patterns of disease over time would still occur, albeit much more slowly, for genetic changes are inevitable and will influence disease. Genetic changes in human populations are very slow. Genetic changes in microbes are, however, fast and infectious disease pattern can change quickly if the virulence of the microbe changes.

Box 3.1 Benefits of studying variations in disease

- What potential benefits are there from investigations of changes in disease frequency?
- Is a decline in disease as worthy of investigation as a rise?

Box 3.2 Reasons for variation

- ◆ Why, in general terms, do diseases vary over time, between places, and between subgroups of the populations?
- ◆ What is the relative importance of genetic and environmental influences in bringing about population differences in disease?

All humans belong to one, in evolutionary terms, young species, with mating and reproduction of healthy offspring occurring between all human populations in natural circumstances, so genetic variation between subpopulations is small. Genetic change arises from a number of processes including genetic drift and genetic mutation, which cause random variation in gene frequency across generations. In small populations genetic drift can lead to important, genetically driven disease differences. These changes might be discernible over a few generations.

In large populations, however, genetic make-up is relatively stable. Changes in disease frequency in large populations occurring over short periods of time, meaning years or a few decades, are almost wholly environmental. There must, of course, be the genetic potential to develop a disease for it to occur. For example, hypertension is extremely common in urban-living Africans, especially those living in wealthy, industrialized countries, but not in rural Africans living in traditional lifestyles. Diabetes mellitus (type 2) is extremely common in urbanized Australian Aborigines, but not in those living traditional lifestyles. The increase in disease prevalence in urban settings is due to changes in environmental circumstances in populations with a genetic potential to develop these diseases. It is self-evident that if some health problem arises, then the population must be genetically susceptible to it. Most diseases result from an interaction of environmental and genetic factors.

Though changes over longer time periods, meaning several hundreds or thousands of years or more, may be due to genetic factors, even they are most likely to be due to environmental ones. The varying genetic potential for disease in different populations is acquired (and lost) over evolutionary timescales—that is, thousands, hundreds of thousands and, for biological traits underpinning disease, millions of years. (The main exception to this principle is infectious diseases, where the genetic change is in the microorganisms—genetic changes in microbes can occur at speed because they reproduce quickly.)

To take an analogy from theatre and borrowing from William Shakespeare, in shaping the pattern of disease in large populations, the environment is the leading player and genetics is the stage. This is not to deny the importance of genetic and hence biological factors in disease occurrence. The main cause of lung cancer is the farming and distribution, and then consumption by inhalation, of tobacco. If humans were not biologically susceptible to the carcinogens in tobacco, then tobacco would not cause lung cancer in populations. In individuals, as opposed to populations, genetic make-up is profoundly important, for genetic variation between individuals is sometimes great. But these differences mostly average out at the population group level.

This is a public health paradox: for populations the environment is the dominant influence on the pattern of disease, while for individuals, genetic inheritance may be equally or more important. Disease is, to repeat, caused by the interaction of the genome and the environment. Nonetheless, the control of disease does not usually involve influencing this interaction, but in choosing between genetic or environmental manipulation, the latter usually being easier than the former. With advances in genetic techniques, genetic epidemiology is advancing, growing, and even dominating the discipline. The next section provides the fundamental biological and epidemiological principles to follow the literature. In Chapter 9, I will outline a study design that utilizes genetics, that is, Mendelian randomization.

As already discussed in section 2.7, in the last few hundred years change in the environment has rapidly and profoundly changed disease patterns, particularly in populations which have industrialized and become wealthy. A decline in birth and death rates has led to the demographic transition and to the epidemiological transition. In a few decades, infectious disease can decline dramatically and chronic diseases such as coronary heart disease, stroke, diabetes and cancers of the lung, breast, and colon, can become dominant. This transition is reversible, for when poverty strikes either as a result of economic or political turmoil or in war, infectious diseases return.

International differences in disease patterns mainly, though not wholly, reflect the fact that the populations are at different stages in the demographic and epidemiological transitions. Some of the differences, however, are due to local environmental factors (e.g. climate) and some to genetic factors (e.g. blood disorders known as haemoglobinopathies). International variations, and ethnic differences within populations, will be much reduced, though not eliminated, as the demographic and epidemiological transitions progress. The same underlying principles apply to differences in disease patterns in other types of subgroups within a geographically defined population. Disease differences between social classes or ethnic groups, within a country for example, largely reflect differences in the environment and not in genetic composition. These differences, too, can be conceptualized as a result of subpopulations being at different stages of the demographic and epidemiological transition. In section 3.3, I provide a simple background for readers not already versed in human genetics, given the rising importance of this subject, and as a prelude to the consideration of Mendelian randomization studies in Chapter 9.

3.3 Introducing human genetic variation and genetic epidemiology

3.3.1 The human genome

The genome, comprising all of the genes and associated material in DNA, is the recipe book for human biology. In humans there are about 24 000 genes, the basic units holding the genetic code. Most of the genes are in the 23 pairs of chromosomes in the cell's nucleus. In addition, there are a small number of genes in the mitochondria, which are cellular components in the cell's cytoplasm, that is, the part outside the nucleus. These mitochondria are remnants of primitive bacteria that perform the crucial task of energy production. They are important to human health but, for simplicity, the remainder of this discussion considers the genes in chromosomes in the nucleus.

Twenty-two pairs of the 46 human chromosomes are called autosomal chromosomes, and one pair the sex chromosomes. One of each pair is inherited from each parent. As implied by the name, the sex chromosomes differ in men and women. Though this is a simplification, men have one sex chromosome called X and one called Y, while women have two X chromosomes. This difference alone determines the biological differences between men and women and it illustrates the power of genetics in shaping biology. Damage to and faults in the chromosomes usually have extremely serious consequences, with survival being imperilled. It is no surprise, therefore, that all human populations are identical in terms of chromosomal number and basic structure. Chromosomal differences are common in different species, and that is a reason why cross-species (healthy) reproduction does not occur in nature.

Each chromosome consists of two chains of so-called bases, like a train track, with a varying number of genes. Chromosomes, and hence genes, consist of deoxyribonucleic acid, or DNA for short. DNA is a double strand of several chemicals, but the genetic code is in the nucleic acids, of which there are four: adenine, guanine, cytosine, and thymine. These are known as nucleotides, and bases. Each of these four chemicals lines up, on this train track, with its natural pair, adenine with thymine, and guanine with cytosine. This pairing is the key to replication of DNA and the creation of RNA (ribonucleic acid), which takes the code to where it is needed in the cell.

The nucleic acids provide the code for amino acids, the chemicals that make proteins. A sequence of three nucleic acids provide a code for an amino acid. A string of such triplets (known as codons) will, therefore, give the sequence for a string of amino acids. Twenty different amino acids make all the thousands of different human proteins, when assembled in a particular order in the cellular machinery. These proteins, in the form of enzymes, structural proteins, receptors, signalling proteins, etc. in turn, function to create all the other compounds required for life.

The 'rail track' of the DNA double strand bases is twisted like a spiral staircase, giving rise to the figurative description of the double helix. The double helix is packed up tightly, and is uncoiled (partially) when a protein is to be made, and uncoiled fully for reproduction.

To make proteins, the DNA structure is used to create RNA (ribonucleic acid), which (unlike DNA) is single stranded. The RNA is transportable, leaving the nucleus to give instructions to the cell's protein-making systems. In RNA, the nucleic acid thymine is replaced by one called uracil. Just as DNA can give rise to RNA, so RNA can be converted back to DNA.

Genes, therefore, contain the code for proteins. Genes also contain a great deal of other code, the function of which is not fully understood. Contrary to long-standing expectation, each gene can make several proteins, depending on needs and circumstances. Genes may vary in their precise composition, while remaining functional, although function may vary too.

Reproduction requires that the DNA in the sperm cell enters the ovum (egg cell). As each cell consist of two chromosomes (including the fertilized egg cell), both the sperm cell and the ovum need to shed one set of chromosomes, leaving 23 rather than 46, prior to such a union. The sperm and egg cells with 23 chromosomes are known as gametes.

In the process of forming gametes, a crucially important process takes place that underlies the concept of Mendelian randomization, which is contributing so much to contemporary genetic epidemiology (see Chapter 9). Essentially, prior to discarding one set of chromosomes, the pairs of chromosomes exchange blocks (or sequences) of genetic code comprising many genes. The gamete consists of a single chromosome, not a pair, but it is now a mix of the former pair. In this way, the single chromosome consists of a mix of the-fetus-to-be's grand-maternal and grand-paternal genes. The process of mixing is essentially, but not completely, random (because the exchange between chromosomes is in blocks of genetic code, and not single genes).

Imagine that in the original pair of chromosomes, the grand-maternal chromosome coded for a gene variant leads to high serum cholesterol level, while the grand-paternal version leads to low serum cholesterol. The fertilizing ovum (or, alternatively, sperm) has a 50:50 chance of containing either grand-maternal or grand-paternal variants.

Only the sex cells, that is, sperm and ova, undergo this process—called meiosis—while all other cells divide by the simpler process of mitosis where all the original 46 chromosomes are in the resulting cell. The union of male and female gametes, therefore, creates a fertilized ovum with 23 pairs of chromosomes formed after Mendelian randomization, one from the sperm (father) and one from the ovum (mother). The children, therefore, inherit more or less equally from the mother and father. If the fertilizing sperm contains the Y rather than the X chromosome, the offspring will be male. Since the X chromosome has many genes, and the Y chromosome few, the male has only one copy (and not a pair) of most of the genes from the sex chromosomes.

From this basic, simplified account, readers should be able to understand the ways that variations in the genome can lead to variations in disease at the individual and population levels, as discussed in section 3.3.2.

3.3.2 Genomic variation as the potential basis of human disease and population variation

As already stated, chromosomal abnormalities such as missing chromosomes, extra chromosomes, or misplaced parts of chromosomes, are extremely serious. Mostly, the fertilized ovum will not progress to a viable pregnancy. Either the ovum will not implant itself in the uterus, or if it does, there will later be an abortion. Some abnormalities of this kind, nonetheless, lead to relatively small effects, for example, an extra X chromosome in a woman or an extra Y in a man. Down's syndrome, or trisomy 21, where three chromosomes are seen at the twenty-first chromosome position rather than two, is one of the commonest chromosomal problems. Epidemiological studies on chromosome level variations are not common and, equally, chromosomal variations are not a major contributor to genetic epidemiology. (They are, of course, of great interest to clinical genetics.) Most genetic epidemiology is currently on variations in gene structure.

Variation in gene structure is easily demonstrated, in both individuals and between and within populations. This variation may cause differences in protein production and structure, which influences either susceptibility to disease, or directly causes diseases. Using the central epidemiological strategy of linking variations in causes (here gene structure) to diseases, or precursors of diseases, epidemiologists hope to understand disease causation.

The structure of genes varies because of mutations. Mutations are changes in the sequence of nucleic acids in the DNA, potentially changing the nature of protein production. They are caused by errors in the process of DNA replication and repair, and mutagens that cause mutations such as radiation, some drugs and chemicals, and viruses. Mutations are central to carcinogenesis, the process underlying cancers. Mutations in cancer disrupt the normal processes regulating cell division and regulation.

Gene function is important in virtually all disease processes at the individual level. From an epidemiological perspective, however, such variations are of value only when they are systematically, and consistently varying in identifiable population groups. This happens when populations are systematically differently exposed to mutagens. So, for example, uranium miners, cigarette smokers, and airline pilots are more exposed to mutagens than the general population and are more likely to have mutations that cause diseases. In these examples, the epidemiological interest is primarily in the causative exposure, here of radiation and cigarette smoke. The removal of the causative exposure will partially remove the population variation in disease. The mutations here are not a fixed and ongoing feature of the population under study although they are permanent for the individual. In these examples, the mutation is in the autosomal chromosome genes.

For mutations to become a lasting feature of populations, they have to be transmitted across generations, and this can only happen if they occur in the sperm cell or the ovum. Mutations in these cells may not be compatible with fertilization or the progression of pregnancy (so-called lethal mutations). If they are compatible with life, they may lead to: (a) no change in function; (b) impaired functioning in relation to the environmental context (perhaps the most likely outcome—and hence the reason why most mutations are not propagated) or; (c) improved functioning. In (a) the mutation will be transmitted to future generations and hence become a normal part of the population. In (b) the recipient's capacity to function, and hence reproduce, will be diminished so the mutation will not thrive and there will be pressures for it to be selected out. In

(c) there may be greater reproductive success and the mutation becomes commoner across the generations.

Mutations are the basis of biological evolution. The theory of evolution predicts (correctly) that inherited changes that increase survival in particular environments underlie all permanent, inheritable biological variation (anatomy, physiology, biochemistry, etc.), within and between species. Unless the theory is overturned, it seems that all life on earth has a common ancestor, seemingly a simple microorganism. Mutations over billions of years have given rise to the variety of life.

The commonest difference among genes is in a single nucleic acid. This is known as a single nucleotide polymorphism or SNP (pronounced 'snip'). The production of SNPs by mutations in cells (most importantly sperm and ova) is, to a large extent, a random process. Over evolutionary timescales, millions of such mutations have occurred and have been retained in the genome, and are observable now. (No doubt many other millions occurred, but were lethal or damaging so were not retained.) Most such mutations are seen in few people. Strictly speaking, the term polymorphism (SNPs are the most common form) is for mutations with a frequency of more than one per cent in the population—an arbitrary distinction that is often ignored. Some are very common, being present in 15 per cent of the population or even more. Some mutations have become normal in some populations, for example, those that led to the capacity for adults to digest milk in adulthood and those that led to loss of pigment in the skin. Both have become the normal variant in Northern European populations. The capacity to digest milk has evolved in the last 7000 years or so.

The epidemiological and clinical significance of the SNP is well illustrated by sickle cell disease. Sickle cell disease is a serious condition where the underlying abnormality is that the haemoglobin, the molecule that carries oxygen in the blood, crystallizes and then distorts the red blood cell with anaemia and other complications. The disease is caused by a variety of SNPs and mutations. For the variant known as haemoglobin S, the SNP in the gene leads to the production of a protein with a different amino acid (valine instead of glutamic acid). This was discovered in 1955. Most SNPs on the gene coding for the proteins that make haemoglobin are harmless. People with this particular SNP on both copies of the genes inherited from their parents have sickle cell disease. Those with the SNP on only one of their two chromosomes have sickle cell trait (called allelic variation). The inheritance follows the so-called Mendelian pattern, after Gregor Mendel. This SNP causes a single gene disorder that is recessive, meaning that the gene variant is expressed only if both copies of the gene are affected. Sickle cell trait, therefore, does not usually cause serious problems. If two people with the trait have children, there is a 25 per cent chance of their child having sickle cell disease.

Sickle cell trait and disease varies greatly across populations. How do we explain this disease variation? The SNPs concerned that cause such diseases (haemoglobinopathies) are very common in the Eastern Mediterranean and Sub-Saharan Africa (affecting up to 30% of the population) but rare in Northern Europe. Why? There must be some evolutionary, reproductive advantage that balances, indeed even outweighs, the disadvantage. The advantage is that people with blood cells with the SNP are more resistant to the malaria parasite, and therefore less likely to acquire malaria and die from it. This is an example of a so-called balanced polymorphism. The problem is that when the environment changes, or people move to a new environment (say, without malaria), the advantage is no longer balanced by the disadvantages. The same principles apply for all common polymorphisms, for example, those that lead to cystic fibrosis, but we may not understand their benefits, even while the clinical problems are clear.

Obviously, mutations at a particular part of the genome occur in a few people. It takes time and evolutionary pressures to select in favour of people with them, thus increasing the prevalence. Polymorphisms that are common are, therefore, ancient. The circumstances that favoured their selection may be long gone and, if not, are likely to be obscure. Disentangling the causes is a high-level epidemiological challenge that requires multidisciplinary work including genetics, evolutionary biology, history, and palaeontology.

While there are currently more than 10 million known SNPs, giving ample variety for epidemiology, the genome is remarkably similar between humans and human population groups—perhaps 199 out of every 200 of the nucleic acids that comprise the DNA are identical in their location (0.5% difference). This testifies to the precision of the mechanisms copying DNA and to the importance of replicating accurately the protein structure to sustaining life.

The SNP is not the only way genes can vary but it exemplifies the principles most clearly. The DNA code for the protein may vary in length (the gene for the lipoprotein called Lp(a) is a good example) as well as in nucleic acid sequence. This will create a different protein, and in the case of Lp(a), a longer one. The code for the protein may be interrupted by non-coding sequences in different ways. The composition of the non-nucleic acid chemicals in the DNA may be different. These differences lead to subtle effects on protein function. The way that non-nucleic acid components change and affect gene function is called epigenetics. This is one way that the environment triggers changes in gene function. The changes triggered may be short term or last a lifetime, and even be transmitted across generations (but these changes are reversible). These epigenetic factors may determine which of the several proteins that the gene can code for it actually produces at any one time, and this may change over time. A chemical reaction called DNA methylation is the best example of epigenetic effects. So, a disease can alter the functioning and structure of the genome, and of course vice versa. Therefore, the concept of reverse causality, whereby the disease outcome alters the risk factor, is applicable to genes (see also Chapters 5 and 9). These epigenetic processes are the fundamental mechanism underpinning gene–environment interactions.

Every cell has (or has had) the entire nuclear DNA. Cells specialize by shutting down some functions, often permanently. This process is controlled by the non-nucleic components of DNA. When such controls break down, serious health problems can occur.

The genetics of diseases caused by chromosomal abnormality and of single gene disorders following Mendel's laws of inheritance are well understood. The current excitement in epidemiology is whether genetics can help us understand and control the complex, chronic diseases, and this is discussed in section 3.3.3.

3.3.3 Susceptibility to diseases, chronic diseases, and genetics

Most health problems, including chronic and infectious diseases, run in families. A family history does not, however, equate to a genetic basis for disease. As with any other association in epidemiology, one with family history raises questions and suggests hypotheses. Before reading on, reflect on the thought exercises in Box 3.3.

A family history may arise from a common genetic heritage, a common experience in the womb (which may have common features across different generations), similarities in lifestyle, and similarities in environment. However, it probably reflects a combination of these and perhaps other

---

Box 3.3 Genetics and chronic diseases

(a) In general terms, in addition to genetics, what else might cause diseases to run in families?

(b) Why might infectious diseases run in families?

(c) Why is it unlikely that chronic diseases are caused by genetic mutations?

factors. Infectious disease may be passed from mother to child and family member to family member. They may flourish in environments that families share. Families may also share genetic susceptibility to some infectious diseases.

Complex chronic diseases such as heart disease, stroke, breast cancer, colorectal cancer, diabetes, psychosis, dementia, and osteoporosis definitely run in families. They also vary hugely in time, place, and by person. It is exciting to believe that the explanations for the causes and variations lie, and will be discovered, in the variation in the human genome. These chronic diseases, however, change their incidence rapidly. Many of them were non-existent or rare in the past, so evolutionary pressures to select for disease genes would have been minimal or non-existent. While we can see (sometimes) the potential benefits of a physiological trait such as the sickle cell variant of haemoglobin, what evolutionary advantage would accrue from a heart attack, stroke, cancer or dementia, or the conditions that precede them? Most of these diseases occur after reproductive age, and so selection through the enhancement of reproduction is not possible. Therefore, the idea of disease genes is misleading in the context of the common chronic diseases (unlike for some infectious diseases that have been present over evolutionary timescales).

The critical issue is whether some gene variants code for protein variants that alter biochemistry, physiology or immunology, and thereby increase susceptibility to the pathological processes that lead to chronic diseases.

Without such susceptibility to the pathological processes, diseases cannot occur in humans. This is easily understood for infectious and like-diseases. The common viral foot and mouth infection that is endemic in many countries and affects animals such as sheep and cattle, does not occur in humans, or is extremely rare. Scrapie, a brain disease, is caused by a prion and it affects sheep but not humans. The closely related disease of cows, bovine spongiform encephalopathy (mad cow disease in popular terms) does affect humans, although rarely and only those with some genotypes. Measles and leprosy are among diseases that are uniquely human.

These susceptibilities are genetic. Here the susceptibility can be thought of as the fit of a lock and key. Without the key, the microorganism cannot unlock the door to the human host. If there is no such susceptibility, the disease cannot occur. Susceptibility can be acquired if there is a genetic change through mutation in either the infecting agent or the human host. HIV and influenza are among the human diseases arising from viruses that usually infect animals, where human susceptibility has been initiated by such changes. A mutation permits the virus to change so that it can now invade the human host and maintain the infection in the population through spread from one person to another.

Rothman has made the surprising statement that diseases are 100 per cent genetic and 100 per cent environmental. The reasoning is easy to understand for infections. Every host must have genetic susceptibility. Equally, the environment must expose every host to the infective agent. By either changing genetic susceptibility or altering the environment (so there is no exposure to the infective agent), 100 per cent of the disease could be removed. Even a fractured skull following a head injury, caused, say, by a fall from a bicycle, can be thought of as both 100 per cent environmental and 100 per cent genetic. Obviously, the bicycle injury is environmental. But what is the role of genetics? Genetics determines the shape, strength, and susceptibility of the skull. Our skulls must be genetically susceptible to a fracture after the kind of injury here. By contrast, our skulls are not susceptible to a fracture when hit by a tennis ball.

The issues in relation to chronic diseases follow similar principles but are much subtler, at least partly because our knowledge base is insufficient at present.

The causes of the chronic diseases are poorly understood but are multifactorial, that is, many factors are statistically associated with the risk of disease. For example, smoking cigarettes, lack of exercise, obesity, diabetes, high blood cholesterol, and high blood pressure each double or triple the risk of a heart attack. These factors work primarily (but not solely) through processes that lead to atherosclerosis, which itself starts through damage to the inner lining of arteries (endothelium). If humans did not have the biological capacity to develop atherosclerosis, this would not happen. There are hundreds of factors statistically associated with either increasing or decreasing the risk of a heart attack, although the evidence base is weak for most of them. Hundreds of SNPs have also been similarly associated, but even all together they do not have the strength of association of even one major non-genetic risk factor.

Cigarettes are a relatively new human invention. Why then do humans react to them biologically, and therefore genetically? Presumably, the genome has evolved to permit the body to react to substances in nature similar to tobacco smoke, for example, smoke in fires, particles in the air, etc. This interaction between the risk factor and biological reaction is mediated by genes, in this case by those in endothelial cells lining the arteries and cells of the immune system that react to the signals sent by the endothelial cells. This reaction is an inflammatory response, which is fundamental to the body's control and repair mechanisms.

Diseases, and precursor conditions that lead to diseases, arise through the effects of their causes on normal biological processes. Processes such as inflammation, cell division, cell death, and cell repair are each governed by many genes. The effects of a single risk factor such as smoking may be mediated by altering the function of dozens or hundreds of genes. Mutagens in the smoke also damage and alter DNA. There are about 10 major (and a multiplicity of minor) environmental risk factors for atherosclerosis. These almost certainly act through hundreds and perhaps thousands of genes. For this reason, the complex traits such as atherosclerosis are potentially alterable by mutations, for it is more likely that one of these many genes will have a mutation than a solitary gene.

These genes not only interact with environmental factors but also with each other (i.e. there are gene-to-gene interactions). This means that when gene A is activated, so is gene B, possibly in a way that differs from the way that gene B would work if gene A were not activated. A gene may also work differently in the presence of one or more environmental exposures.

This account, though complex, is a simplification of the reality and it explains why disentangling the genetic basis of chronic diseases is such a complex task which, despite huge research efforts leading to thousands of papers, has hardly shed new light on the questions of cause and effect in chronic diseases at the population level.

Epidemiologists have focused on gene variants that increase the risk of chronic diseases. This way we find people at high risk (for targeting clinical and public health interventions) and insights into how genes influence the pathological processes leading to diseases. Studying high-risk groups, for example families and isolated small populations, advances understanding of disease mechanisms.

Some gene variants increase chronic disease risk very substantially, for example, the gene variant known as *BRCAI* (one of hundreds of such variants). Women with this gene variant are much more likely to develop breast cancer than other women. Other examples include gene variants that increase cholesterol (familial hypercholesterolaemia) and those that increase the risk of colon cancer. Such gene effects are, however, rare in the population and account for few cases and less than five per cent of the total in the aforementioned examples. Just as the control of heart disease is best done through consideration of a package of risk factors (nine account for about 80–90% or more of cases), so it may be with genes. It may be possible to define a package of gene variants that, in combination, raise risk substantially even though each one only raises risk by a small amount.

Characteristics such as height, skin colour, eye colour, and blood pressure are also controlled by several, not a single, genes. So, if we desire to alter them we will also need to influence a package of genes.

Genetic effects may give important insights on biological pathways maintaining health and causing disease. To be important in public health terms, however, risk factors need to have a big effect (e.g. 50% or more increased risk) and to be common in the population (see Chapter 8, on attributable and population attributable risk). It is clear that the common gene variants (unlike single gene defects that are rare) have small effects, for example, raising the risk of disease by 10–20 per cent, or less. As Yang and colleagues (2005) have calculated, it would take about 20 gene variants that are present in about 25 per cent or more of the population, and which raise the disease risk by 20–50 per cent, to account for 50 per cent of the burden of disease. This is the typical burden accounted for by a few, sometimes only one, of the major environmental risk factors for chronic diseases. This illustrates the formidable task for genetic epidemiology. The tools for the task are being developed, sharpened and widely distributed, as in the mapping of the human genome considered next.

3.3.4 Mapping and manipulating the genome

As discussed in Chapter 9, the study designs of genetic epidemiology are essentially those used by all epidemiologists and the central strategy is the same. The difference is that the risk factors under study are genomic: 24 000 human genes make more than 100 000 proteins, which in turn make innumerable molecules. Each of these millions of factors can be an exposure variable. As just discussed, for a chronic disease, epidemiologists may need to study hundreds of genes found from this larger pool. That is only the first of many steps. How are they to do this?

The 'double helix' structure of DNA was discovered by Watson and Crick in 1953. In 1987 an international collaboration set the goal of mapping the entire human genome (about 3.3 billion base pairs) and in 2002, to worldwide fanfare, the goal was all but achieved. The project focused on mapping the parts of genes that code for proteins rather than the larger amount of DNA that is non-coding (so-called 'junk' DNA). Mapping exercises also focused on SNPs that are used as genetic markers to identify genes, or groups of genes, and their functions.

The technology that has made the task possible is called the polymerase chain reaction, which enables both copying of DNA and producing it in large quantities, so it can be used repeatedly and in several places.

Just as in nature, genes can be snipped out and recombined (as in meiosis in germ cells, discussed previously), so it is in the laboratory. Techniques are available to snip out single genes, or lengths of DNA, and replace them elsewhere (including in different types of cell from different species). These techniques are powerful in cell line and animal experiments. They also permit the study of associations between genes, their location, and their variation in relation to human biological traits (phenotypes) or diseases.

Each person has a unique genotype with the exception of identical twins. Identical twins, especially if reared apart from birth, provide the primary means of disentangling the role of environmental and genetic factors. Such identical twins have an identical genome and a very similar but not identical experience in their mother's womb, but otherwise their environmental exposures differ. This variation between people permits us to use DNA to identify people uniquely, except for identical twins (e.g. as in DNA fingerprints). So, no DNA sample can be truly anonymized, with serious implications for the confidentiality of research (see Chapter 9).

In the next section, we consider the potential role of genetics in explaining population level variation in the pattern of disease, using the example of race.

3.3.5 Population level differences in disease and genetics: the cautionary example of race

For about 200 years the biological concept of race, that is, of human subspecies distinguished by genetically determined physical features, has been one of the important issues in a wide range of scientific disciplines (anthropology, biology, sociology, psychology, and epidemiology). The idea also underpinned much of politics and social relations and, in turn, these social applications reinforced the science.

While a number of religions, philosophies, and societies accepted that humans were one species (ultimately named Homo sapiens sapiens), this was not obvious or easily demonstrable scientifically. The debate on whether humans were one (monogeny) or more than one (polygeny) species was fierce in the eighteenth and into the nineteenth century, when it concluded in favour of monogeny. There are still proponents of polygeny, as a search on the internet will show. The physical differences between humans across the world were painstakingly studied by scientists and used to create several racial classifications. These classifications persist in the categorizations of humans as, for example, White or Caucasian, Black or Black African, Chinese, Aboriginal, etc. Such categories remain a dominant feature in epidemiology, although they are slowly being replaced by ethnic group categories. Ethnicity is a related but different concept, though it is too often treated as a synonym for race.

The physical differences between such human groups underpinning race, for example, skin colour, eye colour, hair colour, type of hair (straight or crinkly), facial shape, etc., are genetic, although environmental factors can influence them.

Epidemiology is one of the sciences that have taken a keen interest in differences between population groups, using race as an exposure variable. Epidemiologists have noted differences in the pattern of disease and in the biological and social risk factors that underpin disease; for example, in the United Kingdom, people of African-Caribbean origin have relatively high rates of prostate cancer and stroke and relatively low rates of coronary heart disease. People of Indian origin have relatively low rates of colorectal cancer and high rates of diabetes. There are hundreds, if not thousands, of such observations on a range of diseases. Equally, there are numerous such observations on intelligence, education, psychological traits, lifestyles, skills, behaviour, and physiology.

The question that has intrigued scientists, particularly in the nineteenth century—the heyday of race science—is whether these wider attributes, especially intelligence, might also be biological, that is, innate and associated with physical features causally. With this reasoning, the forces that shaped the genetic changes leading to difference in physique would also have shaped the susceptibility to these wider attributes.

The particular environmental circumstances of Sub-Saharan Africa, where modern humans evolved about 150 000 years ago, influenced genetic variations that lead to a dark skin and curly, crinkly hair. We can only speculate on the genetic advantages of these traits. We have already seen that in the same place the sickle cell trait in blood cells was advantageous. We can use the observation of dark skin/crinkly hair—common in Sub-Saharan Africa—as a marker (albeit imperfect) of increased likelihood of sickle cell trait and disease. The fair, freckled skin of the White Scottish ethnic group can be a marker for increased risk of skin cancers, cystic fibrosis, and multiple sclerosis. These kinds of associations have potential scientific value (posing questions and providing model populations for study) and public health/clinical value (easing diagnosis, screening, and targeting health care).

The mystery behind the skin cancer/fair skin association and the sickle cell disease/malaria association has been solved. However, the causes of multiple sclerosis, diabetes, pancreatic cancer, and motor neuron disease, for example, are mysterious. If we can use racial (and ethnic) variations in disease to point to these causes that would be potentially of great value. The added benefit of studying racial and ethnic variations is that there is greater variation in disease outcome, and genetic and environmental variability, than provided by most other types of comparisons. Similar arguments have been advanced in relation to outcomes other than disease, for example, educational attainment, criminal tendency, IQ, etc.

The theoretical and actual benefits of this line of reasoning have, unfortunately, been greatly outweighed by the harm. By the 1950s, a series of UNESCO (1952) statements concluded, effectively, that the race concept had little or no utility in science. In section 10.10.3 there is an introduction to some of these harms.

From an epidemiological perspective, we can summarize the problems of research using race as follows:

1. The research was done within a racist context often for racist purposes, for example, to justify colonialism, whether this was covert or overt.

2. The variation between racial groups in the human genome is probably too small and too weakly associated with outcomes to generate variation at the population level in the major chronic diseases.

3. The causes of chronic diseases are largely environmental so seeking causes primarily in the genome was doomed (the current emphasis on gene–environment interactions is more promising).

4. Scientists did not have the tools for the task.

The Human Genome Project, and the new concepts and tools that have made it possible, are reinvigorating the study of race in biology and bioscience, including epidemiology. Among the observations already changing our thinking radically is that there is more between-group variation in the non-gene parts of chromosomes than in the genes, that is, there is more racial variation in the genome than anticipated. I will return to this point in section 10.10.3.

Epidemiologists working in this fraught field of endeavour need to be conscious of its history and take particular care. For reasons discussed in my book *Migration, Ethnicity, Race, and Health in Multicultural Societies* (OUP 2014), the concept of ethnicity is likely to be more useful in epidemiology than race. Whatever the epidemiological variable, or risk factor, we need a logical approach to interpretation of data.

3.4 **Variations and associations: real or artefact?**

When changes in disease frequency are natural, or real, and not just a result of the way diseases are diagnosed or counted, the underlying reasons are often difficult to pinpoint. Real changes are an experiment of nature, posing an explanatory challenge to science.

For understanding disease variation, the first step is to exclude chance, error, or artefact (henceforth, collectively, artefact) as the explanation. The second is to develop a hypothesis stated as an association. The third is to design a test of the hypothesis. The fourth is to assess the results using frameworks for causal thinking. Much of this chapter and Chapter 4 show how artefactual variations and associations occur, are identified and excluded. Assessing the causal basis of remaining hypotheses is considered in Chapter 5.

Demonstrating variation in disease is a first step towards establishing an epidemiological association. It is rare for there to be no demonstrable variation and hence association, but if that were

---

Box 3.4 CHD trends in time—examining the association

In studying the association between CHD and time, over several decades, what approach might you take? Set out, in simple terms, the steps in your approach.

---

true, it would be very important. It would show that the factors we have examined are not likely to be causally related to the outcome. There is a tendency in epidemiology to set aside observations of no association, possibly too readily, before extracting the learning there.

The association is a link (or relationship) between a disease and another factor (called exposure or risk factor), whether this factor is another disease, or a characteristic of the person or population under study. In several industrialized countries, coronary heart disease (CHD) mortality rates rose steadily in the twentieth century until the 1960s/1970s when they declined. Before reading on, reflect on how you might investigate the association between time periods and the rate of CHD. Try the exercise in Box 3.4.

First, we would carefully measure disease rates and demonstrate the association of disease rates and time periods. We would need to ensure the association is not simply a result of chance, error, or other artefacts, for example, changing health-care systems, technologies, and staff to make the diagnosis. Once we are satisfied this is not so, we would generate possible explanations. We would attempt to explain the association using our understanding of social, environmental, and lifestyle changes over time. Then, we would develop and test specific hypotheses. One hypothesis might be that the disease pattern reflects the changing levels of factors that are presumed to cause CHD, for example exercise patterns, consumption of dietary fats and fruits and vegetables, and levels of blood pressure. Studies would then be done to assess how much, if any, of the change in CHD over time can be explained by the changing pattern in these factors.

The association fuels a typical process of analysis and research, which either reaffirms causal understanding or raises new questions by rejecting the hypotheses offered. In this example, the decline in CHD was shown not merely to be an artefact and was too rapid to be a result, solely, of change in the risk factors mentioned. Better medical treatment has contributed and there are other unexplained factors.

The association is usually based on data but it can be based on theory alone, that is, a postulate based on first principles with no empirical backing. This kind of association might be thought of as armchair epidemiology. It is born from the epidemiological imagination. This kind of thinking is important and is sometimes published as a hypothesis. Publication of such associations is difficult because editors and reviewers are not easily convinced so some, even modest, data supporting the hypothesis is usually important. Epidemiologists ought to be mulling over hypotheses and associations, even if they are not to be published. Of the many armchair hypotheses I have generated, and often shared with colleagues, three have been written up, that is, the ideas that the high risk of CHD and diabetes in South Asians might be associated with highly efficient mitochondria; thin, fat-deficient legs, and high heat cooking. It is too early to say whether any of these are valuable observations.

The association may be based on observations of one or a few persons. For example, a doctor may observe a few cases of renal failure in patients taking a particular drug, as actually happened for phenacetin and other anti-inflammatory drugs used for arthritis. This would be considered anecdotal evidence, but it might be important.

The association implies that a disease and risk factors may be causally connected. The epidemiological challenge is to demonstrate what the possible risk factors are, to quantify the association,

Box 3.5 Why variations and resulting association may be artefactual

Consider the possible reasons why a variation in disease pattern might be an artefact rather than real. (You may find 7–10 reasons.) Can you group them into three or four categories of explanation?

to assess whether the association is causal, and, if so, to explain how. Ultimately, the challenge is to understand the mechanisms by which the risk factor affects disease and then use this information to prevent, control, or treat it. Understanding of mechanisms invariably requires collaboration with other laboratory, clinical, and social sciences.

The first and crucial question in the analysis is this: is an association an artefact or real? If it is an artefact, then there is no more to explain. Before reading on, do the exercise in Box 3.5.

Most often disease variations are artefacts, arising from the following:

♦ Chance. The numbers of cases (and disease rates) are varying randomly. We will discuss this in Chapters 4, 7, and 9.

♦ Errors of observation. Biased techniques are the most common and important reason for making erroneous observations, and this is discussed in detail in Chapter 4.

♦ Changes in the size and structure of the population from which the cases arose. This was discussed in the previous chapter (see section 2.6) and solutions will be offered in Chapter 8 (age standardization).

♦ The likelihood of people seeking health care and hence being diagnosed and eventually counted in statistics. This varies with the public's level of knowledge and expectations, and the availability, accessibility, and acceptability of health care.

♦ The likelihood of the correct diagnosis being reached. This is dependent on the availability and use of medical care, the level of the doctor's skill, and the quality of the diagnostic facilities available (Chapters 6 and 7).

♦ Changes in the clinical approach to diagnosis. Diagnosis is subject to changing medical trends, for example, whether wheezing is to be called wheezy bronchitis or asthma (Chapter 7).

♦ Changes in data collection methods. These occur, for example, when computerization of medical records takes place with structured methods of entering a diagnosis and automatic data extraction. The numbers of recorded cases are likely to rise (Chapter 4).

♦ Changes in the way diseases are diagnostically coded. Coding is influenced by both the versions of disease codes used and the interpretation of the disease data by the coder (Chapter 7).

♦ Changes in the way data are analysed and presented. For example, merely altering the 'standard' population used in adjusting disease rates for differences in age and sex (Chapter 8) can spuriously alter disease incidence.

These artefactual explanations, listed in Box 3.6, can be further summarized as: chance; measurement error and bias (including confounding); diagnostic variation; data processing and presentation. The role of chance is assessed using statistical probability methods (see Chapter 8) and measurement and data processing errors by quality assurance methods (see Chapter 4). Errors in population counts may be difficult to find or correct, so the key is a high level of awareness. In the field of race, ethnicity, and migration, differential rates of emigration, in the face of insufficient data, may cause a problem of undercounts in the outcome and overcounts in the population at

> ## Box 3.6 Summary of potential artefactual causes of disease variations and associations
>
> **Chance**
> **Error including bias/confounding**
> **Changes in:**
> Size and structure of underlying population
> Health-care seeking behaviour
> Diagnostic accuracy
> Diagnostic fashion
> Data collection
> Coding
> Analysis
> Presentation

risk (known as salmon bias—as like salmon, people may return to their birthplace for the end of their life). Diagnostic activity can usually be assessed indirectly by observing changes in staffing and diagnostic facilities, or directly by counting the number of tests performed. Where specialists are employed, the number of tests done for the disease that interests them will rise, and the disease frequency will appear to rise. For example, the north-east of England has an extremely high prevalence and incidence of primary biliary cirrhosis, and the prevalence rose dramatically in the late twentieth century. One potential explanation was that the number of gastroenterologists interested in this disease increased. This was indeed demonstrated to be the case.

Diagnostic activity, measured by the number of tests, can be related to the number of cases diagnosed to assess this hypothesis. For example, we might think that a high number of cases reflects excessive diagnostic activity. If so, we would predict a large number of tests for each case diagnosed (high test to case ratio). If, however, there were a high incidence of disease, and no excessive testing, then the test to case ratio would be low. Figure 3.1 illustrates this in a study of Legionnaires' disease.

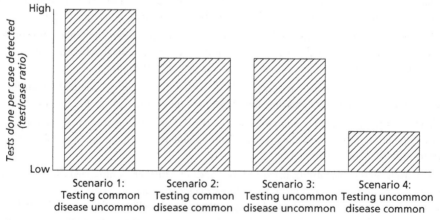

Fig. 3.1 Assessing the effect of diagnostic activity on disease frequency.

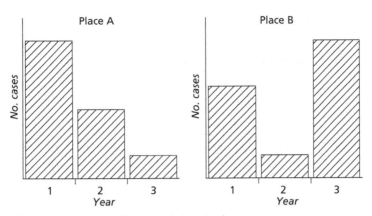

Fig. 3.2 Variations in time masquerading as variations in place.

Reproduced with permission from Bhopal RS. A framework for investigating geographical variation in diseases, based on a study of Legionnaires' disease. *Journal of Public Health Medicine*, Volume 13, Issue 4, pp. 281–9, Copyright © 1991 Oxford University Press.

Geographical variations are particularly likely to be artefact, because clinical practice, and often information systems, vary greatly between places. One real, yet potentially misleading cause of geographical variation, is short-term fluctuation in disease incidence. Figure 3.2 illustrates the point. Over the three-year period, the disease incidence in places A and B was identical. A study done in any one year, however, would have concluded that the incidence of disease varied between places. Short-term changes in disease incidence create geographical variation, when in the long term there is none.

If there are no obvious and important artefacts, and this is difficult to show, the variations in disease are real. Before reading on try the exercise in Box 3.7.

There are numerous explanations for real disease variations; for example, human beings may change their behaviour, their social interaction, or their reproductive patterns. The causes of disease might change; for example, a microorganism might mutate so that it becomes less or more virulent (as happens with influenza) or crosses the species barrier (as has happened with HIV infection and new variant Creutzfeldt–Jakob disease).

The composition of the cause of a disease might change; for example, the reduced tar content of modern cigarettes with filters reduces the risk of lung cancer compared with the high tar, unfiltered cigarettes of the past.

The susceptibility of people to disease may change for reasons including genetic, nutritional, social, and medical factors. For example, measles immunization in childhood led to this disease occurring rarely in childhood, but increasingly in adolescence and adulthood.

Changes in the social, chemical, or physical environment may make a disease easier or harder to contract. For example, a combination of smaller family size, the move from extended

Box 3.7 Explanations for real changes in disease frequency

◆ What explanations can you think of for a real change in disease frequency?
◆ Can you group these into three or four categories of explanation?

Table 3.1 Summary of real explanations of disease variation and examples: the causal triad

Causal triad	Examples
Host	Genetics, behaviour
Agent	Virulence
	Introduction of a new agent
Environment	Housing
	Weather

multigeneration to nuclear single generation families, and more space at home and work, have reduced the incidence of tuberculosis, even when the disease remains endemic and common in some subgroups of the population (e.g. the homeless and some migrant populations). Real changes, as summarized in Table 3.1, are caused by changes in the host (person acquiring the disease), the specific agents of disease, or the wider environment (together known as the causal triad of host, agent, and environment).

The real-artefact framework used in a study of Legionnaires' disease is summarized in Figure 3.3. It can be applied to the systematic analysis of any population variations in disease. Section 3.5 provides the opportunity for you to apply the framework.

3.5 **Applying the real/artefact framework**

Imagine you are the epidemiologist responsible for surveillance of infectious diseases in a city of about one million people. You are examining the statistics in early July 1984 on the numbers of cases of Legionnaires' disease, which is an environmentally acquired bacterial pneumonia with no person-to-person spread. This pneumonia is rare, with a reported incidence rate of about three cases per million in the United States and England and of about eight cases per million in your country.

The main sources of the causative microorganisms, the 'Legionellaceae' or, for short, the legionellas, are complex water systems, particularly cooling towers and hot water systems, which are usually found in large buildings or as part of industrial machinery. The incidence rate varies geographically (between localities, cities, and nations) and over time (seasons and years).

Your surveillance system is based on voluntary reporting by clinical and laboratory colleagues who send you a copy of the laboratory test request form. Your data are entered by a data clerk onto a computer, which provides a list of cases on a week-by-week basis, but your statistical analysis is usually on monthly, quarterly, and annual statistics. The number of cases is based on numbers of reports of laboratory tests compatible with a diagnosis of Legionnaires' disease per month. Your database records the date of onset of illness when this is on the laboratory request form, but this is often missing. You keep the original request forms in paper files.

Examine the surveillance data in Table 3.2 part A and use the framework and aforementioned background information to systematically analyse the pattern. Answer the questions in Box 3.8 before reading on.

Table 3.2 part A shows the number of cases of disease in 1984 per month, and shows a month-by-month fluctuation in the number of cases with an abrupt rise in June. The remainder of the table—part B—provides additional information, but this was not available when you were looking

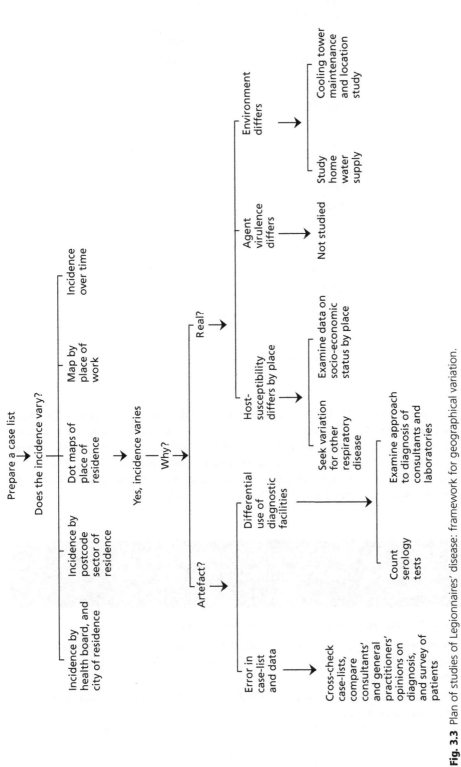

Fig. 3.3 Plan of studies of Legionnaires' disease: framework for geographical variation.

Reproduced with permission from Bhopal RS. A framework for investigating geographical variation in diseases, based on a study of Legionnaires' disease. *Journal of Public Health Medicine*, Volume 13, Issue 4, pp. 281–9, Copyright © 1991 Oxford University Press.

Table 3.2 The number of cases of Legionnaires' disease by month in the city of X in 1984: part A until June and part B until December

Month	Cases
Part A (data available in early July 1984)	
January	0
February	2
March	3
April	0
May	1
June	26
Part B	
July	4
August	4
September	6
October	7
November	7
December	12
Total	**72**

at the numbers in July 1984. The big question is whether the public health department needs to declare an outbreak. You actually need to decide within hours. This is, potentially, a public health emergency and is likely to be major news. You cannot afford to get the decision wrong. Pseudo-outbreaks, including for this outcome, are common and cause fear, waste resources, and are embarrassing. There is no automatic means of judging whether an outbreak has occurred and whether some action is required. Judgement has to be exercised.

Box 3.8 Are the variations in the number of cases of Legionnaires' disease until early July potentially artefactual?

◆ First, describe briefly the nature and content of Table 3.2.

◆ Now, work your way systematically through the factors listed in Box 3.6, and discussed in the text for guidance. What information would help you to decide whether the variations are real or apparent?

◆ Now, make a judgement on whether the findings up until June 1984 represent an outbreak of Legionnaires' disease.

In this case, chance (random fluctuation) seems to be a remote possibility so let us dismiss it. Yet, an outbreak of 26 cases in one month is a major public health problem, with serious social, political, and economic repercussions, so that we must not blunder by declaring an outbreak when there is not one. Even worse than a false alarm, however, would be failing to recognize a real outbreak. We first need to exclude explanations based on artefact.

Was there, for example, a problem in the techniques used to handle laboratory specimens being tested for Legionnaires' disease, thereby leading to false positive results? The issue needs to be discussed with the laboratory staff and, if appropriate, the testing methods and reagents used in tests need to be double checked. Once this is excluded, consider other errors. Two common errors are misdiagnosis and miscoding. On computerized databases, the disease is usually given a code number. Could information on other similar diseases, say pneumococcal pneumonia or influenza, have been miscoded as Legionnaires' disease? A cross-check of the codes against the original report forms, which will have the full diagnosis, will rule out this possibility. These simple checks requiring a little dialogue and data validation will prevent the embarrassment of a lengthy and inappropriate investigation arising from a pseudo-outbreak. We can then assume that no issues arose and so consider other explanations.

Has there been a batch of reports in June, possibly arising from some doctor accumulating reports over some months, or even years, and submitting them to you all together rather than as they arise? Alternatively, someone doing a research project may be re-testing positive specimens from previous years. For research projects, large numbers of blood tests may be submitted as a batch. If the people tested are currently sick, then these explanations can be dismissed. The date of disease onset on the laboratory request form will help to clarify this. If the date of onset varies greatly, say it spans years, then we are not looking at an outbreak. Where the date of disease onset is not given, you should ask the physician in charge. Surveillance systems should analyse cases by date of onset but unfortunately, this information is often not available, leaving the epidemiologist to use the much less satisfactory date of receipt of the specimen. If these investigations do not lead to an explanation, then we move towards non-artefactual explanations.

Has the number of people at risk altered? A change in the size of the population from which the cases are drawn can change the number of cases, though the rate remains the same. This is important for popular tourist areas and sites of religious, musical, and cultural events where the population can increase manifold. If the reputation of the doctors, health-care system, or laboratory becomes enhanced, patients can be referred from a wider catchment area, effectively increasing the population size. This is an unlikely explanation for the data in Table 3.2, the change having occurred so fast. That kind of explanation may be important for other kinds of complex problems, for example, rare cancers.

However, one possibility worth considering for environmentally acquired disease is travel abroad. An increase in international travel can increase the number of cases. Information on the number of travellers is not readily available. The rise in cases in June could reflect a travel-associated outbreak. The cases could be returning from a package tour. You should question the cases about their whereabouts. If these were cases infected abroad it would, in fact, be a real outbreak, but the public health (and media) response would be quite different to one where the cases were infected locally. In fact, the data in Table 3.2 are on locally infected cases only.

Has the likelihood of diagnosis increased, either because of greater vigilance by doctors or of people using the health-care system? A common problem which causes pseudo-outbreaks is the newly appointed doctor who is unusually thorough in reporting certain diseases, either because of a diligent commitment to the concept of disease surveillance or because of a research interest in these diseases. (A fee for notification to a health authority of certain diseases can influence reporting.) This diligence causes problems because the surveillance of disease is normally incomplete, due to a mixture of non-diagnosis and non-reporting. Effective surveillance relies more on stability in the levels of reporting, than on complete reporting. Local knowledge about the doctors and their reporting habits helps you to assess this possibility.

Research projects increase the likelihood of the correct diagnosis being reached, both because of greater awareness of the diagnosis among the doctors involved and more resources and techniques being available to make the diagnosis. As research may be of a personal nature, and may not be recorded in research databases, it may be difficult to detect that this is the cause of an apparent outbreak. The investigator will be alerted to this possibility if there is a predominance of reports from one or a small group of doctors. These kinds of potential explanations are likely to be set aside quickly by an experienced epidemiologist looking at Table 3.2 part A.

Have there been changes in diagnostic fashion or disease definition? Diagnosis is not a fixed or rigid entity but relies on medical knowledge, beliefs about how to manage patients, facilities to practice medicine, and case definitions. The cause of, and diagnostic methods for, Legionnaires' disease were discovered in 1977. Following such a discovery, the incidence of the new disease will inevitably appear to rise and that of the other similar diseases (here, other forms of pneumonia and viral infections such as influenza) will appear to fall. Abrupt changes such as here, with a rise and fall, however, are unlikely to arise merely from changes in diagnostic fashion or disease definitions.

Have there been changes in the completeness of the data collection methods? Change in the process of surveillance will lead to a changed frequency of disease. For example, if following notification of a single case of Legionnaires' disease a microbiologist contacts the reporting doctors to request more information and to discuss the case, the extra education and interest is likely to spur those doctors into notifying and diagnosing Legionnaires' disease in future. More obviously, during the investigation of a declared outbreak doctors are alerted by health officials of the need to report disease and to do the necessary tests for it. The greater likelihood of testing, diagnosing, and reporting is likely to last for a while. In the case of the data in Table 3.2 part A, these explanations seem improbable for the 26 cases in June but are likely to be contributing to the cases after that, that is, part B.

Has there been a deliberate change in the way disease data are coded, analysed, or presented? Disease coding systems change. At the time, as there was no specific code in the International Classification of Diseases (ICD) for Legionnaires' disease, and the codes were probably created locally. In other cases, a new edition of the code book may change the coding rules or codes. For instance, the principal global source of the codes (ICD) is revised every 10 years or so, with new editions more rarely (see World Health Organization 1992). Major fluctuations in the apparent frequency of some diseases occur in the transition period as new editions are adopted. Guidance is available on how to maximize comparability across different revisions of the ICD. These are not plausible explanations here.

The decision on whether a change in disease frequency is real or apparent can usually be taken rapidly. The important thing is to consider the questions systematically and to judge the likelihood of each possibility. In this example, once error is excluded, the date of illness onset in the cases has been checked, and the symptoms and signs found to be of a pneumonic illness, the likelihood is that the rise in case numbers in June is real and there is an outbreak. In this particular outbreak, the public health authorities and the media were alerted promptly and an outbreak control committee met the next day (for which I was privileged to be the apprentice serving on it).

The epidemiological challenge now is to develop a testable explanation, that is, a hypothesis, for the rise in the disease.

Box 3.9 Changes in host, agent, and environment as explanations for the outbreak of Legionnaires' disease

Do changing susceptibility of the local population, changing virulence of the causal microorganism, or changes in the environment explain the occurrence of the outbreak? What might the nature of these changes be?

The rise in locally acquired Legionnaires' disease can be analysed as follows using the host, agent, environment framework (Table 3.2), and the questions in Box 3.9. Reflect on these questions before reading on.

Susceptibility to disease is both genetic and acquired. Genetic factors, immunization, past exposure to organisms, nutrition, general health status, and other relevant risk factors determine the susceptibility of the population. As the susceptibility of the population usually changes over long periods, and in the case of genetic factors over generations, this is not the explanation for the findings in Table 3.2. If the same data were for decades or centuries, not months, such factors might need to be considered.

The virulence of microorganisms is constantly changing but very difficult to determine, and baseline data rarely exist. This is an area of microbiology that is rapidly developing with the recent capability of mapping the microbial genome. These technologies were not available in 1984. Virulent legionellas may have colonized water systems in May or June 1984, possibly replacing other strains, and led to the abrupt rise in disease incidence. In this instance, and indeed in most circumstances, an interaction would be required between the agent and environment. In practice, change in microbial virulence may not be demonstrated and such an explanation will be based on exclusion of other possibilities. A rise in the number of cases could reflect an increase in the level of exposure to the microorganisms, either because the environment has become more hazardous or the contact between the environment and the population has become closer. In our example, the following changes could have occurred:

♦ The weather warmed, leading to the switching on of water systems in air conditioning units that harboured virulent legionellas.

♦ The winds and humidity changed such that virulent organisms could be delivered to a susceptible population at the infective concentration.

♦ Protective mechanisms, such as the drift elimination mechanisms or chemical decontamination procedures in a cooling tower, or temperature control in a hot water system, broke down.

Explanations of this type must be generated and tested. To re-emphasize, the key to a successful epidemiological investigation is the systematic analysis and explicit statement of the possible explanations.

In reality, a rise in cases will be a result of an interaction of factors. Indeed, both real and artefactual factors will be relevant. For example, the rise in Legionnaires' disease shown in Table 3.2 part A probably arose due to environmental changes which permitted a virulent organism to colonize a complex water system and thus permitted the organisms to be dispersed so that many people were exposed, of whom a small proportion (maybe 1%) were susceptible. Once the excess of cases was publicized and case search procedures started, cases were notified which normally would have remained undiagnosed (e.g. patients originally diagnosed as pneumonia or influenza being re-tested for antibody to legionellas, even after they have recovered). This enhanced surveillance will lead to a lasting excess of cases, as seen in Table 3.2 part B.

The story of the investigation of this Legionnaires' disease outbreak has been published (Ad-Hoc Committee 1986). I observed and participated in this investigation, and then proceeded to consider the data from Table 3.2 part B, and beyond that. The weather in Glasgow was very warm and winds were unusually light. These are conditions favouring the movement of aerosols contaminated with legionella bacteria. The investigation led to the discovery of a cooling tower in the postulated area that had mechanical faults and was not properly maintained. While cause and effect could not be proved, the conclusion was that the outbreak investigation could be ended because this was the best of the explanations available.

In practice, teasing out the different explanations is a complex task. In continuing studies of the geographical epidemiology of Legionnaires' disease in Scotland, 1978–1986, I prepared a case list of all 372 potential cases diagnosed over the period. The explanations for geographical variation are listed in column one of Table 3.3. The solutions generated to provide evidence to choose between the explanations are in the second column. The chart showing the plan of the studies is in Figure 3.3. The plan clarifies which hypotheses need exploring, the studies that are to be done,

Table 3.3 Summary of explanations for (geographical) variation in disease with approaches to their study solutions adopted in a study of Legionnaires' disease in Scotland

Explanations	Approaches to study variations adopted
Time variation	
Geographical variation results from varying incidence in time, rather than being geographical per se	A reasonably long time period was studied (1978–1986)
Artefact	
Differences in case definition	Standard case definition applied
Missing cases/incomplete surveillance	Cross-checked case lists; used data from several sources
Errors in address data/postcodes (zip codes)	Addresses checked against medical records; all post codes confirmed using postcode directory; living patients and relatives asked to check basic details
Differential hospital admission rates	Examined hospital admission rates for other diagnoses (effect would be non-specific); compared travel and non-travel-related Legionnaires' disease cases
Differential use of diagnostic tests	Ratios of serology tests to pneumonia and serology tests to Legionnaires' disease used as an indicator; consultants' and laboratories' approach to diagnosis surveyed
True variation	
Host susceptibility differs	Assessed whether geographical variation existed for other diseases which share risk factors; assessed whether populations differed in terms of socio-economic status
Agent virulence differs	Not studied
Environmental factors differ	Developed hypotheses on most likely sources focusing on cooling towers; collected new data on location and maintenance of cooling towers and did association studies

and indeed which explanations remain untested. Such an overview is highly advised in all investigations of disease variations, both as a guide to the actions needed and as a means of data interpretation. The kind of reasoning illustrated here applies to all conditions and all epidemiological investigations of variation.

3.6 Disease clustering and clusters in epidemiology

According to the *Oxford English Dictionary*, a cluster is a collection of things of the same kind, a bunch, a number of persons close together, a group or crowd. In epidemiology, according to *A Dictionary of Epidemiology*, a disease cluster is a greater than expected aggregation of relatively rare events or diseases in time or place, or both. The terms cluster and clustering are not used either for common diseases because clustering is inevitable due to chance alone, or for infectious diseases that spread from person-to-person where clustering is the norm. A disease cluster in epidemiology is a mini-epidemic of a rare event.

The cluster is a special instance of disease variation. Typical examples might be four cases of leukaemia in one street, or three cases of primary biliary cirrhosis in a single nursing home, or five cases of Legionnaires' disease in a factory. Once observed, such a cluster cannot be ignored, and presents a difficult epidemiological puzzle. From a scientific perspective, if the factors that led to the cluster can be identified, then the cause of the disease might become clearer. The cluster is a potential causal goldmine but the yield is usually poor. From a public health perspective, the fear is that unless the cause of the cluster is discovered and preventive action taken there may be further cases. The cluster may herald a large outbreak or even widespread epidemic. Clusters are an especially difficult problem in epidemiology, for the causes are rarely discovered so the difficulties of judging the appropriate public health action remain. Epidemiologists should be cautious in mounting detailed and costly investigations into disease clusters, as very often the explanation will not be found. A brief investigation as a prelude to a decision on detailed investigation is wise.

Typically, clusters are identified by a member of the public or a local health professional observing an excess of cases in a locality or over a short time period. For example, McAlister N. Gregg observed that in 1941, cases of cataract in newborn babies, an exceptionally rare problem, far exceeded the usual. He saw 13 cases of his own, and seven of his colleagues. He hypothesized that this cluster was associated with a preceding outbreak of German measles (rubella) in 1940. He was correct and rubella syndrome was discovered.

This is a classic example of one of the greatest advances spurred by investigating a disease cluster, in this case with the focus on events occurring over a period of time. Of course, it is also a cluster characterized by the people affected (babies in the womb) and in a place (Sydney, Australia). It is noteworthy that, as with most studies of clusters, Gregg simply reported a case series (see also section 9.3.1). In addition to tracking down the cause of a previously baffling problem of congenital defects of cataract, hearing loss and heart problems, Gregg's work showed for the first time that virus infections in the mother could be transmitted to the fetus through the placenta. The other inspiring and noteworthy fact is that Gregg was an ophthalmologist (eye surgeon). Gregg's conclusions were corroborated independently in 1943 (with another case series). Nonetheless, in 1944 a Lancet editorial concluded the evidence was weak—a judgement that history overturned. In Chapter 9 I will look at case series especially carefully, given there is a modern view that the evidence they produce is weak.

Clusters may also be identified through examining routinely collected surveillance data, and this becomes easier if cases are mapped, or plotted over time. The opportunities to seek clustering of disease are expanding with automated searching on large data sets. Geographical information systems (GIS) make it easy to examine the space and time location of cases. The key data for seeking clusters are spatial coordinates usually obtained from postcodes (zip codes), time (usually date of onset of disease), and personal characteristics of the case such as age, sex, and occupation.

Identification of a cluster of cases is not the solution to a problem, but rather the beginning of one, that is, the problem of explanation. Leukaemia clusters have been observed for over 100 years, but explaining them has been extremely difficult. Clustering usually points to environmental causes. Clustering of childhood leukaemia around nuclear power stations occurs commonly. Intuitively, the explanation would be expected to be exposure to low levels of radiation. The radiation hypothesis for such clustering has not held despite much investigation. Another hypothesis is that leukaemia is one rare outcome of a common childhood infection. Leukaemia clusters are possibly a consequence of a change in the pattern of such an infection resulting from the migration and population mixing that occurs when a nuclear power plant is built and put into operation.

As clustering is merely a specialized variant of disease variation, its analysis follows the principles in section 3.6. Clusters may arise from data error, or chance. One potential problem is of investigators selecting cases by focusing on those that are in a cluster and ignoring others. This can be done by choosing time periods or geographic boundaries selectively. This is the so-called 'bull's eye' or 'Texas Sharpshooter' effect. Here the observer only looks at the shots that cluster, especially around the target, and ignore all the other shots that went astray. To avoid this problem, the cases in the apparent cluster should be studied as part of the series of cases that occurred in the population, say over a three-year period in a city or region with a population of a million people or so. As clusters, by definition, are of rare events, only by adopting this kind of approach can we place the cluster under investigation into a context, starting with the question of whether the observed cluster is unexpected.

Most of the discussions of clusters point out that too many are notified and investigated for little benefit. Clusters are, however, often missed in clinical practice and even by routine surveillance systems, either because of incomplete data (e.g. the date of disease onset is missing), or the insensitivity of data presentation and analysis methods. With the routine computerization of health data, linkage across data systems, larger and more comprehensive data sets and the availability of software for analysis, the issues around both detection and correct interpretation of disease clustering are growing.

The concept of a cluster in epidemiology goes beyond that of merely a group of cases; that is, beyond the statistical concept, as shown in Figure 3.4, using the analogy of grapes. Do the exercise in Box 3.10 before reading on.

The five grapes seem to be a cluster. They look the same and are close together spatially. The fact that they look equally fresh suggests that they share a common origin in time. If two of the grapes

Is this a cluster?

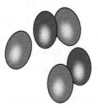

Perhaps. The challenge is
statistical and causal

Fig. 3.4 Clusters I: are these grapes in a cluster?

Box 3.10 Do the five grapes make a cluster?

Reflect on whether the five grapes in Figure 3.4 make a cluster. What characteristics make you think that they may be a cluster? What information would lead you to change your mind?

had been red and three green, one was a plastic replica and one dried and shrivelled, we would not have perceived them as a cluster.

So, we would probably conclude that the grapes in Figure 3.4 are part of a cluster. The next step is to show that the number of grapes in this space and time was unexpectedly high. We have already observed that this requires us to set this cluster in a wider context. Imagine, instead of grapes, five cases of acute leukaemia are reported by a member of the public from a single street in a small town. The first action is to verify this observation. If all five cases are truly recent cases of acute leukaemia, we would be inclined to judge this as a cluster. If one turns out to be a misdiagnosis (say anaemia), one occurred 15 years ago, one was chronic myeloid leukaemia, and only two were acute leukaemia in childhood, we would not perceive them as a cluster. A mixed bag of diagnoses makes an unconvincing cluster, exactly as does a mixed bag of red and green grapes. Let us assume that the five cases were all acute leukaemia.

The epidemiological challenge is to discover how the cluster came together. Do the exercise in Box 3.11 before reading on.

Evidence that the grapes had one stalk or even that they came from the same vine would be compelling. For diseases the common factor, which holds or brings the cluster together, provides this compelling evidence. Diseases have a background rate of occurrence. Five cases of leukaemia close together in time and place could occur by chance. Statistical tests utilizing data from several years in a larger population in this small town and its surroundings would help to assess the role of chance. The close occurrence of leukaemia cases could be an artefact. Just as the grapes may have come from several bunches and have been placed together, so the cases of leukaemia may come from several localities. For example, a children's hospice will bring cases together. An even more mundane explanation would be a coding error in residential postcode, so that cases are wrongly being given the same but erroneous postcode (zip codes). I once observed a set of postcodes on the wall of a coding clerk's office. I asked why this list was on the wall, and I learned that when the real code was missing from the records, one was randomly chosen from the list, as the record could not be submitted without one. These are the kinds of practical behaviours that epidemiologists should be aware of when interpreting others' data, particularly routinely collected health service data.

Box 3.11 Assessing whether the cluster of grapes and of leukaemia are artefacts or whether there are common causes

Reflecting on both the cluster of grapes and five cases of childhood leukaemia, what evidence would you seek to help you to exclude artefact and to ascertain a common cause? What would provide irrefutable evidence that the grapes are part of one cluster? It is possible to produce such strong evidence for leukaemia?

Is this a cluster?

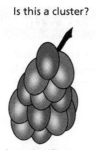

Yes, but, significance unclear
i.e. how or why the grapes
are together
The challenge is biological and causal

Fig. 3.5 Clusters II: what is the significance of this cluster? How did it come about?

Figure 3.5 shows the grape's common stalk and leaves no doubt that the cluster is real. Similarly, if our investigation of leukaemia cases had shown that these were bound by common factors such as type of leukaemia, age group, residence, time of disease onset, and exposures to known or potential causal factors we would think the cluster is real. The next step is to explain mechanisms. This is easy for grapes; we simply study the mechanisms by which grapes grow on vines (Fig. 3.6) as clusters. For diseases, the processes are far more difficult to study. Nonetheless, the guiding concepts are similar. The investigator's job is incomplete unless these steps are achieved—but it is rare to explain why and how the cluster arose. To achieve such understanding requires epidemiology to work with sciences that study mechanisms. We now return to Legionnaires' disease.

Is this a cluster?

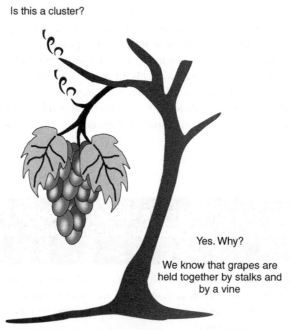

Yes. Why?

We know that grapes are
held together by stalks and
by a vine

Fig. 3.6 Clusters III: explaining the cluster—the vine.

Table 3.4 Number of non-travel, non-outbreak cases of Legionnaires' disease in Greater Glasgow Health Board by year and month

Year	Jan	Feb	Mar	Apr	May	Jun	Jul	Aug	Sep	Oct	Nov	Dec	Total
1978			1	1			1			1	3		7
1979				3			2	4	3		3		15*
1980	1							1	2		1		5
1981	1			1		1			1	1			5
1982						1	1			1			3
1983	2	2					1	1	3		6	1	16
1984		1	2			2	1	3	2	7	6	12	36
1985	4	7	1	2	1	1	1		1	3	4	4	29
1986											1	1	2
Total	8	10	3	4	5	5	7	9	12	14	24	17	118

*For one case neither the month of onset nor the date of serological testing was known.

Reproduced with permission from Bhopal RS, Diggle P, and Rowlingson B. Pinpointing clusters of apparently sporadic cases of Legionnaires' disease. *British Medical Journal*, Volume 304, Issue 6833, pp. 1022–27, Copyright © 1992 BMJ Publishing Group.

Legionnaires' disease cases may occur in outbreaks, or in solitary or sporadic form. The cause of outbreaks has often been tracked to cooling towers or complex hot water systems, as the sources of infective aerosol. What of sporadic cases? By definition, these are solitary cases, unconnected in space and time to others. The source of infection for such cases is harder to study, but epidemiology has a role to play. I studied non-outbreak, non-travel Legionnaires' disease in and around the city of Glasgow 1978–1986. The results are shown in Table 3.4. Before reading on, do the exercise in Box 3.12. Remember, the number of cases expected in a year at this time was about eight.

As these were apparently sporadic cases no clustering was expected, but there clearly was some. Nine cases occurred in July–September 1979, six in November 1983, and 36 between October 1984 and February 1985. The next step was to see whether there was clustering in space too. Table 3.5 shows these cases by postcode, the number of hospitals and the number of hospital consultant physicians in charge of each cluster, and Figure 3.7 shows similar data on a map.

These data indicate that some supposedly sporadic cases were actually part of space–time clusters. Questions that arise include these: why were these clusters missed, and what is their cause? The findings showed that clusters can be easily missed in clinical practice, possibly because of the dispersion of small numbers of patients to several hospitals and physicians, and because of incomplete data. For example, the six cases in postcode sectors G31.4, G31.3 and G31.1 in October 1984–November 1995 were spread over time, admitted to two hospitals and cared for by four

Box 3.12 Defining and assessing clusters of Legionnaires' disease

- On first principles, what would you expect the distribution of cases to be like in time? What possible clusters do you see in Table 3.4?
- What additional information would you like to assess these?

Table 3.5 Clusters of apparently sporadic cases of Legionnaires' disease by area of residence, date of disease onset, and numbers of hospitals and consultants (hospital specialists) involved

Health board and postcode sector of apparent cluster*	No. of cases	Date of onset	No. of hospitals	No. of individual consultants in charge of each group
Greater Glasgow				
G5.0	3	Oct, Nov 1978	2	3
G21.1, G21.3	2	Nov 1983	2	2
G11.5, G12.8	2	Nov 1983	2	2
G4.0	2	Aug, Nov 1983	1	1
G33.5	2	Sep, Dec 1983	1	2
G4.0	5	Mar, Jun, Aug, (2 cases), Oct 1984	2	5
G31.4, G31.3, G31.1	6	Oct, Nov 1984; Jan, Feb, Apr, Nov 1985	2	4
G33.3	3	Jul, Oct, Nov 1984	2	3
G13.4, G13.3	2	Sep, Dec 1984	2	2
G72.8	3	Nov, Dec 1984	2	3
G5.8, G5.9	2	Feb 1985	2	2
G21.2, G22.6, G21.4	5	Jan, Feb, Oct 1985	3	6

*Postcodes in a row are adjacent areas.

hospital consultants. The routine surveillance system's data on postcode and date of onset were, in fact, incomplete. (I had to communicate with patients and doctors and examine medical records to extract much of the necessary information.) In these circumstances, identification of clustering is problematic. Effective surveillance requires proactively seeking, completing, and analysing data to find patterns of disease. The final step of ascertaining cause requires us to develop and test hypotheses, here, as to why some apparently sporadic Legionnaires' disease cases come in clusters. Aside from artefacts, the principal three hypotheses generated were these:

1. People living in different parts of Glasgow are differentially susceptible to Legionnaires' disease. This seemed highly unlikely.

2. The clusters reflect the intermittent virulence of Legionella. This hypothesis seems unlikely and is extremely difficult to test.

3. That sporadic cases are either part of larger outbreaks, or are mini-outbreaks, arising from the same general sources of aerosol as for most outbreaks. This was tested by seeking an association between the location of Glasgow cooling towers and residence of cases, as shown in Figure 3.8. Table 3.6 summarizes these data and shows that living near a cooling tower was associated with a greater risk of sporadic Legionnaires' disease. This pattern was not present for travel-associated disease or lung cancer (data not shown; available in Bhopal 1991). This work, therefore, provided a general explanation for the phenomenon of clustering, but it did not provide a specific explanation for each of the many clusters, that is, which cooling tower was involved for each cluster. That is often the best that can be accomplished epidemiologically, especially retrospectively.

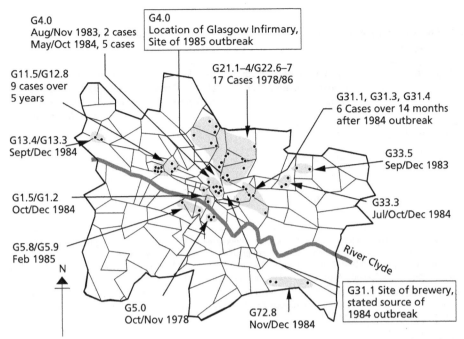

Fig. 3.7 Community-acquired, non-travel, and apparently sporadic cases of Legionnaires' disease in Glasgow suspected to constitute a space–time cluster.

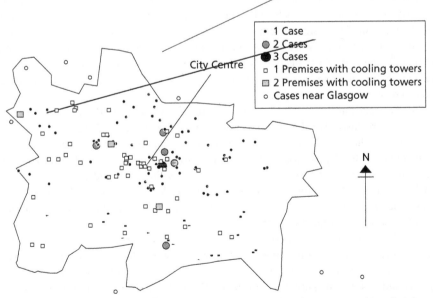

Fig. 3.8 Clusters: map of the location of cooling towers in the city of Glasgow and in relation to the residence of non-travel, community-acquired, non-outbreak cases of Legionnaires' disease.

Table 3.6 Relation between distance of patients' homes from cooling tower and risk of Legionnaires' disease

Study group	Distance of home from nearest cooling tower (km)*	No. of cases observed (no. expected)	Relative risk of disease compared with group living >1.0 km from nearest cooling tower
Legionnaires' disease: no history of travel abroad (n = 107)	≤0.25	12 (4.4)	3.89
	>0.25 to ≤0.5	28 (13.2)	3.00
	>0.5 to ≤0.75	15 (17.9)	1.19
	>0.75 to ≤1.0	14 (17.9)	1.11
	>1.0	38 (53.7)	1.00

*The denominator population living within each distance category varied from year to year owing to the varying numbers of cooling towers in each year. The average denominator populations were as follows: 404 431 people lived more than 1 km from a cooling tower; 116 339 lived between 0.75 and 1 km away; 114 886 lived between 0.5 and 0.75 km away; 84 466 lived between 0.25 and 0.5 km away; and 27 884 lived less than 0.25 km away.

Adapted with permission from Bhopal RS, Fallon RJ, Buist EC, Black RJ, and Urquhart JD. Proximity of the home to a cooling tower and risk of non-outbreak Legionnaires' disease. *British Medical Journal*, Volume 302, Issue 6773, pp. 378–83, Copyright © 1991 BMJ Publishing Group.

3.7 **Applications of observations of disease variation**

Variations in disease patterns are of practical value in helping the clinician in both the diagnosis and management of disease. For example, the diagnosis of myocardial infarction (heart attack) is much more likely to be correct in a man of 70 years complaining of chest pain than in a woman of 30. This is based on age and sex variations in heart attack. Clinicians can also make use of seasonal variations and of variations by ethnicity, geographical origins, occupation, and pattern of travel. So, for example, Muslim patients with diabetes mellitus are most likely to have problems with control of their disease when fasting during daylight hours in the month of Ramadan than at other times of the year. Most infections have a distinct seasonal pattern; for example, influenza is more common in winter and gastroenteritis in summer. Outbreaks and clusters alert clinicians to consider a diagnosis even of rare diseases.

Long-term trends are important to clinical practice; for example, the changing nature and decline of tuberculosis over the last few hundred years has led to a change in the differential diagnosis (the preliminary list of possible diagnoses) of symptoms such as coughs and fever. It is likely that within 10–20 years, assuming that the recent rise and decline in CHD continues, the differential diagnosis of chest pain will also alter. Certainly, doctors in India and other developing countries, where CHD is on the rise, will be much more alert to this diagnosis than hitherto. By contrast, doctors in the United Kingdom or United States may be looking for other commoner causes of chest pain; for example, gastritis.

For health policy decisions, disease variations over decades (known as secular trends) are of special importance in setting priorities and for evaluating whether health objectives have been achieved. Variation in disease by place and by socio-economic status is a guide to the level of inequality and possibly inequity in health status. The health-care planner uses disease variations to match resources to need. One simple example is the prediction, based on long-term surveillance data, that in winter emergency admissions to hospital will rise, especially when there is an epidemic of influenza, and hence there will be fewer beds available for elective, non-emergency admissions. Non-emergency admissions can, therefore, be re-scheduled for other parts of the year.

The health promoter can tailor both the timing and the content of interventions. For example, an educational campaign on the perils of drinking and driving could be timed using information on alcohol consumption patterns by day of the week, week of the year, and the peak incidence of road traffic accidents.

Spatial variations in health behaviour and disease patterns can help in assigning staff and resources to particular places; for example, community health staff may spend more time in geographical areas with low breast feeding rates.

Analysis of disease variation is, therefore, both the prime source of information to spark hypotheses on causation and also at the heart of applied health care and public health epidemiology.

3.8 **Epidemiological theory underpinning or arising from this chapter**

Disease variation arises because of (a) changes and subsequently differences in either or a combination of the host, the agent of disease, or the environment; or (b) changes and then differences in interaction between the host, agent, and environment. As these changes occur at a different pace in different places and subpopulations, disease variations are inevitable. In studying these variations in epidemiology, we are seeking to uncover the natural forces that caused them (I will focus on this in section 10.2). (The first step, however, is to ensure that variations are not merely artefacts, which is examined in Chapter 4.)

3.9 **Conclusion**

The interpretation of change in disease frequency and subsequent variation is difficult. Erroneous conclusions arise easily. Therefore, to avoid the twin and opposite pitfalls of (a) false alerts or (b) missed clusters, outbreaks, epidemics, and health inequalities, a systematic approach to the collection and interpretation of data is necessary. The approach outlined here provides a structure for the investigator's thoughts. It places heavy emphasis on artefactual causes of changes in disease incidence. These artefacts and related biases are discussed in more detail in the next chapter. The study of variation lies at the heart of the epidemiological strategy. It is a fundamental bedrock of observational epidemiology. It is in this kind of work where new ideas are generated and where great discoveries (whether practical or theoretical) start. Yet, this kind of work is out of fashion, a

Table 3.7 Summary of key results relating to Tobias *et al.*'s (2009) hypotheses

Hypotheses	Some of the evidence in support
1. Ethnic inequalities altered in response to economic policies	1. The long-term decline in the gap in life expectancy reversed from 1986 to 1996 and then again declined 2. There was an increase in mortality rate ratios from 1986–1989 to 1996–1999 after which the rate ratios stabilized
2. Changes would be specific to conditions affected rapidly by socio-economic change	1. In males both actual and relative inequality increased. In females actual mortality difference declined while relative inequality increased 2. Suicide rates were lower in Maori at the beginning of the period but by 1996–1999 were higher than in European/other group. Then the rates fell fast from 2001–2004

Source: data from Tobias M, Blakely T, Matheson D, Rasanathan K, and Atkinson J. Changing trends in indigenous inequalities in mortality: lessons from New Zealand. *International Journal of Epidemiology*, Volume 38, Issue 6 pp. 1711–1722, Copyright © 2009 Oxford University Press.

trend that has accelerated in recent years. There is no logical reason for this. Currently, the fashion favours trials (experiments), and meta-analyses/systematic reviews. However, globally huge investment is underway to build very large data sets—and the concomitant result of this will be fresh data sets and ways of tackling the study of variations. Exemplar 3.1 illustrates the power of this kind of work.

Exemplar 3.1: Tobias, M., Blakely, T., Matheson, D., Rasanathan, K., and Atkinson, J. (2009) Changing trends in indigenous inequalities in mortality: lessons from New Zealand. *International Journal of Epidemiology*, Volume 38, Issue 6, pp. 1711–22

The background

In this chapter, I have explained that the description of health data in time, by place, and by population groups is at the heart of epidemiology. I noted both that this kind of work has gone out of fashion recently and, given the massive data sets being collected and the power of data linkage, it is likely to be resurgent in the future. This paper exemplifies the power of descriptive epidemiology in every respect, including causal analysis. It focuses on, arguably, the greatest modern public health challenges—inequalities in health status, which are, of course, described using epidemiology.

The study aim and methods

The authors described trends in mortality comparing indigenous Maori and non-Maori, mainly of European origin, populations in New Zealand.

They used a linked data set whereby the five New Zealand censuses from 1981 to 2004 were linked to death records. They included people aged 1–74 years of age who died within three years of any of these censuses. The two data sets were linked using a technique called probability linkage (see also Exemplar 7.1 and Exemplar 8.1 for a similar Scottish linked cohort). This created five retrospective cohort studies (see Chapter 9). The linkage ranged from 70.9 to 79.6 per cent.

The ethnic group was from the census. Maoris were people who included this category in their self-identified responses and the reference group were not in the categories Maori, Pacific, or Asians. The causes of death were coded from death certificates using The International Classification of Disease (see Chapter 7).

Using a standard population structure (world population) to age standardize (see Chapter 8), rates and the ratios of these rates were calculated. Some specific causes of death were examined. The possible role of some social and economic variables in the found differences were examined in the age group 25–59 years.

Life expectancy data were also examined between 1951 and 2005. Given that Maori ethnicity is not always accurate on the death certificate and correction of estimates was not possible until 1981, the authors urge special caution in interpreting early data.

The study hypotheses

There were two major hypotheses which I have summarized as: (i) that during 1984 to the early 1990s, ethnic inequalities would have widened and narrowed again later in the 1990s, in response to changing economic policies; (ii) the changes would be most evident for causes that respond to socio-economic changes.

Results

The data are complex (five figures and two tables in the main text), not least because the authors have presented both the measures and ratios of rates. I have summarized the results in relation to the two hypotheses in Table 3.7.

Tobias *et al.*'s conclusion

The general pattern showed ethnic inequality widening in 1986–1996. The authors judge that this was plausibly, partly causally related to the economic changes introduced between 1984–1993. These changes affected the Maori population much more adversely than the European/other New Zealand population. The result was clearer for Maori men than women. The authors think that economic reforms affect men more than women. The ethnic inequality narrowed when there was an economic recovery and changes in economic, social, and health-care policy.

The authors acknowledge the following limitations of their study:

♦ incomplete linkage of data;

♦ changing definitions of ethnicity over time;

♦ missing data;

♦ the possibility the then contributing effects of socio-economic variables were not fully and accurately captured.

Concluding remarks

This is a study of variations in time and person (ethnic group and sex) in one place. It is a rare and remarkable example of a study relating important health outcomes to assess the potential causal effects of macroeconomic policy, and health and social care reforms.

It shows what descriptive epidemiology can contribute, outlines powerful methods, and sets out the difficulties of determining whether the associations are real and causal, or artefact. I recommend that you read this paper carefully after you have studied Chapters 7, 8, and 9.

Source: data from Tobias M, Blakely T, Matheson D, Rasanathan K, and Atkinson J. Changing trends in indigenous inequalities in mortality: lessons from New Zealand. *International Journal of Epidemiology*, Volume 38, Issue 6, pp. 1711–1722, Copyright © 2009 International Epidemiological Association

Summary

Diseases wax and wane in their population frequency. The underlying reasons are often diffi-cult to detect and may remain a mystery. On the occasions when the mystery is solved we tend to gain huge insights, both scientific and practical, to help in disease control. There are three principal reasons for investigating variations in disease frequency. First, to help bring under con-trol an apparent abrupt rise in disease incidence (a suspected epidemic, outbreak, or cluster, the commonest public health emergency). Secondly, by understanding the factors that changed the disease frequency, to gain insight into the causes of disease. Thirdly, to use the knowledge of the disease trend and its causes to make predictions and plans, both in terms of health policy and health care, and the frequency of disease.

Disease variations are often, however, artefactual, and arise from data errors. A systematic approach to the analysis of variation in disease begins by differentiating artefactual change from real change. Artefactual change can be analysed as chance, error, changing population; and changing approaches to health care, diagnosis and data collection, analysis, and presentation.

Real change results from changes in host susceptibility, in the agent's capacity to cause disease, and in the influence of the environment. Changes in the human host may be genetic (biological), epigenetic, or through culture and behaviour. Genetic changes at the population level occur over multiple generations, while epigenetic changes can be transmitted across generations. Cultural and behavioural changes occur remarkably fast in the modern world and at a different pace in different populations. External agents of disease can change fast and in microorganisms, these rapid changes include genetic mutations altering virulence. The environment may also change fast and unpredictably with vast consequences, for example as in a drought. The epidemiological challenge here is to pinpoint the causal factors.

The principles behind the investigation of clusters, outbreaks, epidemics, and inequalities in both of communicable and non-communicable diseases, are similar.

Sample questions

Question 1 Define what is meant by a disease cluster and describe the factors that you would take into account when determining whether an alleged cluster (e.g. of childhood cancer in pupils of a primary school) is likely to be real.

Answer A disease cluster can be defined as a higher than expected number of cases of a relatively rare health event or disease, where cases are aggregated in time or place or both; for example, an unusually high number of cases of lymphoma occurring in residents of a small village over a period of five years.

The following factors should be taken into account when determining whether an alleged disease cluster is likely to be real:

◆ Are the cases all of a similar clinical problem?

◆ Are the cases all real, that is, correctly diagnosed, meet a sensible case definition, and correctly coded and recorded?

◆ Do formal statistical tests confirm that the incidence of disease in the locality/time period of interest is likely to be genuinely higher than background expected levels, that is, that such a finding is statistically unlikely?

◆ If the cause of the condition is understood, is there a plausible explanation of how a cluster could have arisen, for example, known or possible exposure of the local population to accepted risk factors?

Question 2 Why do virtually all diseases vary in incidence over time, between places and between populations?

Answer The causes of disease are constantly changing, for example, over time we see changes in, weather, quality of housing, etc.; in place: by quality of water, food, man-made environment, etc.; between populations: we see variations in health-related lifestyles and behaviours such as smoking and alcohol drinking. Over short periods, there are changes in the genetic make-up of microbes that can increase or decrease their virulence as human pathogens. In humans, genetic changes have occurred over long time periods and these influence some disease patterns.

References

Ad-hoc Committee (authors: Fallon, R.J., Reid, D., Donaldson, J.R., Wilson, T.S., Jackson, J., Donaghey, M., and Bhopal, R.S.). (1986) Legionellosis—a combined study of a community outbreak. *Lancet*, **ii**, 380–2.

Anonymous. (1944) Rubella and congenital malformations. *The Lancet*, **316**.

Bhopal, R.S., Diggle, P., and Rowlingson, B. (1992) Pinpointing clusters of apparently sporadic Legionnaires' disease. *British Medical Journal*, **304**, 1022–7.

Bhopal, R.S., Fallon, R.J., Buist, E.C., Black, R.J., and Urquart, J.D. (1991) Proximity of the home to a cooling tower and the risk of non-outbreak Legionnaires' disease. *British Medical Journal*, **302**, 378–83.

Bhopal, R.S. (2014) *Migration, Ethnicity, Race, and Health in Multicultural Societies*, 2nd edn. Oxford, UK: Oxford University Press.

Gregg, N.M. (1941) Congenital cataract following German measles in the mother. *Transactions of the Ophthalmological Society of Australia*, **3**, 35–46.

Tobias, M., Blakely, T., Matheson, D., Rasanathan, K., and Atkinson, J. (2009) Changing trends in indigenous inequalities in mortality: lessons from New Zealand. *International Journal of Epidemiology*, **38**, 1711–22.

UNESCO (1952) *The Race Concept: Results of an Enquiry*. Paris: UNESCO.

Watson, J.D. and Crick, F.H. (1953) Molecular structure of nucleic acids. *Nature*, **171**(4356), 737–8.

World Health Organization (1992) *ICD-10 - International statistical classification of diseases and related health problems*. Geneva, Switzerland: World Health Organization.

Yang, Q., Khoury, M.J., Friedman, J.M., *et al.* (2005) How many genes underlie the occurrence of common complex diseases in the population? *International Journal of Epidemiology*, **34**, 1129–37.

Chapter 4

Error, bias, and confounding in epidemiology

Objectives

On completion of the chapter you should understand:

- that error in measurement is crucially important in applied sciences such as epidemiology, especially when studying free-living, human populations;

- that bias, considered as an error which affects comparison groups unequally, is particularly important in epidemiology;

- the major causes of error and bias in epidemiology can be analysed based on the chronology of a research project;

- that biases in posing the research question, stating hypotheses, and choosing the study population are important in epidemiology;

- that errors and bias in data interpretation and publication are particularly important in epidemiology because of its health policy and health-care applications;

- that confounding is the mismeasurement of the relationship between a risk factor and disease, which potentially arises in comparisons of groups that differ;

- that different epidemiological study designs share many of the problems of error, bias, and confounding.

4.1 Introduction to error, bias, and confounding in epidemiology

An error is an act, assertion, or belief that is not right. In mathematics, an error is the difference between a computed or measured value, and a true or theoretically correct value. For example, a metre is a length fixed by agreement, but in different ways at different times and currently as the path travelled by light in a vacuum in a particular time. The metre is arbitrarily decided by agreeing a definition, which is the then truth.

In health and disease, the truth is unknown and cannot be either defined or computed unequivocally. There is no 'right' body shape, height, or weight. There is no 'truthful' measure of asthma, heart disease, or irritable bowel syndrome. Even agreed definitions on diseases change periodically as knowledge advances (Chapters 1 and 7). In health and disease research, including epidemiology, errors are common. If not recognized, errors generate false knowledge. Of course, all human endeavours and certainly all sciences have errors, but they have a particular importance in epidemiology for the reasons discussed below. Bias is common and important too. Before reading on, reflect on the exercise in Box 4.1.

Box 4.1 Error and bias

Reflect on the word bias. What is the difference, if any, between error and bias? Why might error and bias be particularly important in epidemiology?

A bias is a subtle kind of error and is a preference, especially one that inhibits impartial judgement or leads to unfairness. In science, including epidemiology, error, and bias are frequently used as synonyms. Bias is the usual term applied to a range of errors in science (usually excepting random statistical error). It is subtler and more diplomatic to say the study was biased than that it was erroneous or simply wrong, though all these descriptions mean the same. There is a famous and widely used diagram to illustrate the difference between error and bias using a bull's eye target. This is shown in Figure 4.1. I have simplified this to illustrate the point. Imagine a study makes a measurement and if it is correct then we illustrate that with an 'x' in the bull's eye, as in Figure 4.1.

We would accept that the measurement is about correct in (a) but incorrect in (b). In research including epidemiology (unlike clinical practice), we like to make multiple measures especially when testing our methods. We will show five measurements in the same person. It is clear in (c) that although the measurement differs slightly we can conclude that, overall, our method is both reasonably accurate and precise. By contrast, in (d) the method is neither particularly accurate nor precise. Figure (e) shows the measurement to be incorrect but reasonably precise, while (f) shows inaccuracy and imprecision. It is commonly stated that (d) shows error (perhaps qualified as random error) while (e) shows bias. In fact, (e) shows a serious error, more so than (d), and is the kind of error that we call bias. We also call this a systematic error, which is a good phrase. Since so much of epidemiology is concerned with comparing groups, in this book bias in epidemiology is conceptualized to be error, which applies unequally to comparison groups.

We can see that in comparing two or more groups we must avoid all error, but especially systematic error. Before reading on do the exercise in Box 4.2.

The measures are likely to show a fair bit of variation, simply because it is difficult to standardize even on the same person. The result might be somewhere in between Figure 4.1(c) and Figure 4.1(d). Of course, we do not know where the bull's eye, or correct measure, actually is. Let us plot the results from the morning first, setting this researcher as the 'gold standard'. Where are the second researcher's results likely to lie? The waist gets bigger as the day goes on, and varies with meals. It could reasonably be said that the morning values are more accurate. Figure 4.2 plots what we are likely to see, with the morning measures as X's and the evening measures as circles.

Figure 4.2 shows some random measurement error (much the same for both researchers) but also a systematic error. In this case, we would conclude that both affected the study. This is normal!

Whether science is estimating the age of the Earth, calculating the speed of light, achieving cold fusion in the laboratory, or assessing when humans first started using weapons, errors and corrections are the norm. Epidemiology is no exception. The provocative Popperian view is that science progresses by the rejection of hypotheses (by falsification) rather than the establishment of so-called truths (by verification) (Popper 1989). Epidemiologists must accept errors, except those that are deliberate, or a result of shoddy work and thus preventable.

Research on living beings is difficult because of the complexity of life, and because of natural variations; for example, those arising from circadian (24-hours) rhythms. In addition, measurement techniques in epidemiology are usually limited by technology, cost, or ethical considerations. In human studies, especially those using large community-based populations, these difficulties

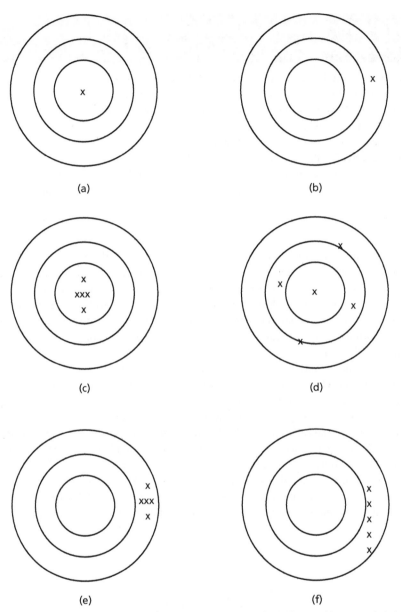

Fig. 4.1 Illustrating error and bias using the archery target and the bull's eye (the central circle).

are compounded by the rules on what measurement is ethical and what humans are willing to consent to. To take an example, the best way to make a diagnosis of Alzheimer's dementia is brain biopsy, and this may be done after death. This 'gold standard' test would not be possible in an epidemiological study to measure the prevalence of dementia in the population. We accept the error for ethical and clinical reasons. Other methods of diagnosing Alzheimer's disease, mainly based on clinical assessment and brain imaging are used, and we forego the brain biopsy test.

Experimental manipulation to test a hypothesis is usually done late, and observation, without deliberate intervention by the investigator, is the dominant mode of investigation in human

Box 4.2 Error in the measurement of waist circumference by two observers

Imagine you are studying the size of the waist in people 65–74 years of age in one city. You employ and train two research staff to do this using a tape measure. As a check on your measurement methods, you ask your researchers to visit one willing volunteer and making measurements with a tape measure using a standardized protocol. You leave it to the discretion of each member of staff to schedule the timing of the exercise. You simply specify the day that you have agreed with the volunteer. One researcher takes the measures in the morning at 11 am, the other in the evening at 8 pm. What are the likely findings in relation to error? Bear in mind that the measurement of the waist, even with a standardized measurement protocol, is difficult.

epidemiology. The usual explanation for the late conduct of trials, ethical constraints, is only partially true. Commonly, experiments are neither warranted nor needed to substantiate the hypothesis. Even more fundamentally, we can only design trials once our knowledge is advanced, and even then, it may prove impossible to implement a trial (Chapter 9 will consider these matters in detail). Moreover, epidemiology is primarily interested in health and disease in human populations living normally in their natural environment, not in laboratory or institutional settings (or even clinical trial settings).

Most discussions of bias in epidemiology are simplified to: (a) selection (of population); (b) information (collection, analysis, and interpretation of data); and (c) confounding, although this latter phenomenon is sometimes considered as separate from bias. The important question of error and bias in research questions and hypotheses is too seldom raised. For example, are the questions of sex or racial differences in intelligence, disease, physiology, or health, biased questions? A long history of misleading and damaging research would have been avoided if questions about racial and sex differences had not been posed in the way they were. The Tuskegee Syphilis Study of the United States Public Health Service (see Jones 1993), for example, followed up 600 African American men for some 40 years, to assess the natural history of disease (see also sections 6.1 and 10.10.3). The underlying question was: does syphilis have different and, particularly, less

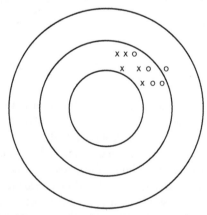

Fig. 4.2 A plot of the morning (x) measures and evening measures (o).

serious outcomes in African Americans than Americans of European origin? (I have modernized the race terminology.) The study was based on a premise that races are biologically different. This premise has repeatedly been shown to be in error. In retrospect the study question was wrong, biased, and unethical. The process of defining, selecting, and funding research questions deserves much more attention in consideration of errors and bias in epidemiology. This is not to advocate no-go areas, but to advocate carefully constructed bias-free questions (section 4.2.1).

Much of epidemiology is concerned with comparison between populations. Even when an epidemiological study is of a single group, its interpretation usually rests on an understanding of, and inference about, how the group compares with the population from which it was selected. The scientific value of the work, in the sense of generating understanding about disease patterns in populations, arises from its generalizability. Furthermore, to make sense of most studies where the data have only been collected from a fraction of the population of interest, sometimes due to non-response by study subjects, the interpretation rests on the assumption that the results apply, by and large, to the whole group as originally chosen. Only in recent decades have medical sciences, including epidemiology, moved away from mainly studying White European-origin, adult men, and assuming that the understanding so generated can be applied to women, other ethnic groups, and other age groups. This assumption of such generalizability has now been shown to be over-optimistic, although it often holds. The choice and composition of study population is, therefore, a crucial matter in avoiding error and bias.

One conception of bias in epidemiology, and which is close to the everyday usage of the term to mean discrimination against individuals and groups because of prejudice, is error which affects population or study subgroups unequally (the way it is usually used in this book).

This leads us to so-called differential errors, that is, errors that differ between groups. This kind of error is usually far more serious than so-called non-differential error, which is error that is similar between groups (section 4.2.7). Figure 4.3 uses the scales of justice to symbolize and illustrate the concept of bias as unequal error in compared populations, which may lead to wrong conclusions.

Error control requires good technique. Bias control needs equal attention to error control in all the population subgroups. As error and bias cannot be fully controlled, the most important need is for systematic, cautious, and critical interpretation of data (Chapter 10, sections 10.10–10.13).

4.2 **A classification of error and bias**

Epidemiologists have been creative in identifying and naming biases, and there are lengthy lists of hundreds of unconnected biases. The *Dictionary of Epidemiology* defines a selection of more than 30 of the many biases in the literature. It is not appropriate for the reader to learn all biases: it is better to develop an understanding of their nature and effects. Errors and biases can be analysed logically by using the concepts in section 4.1 and a framework. It is a good idea for each reader to think through this matter, by trying the exercise in Box 4.3, and using the chronology of a research project. Then, look at Table 4.1 and the following.

The common grouping of selection bias, information bias, and confounding is incomplete, and hence too simple. In Table 4.1, this grouping is shown in the broader context as discussed next. There are many other biases which will be considered later, for example, lead time and length bias (Chapter 6 in relation to screening).

4.2.1 **Bias in the research question, theme, or hypothesis**

Scientists may have strong views, generated both through and independently of their research. Science is as much about generating imaginative ideas, and collecting data to test them, as about

(a)

- Error is normal in science
- Researchers have their human foibles
- In epidemiology bias is unequal error in comparison populations
- Bias creates false patterns and misjudgements—either differences where none exist (a) or failure to detect differences (b)

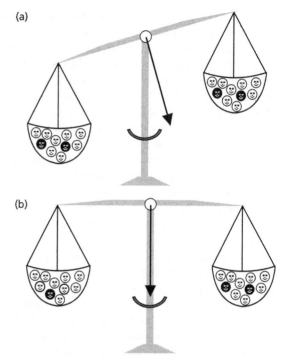

(b)

Fig. 4.3 Bias: a picture illustrating unequal (systematic) errors in compared populations. (a) Error is unequal in one of these identical groups, leading to falsely detecting differences; (b) error is unequal in one of these groups leading to a failure to detect differences. (Each circle is a person—shaded circles represent cases of a disease.)

looking to data to inspire ideas. Scientists become attached to their ideas, which they hope to support (and very reluctantly, if at all, reject) through their research. They share in the social values and beliefs of their era, including those that may, in retrospect, be considered unworthy such as class, racial, religious, and sexual prejudice.

It is worth reflecting on whether a scientific question or even a research theme can be inherently biased. (Surprisingly the *Dictionary of Epidemiology* has no entry on research question or question bias.) In epidemiology, a biased question might favourably or adversely affect one group more than another. The question 'Are men more intelligent (or healthy) than women?' could be considered biased, for there is a presupposition in the way the question is written that there is a case to be answered. Otherwise, the question could have been whether women are more intelligent than men, which might be biased in the opposite direction. The apparently neutral hypothesis here would be that there are no sex and/or gender differences in intelligence. If the underlying values of the researchers are that men are more intelligent than women (a widely held view through history

Box 4.3 Towards a classification of errors and biases

Think through the main steps of a research or related data collection project and consider how error and bias might arise at each step. Develop a set of three to six broad categories for all the errors and biases you list. In doing this task, consider in what ways two groups of the population might be affected unequally.

Table 4.1 A classification of non-random error and bias (including confounding*) based on the chronology of a research or related data collection project

Potential cause of bias	Example	Specific technical terminology	Broad general category of bias
1. Research theme, question or hypothesis is written in a way that prejudices the work	Posing a question or hypothesis in a way which shows one population in a poor light, and creating a sense of superiority and inferiority	None agreed (but question bias seems sensible)	The terms assumption or conceptual bias are close matches. My recommendation is research question bias
2. Falsification of data	Deception by study subject, investigator, or diagnostician, with wrong or even fabricated data	Misconduct	Misconduct or fraud
3. Choice of populations to study is discriminatory	Sampling based on convenience, or preferences of researcher	Population bias (volunteer bias, sex, race, or age bias)	Selection bias
4. Participation in a study is variable	Hospital populations studied where two or more associated problems increase the chance of hospitalization Unequal time and effort spent in the invitation leading to unequal participation, or unequal interest or motivation	Berkson's bias Response bias	Selection bias
5. Mismeasurement of disease, and factors which could cause disease	Diagnostic effort, skill, and facilities unequal Measurement imprecise or unequal In reporting, there is unequal memory of the problem in minds of doctors Effort, skill, and facilities to collect data unequal in comparison groups Interviewer extracts information differently in different groups Unequal effort made to maintain contact by investigator or subject Unequal proportion of subjects drop out Intervention in health care not equal	Measurement error Recall bias Work-up bias Interviewer bias Response bias Treatment bias	Information bias

(continued)

Table 4.1 Continued

Potential cause of bias	Example	Specific technical terminology	Broad general category of bias
6. Participation, itself, influences risk factors and outcomes	Participation in study alters behaviour unequally in different groups	Hawthorne effect Placebo effect	Intervention or participation bias
7. Analysis and interpretation of data	Preferred outcome in mind of investigator	Conceptual bias Interference bias	Interpretation or presentation bias
8. Comparing populations which differ	Study population is older than the comparison population, leading to a false interpretation that there are differences in disease rates other than those caused by age	Confounding	Confounding*
9. Selected findings reported	Reporting interesting findings, usually findings of difference between groups (i.e. positive results) Reporting publishable findings	Various	Publication bias
10. Interpretation, judgement, and action by readers and listeners	Reader and listener interpret data in a way that suits them	No specific name	Interpretation or interpretive bias

*Confounding is a phenomenon now seen as being separate from bias, but it is conceptually convenient to consider it here.

that is now undermined, although it persists) then the bias will remain. Researchers' beliefs, values, and hopes do influence the conduct and reporting of research.

This issue demands more attention in epidemiology. It is problematic to describe difference without conveying a sense of superiority and inferiority. Stigmatization may be an inevitable outcome of epidemiology, for example, in demonstration of the association between HIV and homosexuality, and cigarette smoking and disease. This potential harm has to be balanced against the potential benefits. This is not to say we should not study these matters, but that we should also study the consequences for the people involved. This problem is discussed further in Chapter 10 in the context of race, ethnicity, and health.

4.2.2 Choice of population—selection bias, and the benefits and disbenefits of representativeness

Bias can result from the choice of populations to be studied. This is known as selection bias. (These biases are also known as collider stratification biases, in the language of the directed acyclic graph introduced in Chapter 5.) Investigators are prone to include or exclude individuals and populations for reasons of convenience, cost, or preference rather than for neutral, scientific reasons. Volunteers are popular. The problem is that volunteers tend to be different in their attitudes, behaviours, and health status compared with those who do not volunteer. Men have been selected more often than women, for example, in studies of coronary heart disease. Sometimes investigators want to avoid the ethical and other problems posed by the possibility of pregnancy

- Ignoring populations
- Questions harming one population
- Measuring unequally
- Generalizing from unrepresentative populations

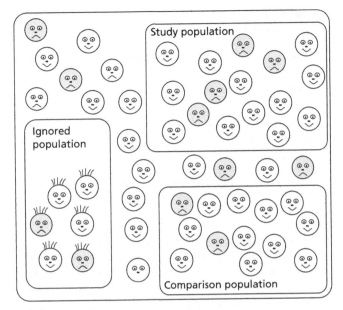

Fig. 4.4 Bias in epidemiology: population concept.

during the study, but sometimes the problem under study is seen as less relevant to women. Ethnic minority groups are much more likely to be excluded from major studies than the ethnic majority. These observations led to laws requiring the main United States research funding agency, National Institutes for Health (NIH), requiring investigators to include women and ethnic minority groups, or provide a reasoned justification.

Selection bias is affected by how a study population is found. For example, the telephone directory and the register of licensed drivers are both popular sources to identify study populations in the United States of America. Those without a telephone or a driver's licence are excluded from these studies. In the United Kingdom, the electoral register and those registered with a general practitioner in the National Health Service (NHS) are popular, but these exclude those not eligible to vote (or unwilling to divulge their details), or those not registered with the NHS, respectively. Figure 4.4 illustrates these points. In addition to the ignored population (e.g. those who do not speak English or are not on the list from which the sample is drawn), others are missed, for example, because they do not receive their invitation or decide not to participate.

Populations in workplaces and institutions (schools, prisons, universities, hospitals) are popular choices for study. Some such populations may be fairly representative of their age group (e.g. schoolchildren), or others not at all (e.g. university students). The attention given to these populations means that research effort is deflected away from other less accessible populations. Extrapolation of results beyond those studied is the norm rather than the exception. Indeed, investigators may even explicitly compare populations derived in different ways. One example is the groundbreaking survey of health and health behaviours by the Health Education Authority (HEA) (1994), which studied ethnic minority groups in the United Kingdom. Typical results are given in Table 4.2. The ethnic minority groups were shown to be different compared with the UK population in several indicators. The emphasis in interpretation fell on those issues where the ethnic minority groups were worse off, thus leading to perceptions that the health of ethnic minorities was impaired, a view propagated in professional journals and newspapers. The comparisons were, however, not easy to interpret because the ethnic minority groups were drawn from areas where at least 10 per cent of the population was

Table 4.2 Selected data, standardized for age and sex, on health and related factors from the HEA's report on black and Asian minority groups (figures are percentages)

Topic	African Caribbean	Indian	Pakistani	Bangladeshi	UK population
Describe health status as poor	17	16	20	29	8
Suffered high blood pressure	16	8	8	10	14
Current smokers	22	10	16	22	28

Source: data from Health Education Authority. *Health and lifestyles: black and minority ethnic groups in England.* London: Health Education Authority, Copyright © 1994 Crown Copyright.

born in six overseas areas of the world (e.g. India, the West Indies). Such places would almost invariably be in the inner city, places where the poorest people live, while the comparison 'UK' population included all areas, not just inner city ones. Irrespective of this bias, the study was at the time of value and interest, but the interpretation was potentially biased. Even although this kind of bias is well known, it is still a common and accepted limitation—sometimes non-comparability is the price paid for achieving feasibility, that is, achieving the study at all. It is better, mostly, to have data that require care in interpretation than none at all. (Prior to the publication of the report I was asked to advise the HEA on this very issue—my advice is summarized in the previous sentence.)

Berkson's bias is an example of how subtle selection bias can be. It specifically refers to a bias in the interpretation of hospital-based case–control studies (see Chapter 9). It arises because hospitalized cases of a disease are not usually a representative sample of cases. In fact, they tend to be the more complex ones, often with other health problems. For example, a man with influenza is more likely to be admitted to hospital if he has chronic bronchitis. In comparing people admitted to hospital, an association between influenza and chronic bronchitis is inevitable because of this selection effect.

Selection bias matters much more in epidemiology than in biologically based medical sciences. Biological factors are usually generalizable between individuals and populations. For example, if an anatomist describes the presence of a particular muscle, or cell type, based on one human being, it is likely to be present in all human beings (and possibly all mammals and even other animals). The anatomist is likely to check that the finding applies to a few other individuals and, if so, will rapidly conclude that it applies universally. By contrast, epidemiological findings usually concern the interaction of social and biological factors. Because societies are made up of highly variable individuals and population groups, the outcome of the biology–environment interaction is variable and context-dependent. The result is crucially dependent on the choice of study population and the interpretation depends on proper understanding of its circumstances. For example, in nearly every population, blood pressure rises with age. It would be easy to conclude that this is a generalizable finding, possibly based on the biology of the ageing process. However, this assumption and generalization needs serious qualification, because in nomadic populations living in traditional ways in the rural areas of countries such as Kenya, there is little or no association between age and blood pressure. Given this caveat, it is reassuring that causal links between exposures and diseases tend to be generalizable, although the strength of the association varies.

Recently, there has been an interesting debate on whether representativeness is necessary in epidemiology, or whether it is better for investigators to seek highly selected populations. The proponents of the latter are discussing this in the context of epidemiology that is trying to understand the cause of a health phenomenon (as it is agreed that representativeness is necessary in descriptive studies on the frequency of disease). The debate is especially important given the increasing difficulty in recruiting representative populations. There is no simple answer to this matter, as it depends on the research question or hypothesis under investigation. It also depends on whether only one study is to be done or whether there is an option to check out the findings from a highly selected sample on other populations (whether representative or highly selected). If the phenomenon under investigation is veering towards biology, then results from highly selected populations may well apply generally (as with the example of a muscle discovered by an anatomist). If the phenomenon under examination is social (e.g. skin colour, assigned race, and mental health), it is most unlikely that the results will generalize. That does not preclude the study of such a phenomenon in a selected population as a test of a concept, and then corroborating the results in other populations. The benefits of this approach is smaller, more focused, and quicker and cheaper research. This approach still requires investigators to find and recruit relevant populations and not just convenient populations. It requires getting high rates of participation from the targeted group as considered below.

4.2.3 **Non-participation: non-response bias**

Some people chosen for and invited to a study do not participate. This causes non-response bias, which is a type of selection bias. In studies of randomly sampled populations the non-response rate is typically 30–40 per cent, and sometimes much higher (even 90%). The response rate in developing counties has been dropping fast, for reasons that are unclear—possibly people are bombarded with requests, given the rise of feedback questionnaires in all walks of life. High response rates—approaching 100 per cent—are still being achieved in the developing world. Before reading on, reflect on why this non-response phenomenon causes bias.

It is likely that non-responders differ from responders. For example, in a written questionnaire study, well-educated people may be more likely to respond than those who have difficulty in reading and writing. Educated people tend to have fewer risk factors and less disease than those who are not educated.

The effect of non-response bias can be partly understood if some information is available on those not participating, such as their age, sex, social circumstances, and why they did not respond. Investigators should seek this information as a high priority. Usually, such information is not available, enticing investigators to assume, wrongly, that the non-responders were not atypical. A similar problem arises in studies of health records when some records are inaccessible to the investigator. The problem is compounded when the non-response rate differs greatly in two populations that are to be compared; for example, men and women (the latter often have higher response rates), groups in different social classes (higher response in well-off people), or ethnic groups (response rates may be very low in minorities for self-completion questionnaires).

Investigators should ensure that the time and effort spent in recruitment meet the need, so that comparison populations have similar response rates. The strategies for recruiting comparison populations may well, indeed, need to differ but, ideally, the type of people participating and the level of non-response should be similar. A degree of non-response bias is, however, an intrinsic limitation of the survey method and hence of epidemiology.

Formal studies of responders and non-responders have shown that the differences are usually important but seldom so great that the study cannot be interpreted. Investigators must consider, at least informally, the effects of this bias on data interpretation. Ideally, the implications of non-response should be considered quantitatively. This is a good time to consider confounding, which may be a consequence of incomplete and differential response rate.

4.2.4 Comparing disease patterns and risk factor–disease outcome relationships in populations which differ (context for confounding)

Confounding is a difficult idea to explain and grasp (and the reader may wish to return to this section again, after reading the remainder of the book). The word confounding is derived from a Latin word meaning to mix together, a useful idea, for confounding mixes us up about causal and non-causal relationships. The word's meaning in everyday language, to confuse or puzzle, is also helpful. This difficulty is reflected in the many definitions and accounts of the concept in the statistical, epidemiological, and causal theory literature. The concept and the ways to handle it are still evolving. One current driving force readers might examine is the increasing use of the techniques, language, and concepts of causal graphs (see Chapter 5). There are nine entries in *A Dictionary of Epidemiology* that readers might examine.

Confounding has, traditionally, been treated as a bias, and *A Dictionary of Epidemiology* calls it confounding bias. It is not, however, either a systematic error or an error that affects groups unequally. It is a causal, not statistical, concept. Confounding is an error of data interpretation, and as such it belongs to this chapter as a prelude to the discussion of causality in the next. Arguably, confounding is the causal epidemiologist's greatest challenge.

As stated in Chapter 1, no variable has any intrinsic epidemiological qualities, so there are no variables that are confounding variables in themselves. There are only variables that in some instances the investigators assign as potential confounding variables. This decision is a major one, and needs a great deal of thought because it has serious consequences. Once assigned the label confounder, that variable ceases to contribute to its other potential roles as exposure, mediator, or outcome in the analysis (of course, the analysis can be separately run in another way).

In epidemiology, confounding refers to the error made in estimating the measure of association between a risk factor and disease, which may arise when there are differences in the comparison populations, other than in the risk factor under study. In this circumstance, confounding might occur, but it is not inevitable. These differences must include one or more variables that are associated both with the disease and the risk factor under study for confounding to be present. These differences may not have been measured or they may have been measured imprecisely, so controlling for confounding may be impossible or incomplete.

Confounding is both a major problem in epidemiology, and difficult to understand, show, and counteract. The potential for it to occur is there whenever the cardinal rule of science, 'compare like-with-like', is broken. The only way to achieve this ideal comparison, conceptually, is simultaneously to compare population X with the risk factor, and the identical population X, but this time without the risk factor. This is impossible and theoretical and hence is called a counterfactual condition. However, if we relax this rule to compare approximately alike with approximately alike, it is achievable (see also Chapter 5, section 5.6.2). In experimental research where study subjects can be randomly allocated to one group or another, a technique that employs the laws of chance to create comparable groups, and where the study is large, the randomized populations will be similar. Even with randomization, however, there is no certainty that the groups are comparable, especially in subgroup analysis (see Chapter 9, randomized trials). If they are, we can think of the two groups as being exchangeable. The degree of confounding can be thought of as the difference between the measure of risk when the study group is compared with a counterfactual population, which can never be known, and that difference seen in real data.

Mostly, we counter the degree of confounding by careful study design and pragmatic statistical techniques, as discussed below and in Chapter 9. The concept of confounding is best explained by examples (Table 4.3) and by illustrations, as in Figures 4.5 and 4.6. Before examining these tables

Table 4.3 Examples of confounding

The confounded association	One possible explanation	The confounded factor	The confounding (possibly causal) factor	To check the assumption (example of type of analysis)
(a) People who drink alcohol apparently have a raised risk of lung cancer	Alcohol drinking and smoking are behaviours which go together, and smoking may be the real reason for the association	Alcohol, which is a marker for, on average, smoking more cigarettes (on our reasoning)	Tobacco, which is associated with both alcohol and with the disease	See if the alcohol–lung cancer relationship holds in people not exposed to tobacco: if yes, tobacco is not the confounder here (stratified analysis, see Chapter 7)
(b) People living in an affluent seaside resort apparently have a higher mortality rate than the country as a whole	A holiday town attracts the elderly, so has a comparatively old population, which will have high mortality	Living in a resort is a marker for being, on average, older	Age, which is associated with both living in a resort and with death	Look at each age group specifically, or use age standardization to take into account age differences (for stratified analysis and standardization, see Chapters 7 and 8)
(c) African Americans are apparently heavier users of crack cocaine than White Americans	Poor people living in the American inner city are particularly likely to become dependent on illicit drugs and many African Americans are in the inner city	Belonging to the racial category African American	Poverty and the pressures of inner-city living, including the easy availability of drugs	Use statistical techniques to adjust for the influence of a number of complex socio-economic factors (for multiple regression, see Chapter 8)

and figures and the next three paragraphs here, reflect on the examples and questions in Box 4.4. We are witnessing the rapid emergence of causal graphs, especially the directed acyclic graph (DAG) as a tool for causal thinking and the potential role of variables. This edition incorporates an introduction to the DAG in Chapter 5 and we will return to this topic again there.

In studying the association between alcohol and lung cancer we can neither observe the same people without the risk factor (the counterfactual approach), nor for ethical and other reasons randomize people into alcohol use/non-alcohol use groups, that is, impose an intervention that will need to last 20–40 years. We use, instead, a comparison group to put the results of the study group into context. A group of people who do not drink and are of the same age and sex provide the pragmatic (not counterfactual, and not randomized) comparison group. The study finds that lung cancer is more common in alcohol drinkers; that is, there is an association between alcohol consumption and lung cancer. The researchers have not, however, compared even approximately like-for-like. For example, it is general knowledge—corroborated by research—that health risk

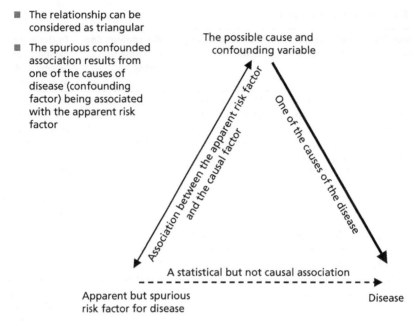

Fig. 4.5 Confounding variable: a pictorial representation.

behaviours go together. So using our causal understanding of the world around us—not data per se and certainly not data in our specific study—we should postulate that alcohol drinkers might smoke more cigarettes than non-drinkers. Cigarette smoking is a powerful causal factor for lung cancer. As part of the study design, the researchers should have identified cigarette smoking as an important confounding factor, and assigned this role to this variable. If they failed to collect accurate data on this variable, the study would be without value from a causal

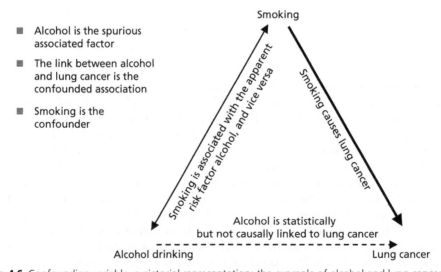

Fig. 4.6 Confounding variable, a pictorial representation: the example of alcohol and lung cancer.

Box 4.4 Some examples and questions to assess confounding

Example 1

Researchers want to know if alcohol drinking might cause lung cancer. They follow-up a group of people who drink alcohol regularly. They find people who do not drink alcohol regularly, who are exactly the same age and sex for comparison. They observe the two groups over some years and count the number of cases of lung cancer in each. They find that alcohol drinkers have more lung cancer than non-drinkers.

Example 2

Researchers are examining mortality rates and discover that mortality risk is greater in an affluent seaside resort than in the country as a whole.

Example 3

A study finds that African Americans are more likely to use crack cocaine than White Americans.

In each of the above examples, ask these questions:

♦ Have the investigators compared like-with-like?

♦ Is a counterfactual comparison group or randomization of the risk factor possible?

♦ In what ways that are associated with both the exposure/risk factor and disease under study might the two comparison populations differ?

♦ What are the potential explanations for the findings, other than the self-evident ones (i.e. alcohol causes lung cancer, living in an English seaside resort is a risk, and African Americans are prone to the crack cocaine habit)?

♦ What is the confounding factor?

♦ What is the confounded, exposure/risk factor?

♦ How can we check out that our understanding is correct?

perspective, even though it may be in itself correct. Examine Table 4.3 part (a) for how to check our confounding assumption.

Investigators find that mortality rates in a seaside resort are higher than in the country as a whole. Why might this be so? Is it something to do with the environmental or social conditions associated with living in the resort, or is there another explanation? In what ways might the population of the resort differ from the country as a whole and in a manner that affects mortality? In posing the question of whether people who live in seaside resorts are approximately like the people who do not, researchers should know, again from general knowledge, that people tend to retire to such resorts, so the average age of their populations tends to be high. Age is associated with both living in such resorts and risk of death. See Table 4.3 part (b) for a way to check the assumption. The observation is of no causal value, even though it is in itself correct, if this confounding assumption cannot be checked.

African Americans were demonstrated to be more likely to use crack cocaine than White Americans (see Lillie-Blanton *et al.* 1993). Is this a racial or ethnic difference in attitudes or behaviour in relation to this drug? In what ways relevant to this observation might the two populations differ from each other? Have these observations been based on comparing African Americans who are approximately alike White Americans (except of course in the race or ethnic group, the exposure variable)? One potential confounding factor is poverty and especially inner-city poverty. This factor is associated with both the exposure (here African American race or ethnicity) and the outcome, crack cocaine use. It would be seriously damaging to the social standing of the African American population if attention was drawn to their race or ethnicity if the causal factor was, instead, poverty or inner-city living. This is a reasonable hypothesis that thoughtful and knowledgeable researchers should have considered in the design and analysis (but did not, until Lillie-Blanton *et al.* 1993 re-examined the data).

In all three examples, the problem confounding causes is in the correct interpretation of the potential causal relationships between the variables. In all three examples investigators need to think through the issues in advance, because if they do not they may not collect the necessary data, or not at the necessary level of detail and quality.

Figure 4.5 offers a pictorial representation of confounding. The relationship between disease, the associated risk factor under study, and the confounding factor is shown as a triangular one. The confounding factor, shown at the apex of the triangle in Figure 4.5, is associated both with the factor being examined and the disease. The right-hand line is shown in bold to signify the solidity of this link. Note that the arrow on the left-hand line points in both directions, showing a relationship in both directions. The arrow in the right-hand line points in one direction because we believe that the confounding factor is somewhere on the pathway that causes the disease, but not vice versa. The arrow at the bottom is a broken line to symbolize (in our view) the non-causal, confounded nature of the relationship. Figure 4.6 illustrates this with the example of alcohol, smoking, and lung cancer. (As these diagrams show two-way associations, they are not DAGs—see Chapter 5.) There is an association between the confounding (smoking) and confounded (alcohol) factor. Do the exercise in Box 4.5 before reading on.

In the association between living in the seaside resort and mortality, age (confounding factor) would be at the apex and living in the resort at the left-hand angle. In the association between African American race and crack cocaine use, socio-economic status would be at the apex and race at the left-hand angle. These interpretations are alternative and simplified explanations of a complex reality and, in turn, need to be subjected to test. This is considered in Chapter 5 in more detail.

The first key analysis in all epidemiological studies is to compare the characteristics of the populations under study, paying particular attention to factors that are thought to be on the disease's causal pathway. Simply because the groups are similar on the characteristics actually measured does not imply they are similar on all relevant characteristics. For example, two groups may be comparable on age, sex, smoking, and exercise habits but differ in the type of housing they live in, a variable on which data are often not collected. If the study is of accidents, infections, or respiratory disease, for example, differences in type of housing may matter greatly.

Box 4.5 Pictorial presentation of associations in Table 4.3

Draw and analyse the associations (Table 4.3) between living in a seaside resort and high mortality, and between being African American and using crack cocaine, using the approach shown in Figures 4.3 and 4.4. What is the nature of the relationship between confounding and confounded factors here?

This same principle applies to all subgroup analysis. A comparison of two populations may show that they are virtually identical in age structure. The investigator may wish to examine the disease experience of men and women separately. The age structure of each sex must again be shown to be similar and this must not be assumed.

Serious problems with confounding are likely if it is not considered at the stage of thinking out the causal relationships, designing the study, analysing the data, and interpreting the findings. A combination of methods is usually applied to handle confounding. It is best to consider it at each stage and take one or more of the appropriate actions as shown in Table 4.4. Whatever is done the possibility of confounding cannot be dismissed and, along with chance, it usually remains an alternative interpretation of epidemiological findings.

We will look at confounding factors in the context of causality and DAGs (Chapter 5) and age standardization in Chapter 8.

4.2.5 Measurement errors and natural variations

Differential mismeasurement

Measurement errors and biases fall into the huge general category of information bias. Before reading on you may wish to reflect on the questions in Box 4.6 on measurement errors in epidemiological research.

Unlike measuring the length of a red cell, an atom, or even the orbit of the moon, which are also error-prone goals, measuring or assessing disease in living humans requires a judgement. It is a subjective judgement, aided by imprecise measures of biological indicators and information provided by the patient or study subject. Medically qualified readers know this already, but others may not—often even all this information does not provide any diagnosis at all. Commonly the information is compatible with several diseases. One of the commonest examples of this is working out whether pain in the lower chest and upper abdomen (like indigestion) is heart disease or intestinal disease. After death the accuracy of the diagnosis can be improved or verified by autopsy but the patient is no longer available for questioning, and some tests, particularly dynamic ones (e.g. an exercise electrocardiogram for heart disease) are no longer possible. A combination of clinical and autopsy data is sometimes essential to reach a diagnosis but even this may be inconclusive.

Similar problems apply to most measurements of exposures and confounding factors. For example, measuring socio-economic circumstances, ethnic group, cigarette smoking habits, or alcohol consumption are complex matters. Even measures such as height, weight, and blood pressure are difficult, particularly in large studies where numerous people may be making measurements in different places, possibly even with different equipment. Accuracy in biochemical and other laboratory tests is also problematic. Issues such as the quality of the specimen, and changing laboratory reagents and techniques come into play. In studies in many places, specimens may be transported to one central laboratory and delays, among other factors, may make the results erroneous and biased.

Measurement error is compounded by biological variation, which is not error but may be confused with it. For example, blood pressure varies from moment to moment in response to stress, posture, and activity, in a 24-hour (circadian) cycle with lowered pressure in the night, and with the air temperature. To examine the relationship between blood pressure and disease, we need a meaningful and true summary estimate. There is, however, no readily available estimate. The usual compromise is taking the blood pressure in standard conditions, measuring it on several occasions, and taking an average of the readings. The resulting value is useful in clinical practice and epidemiology for predicting disease outcomes, but it is not an accurate summary of the

Table 4.4 Possible actions to control confounding

Possible action	Example	Benefit	Cost/disadvantage
Literature review or creative thinking: define causal structure of relationships, as a causal graph if possible	See Chapter 5	Potential confounders (and non-confounders) identified	Need to know the state-of-art knowledge, but this may be insufficient too so there may be unknown confounders
Study design: randomize individual subjects or units of populations, e.g. schools	To determine the effectiveness of sex education in schools in reducing the incidence of teenage pregnancy, half of the schools in a city could be in the intervention group, the other half in a control group. The allocation of the group would be determined by chance (see Chapter 9, section 9.7)	Selection biases bypassed Avoids schools selecting themselves into the intervention group, for they would be different from those that chose the control group	Limited to research questions where randomization is possible, and acceptable to subjects and professionals Comparability may not be achieved, especially in small samples Effective only in large studies
Study design: select comparable groups/restrict entry into study	Study only subjects who are 35 years of age Study non-smokers only, e.g. in studying the health effects of air pollution	Vagaries of chance and selection bias bypassed	Creates extra work in finding the chosen population Findings may not apply to populations not studied Erroneous conclusions may be reached, e.g. air pollution has no effect on health when it might affect smokers but not non-smokers Practical applications of findings in health policy, etc. are reduced
Study design: match individuals or whole populations	Select subjects and controls on pre-determined criteria, e.g. age, sex, race, smoking Select populations on basis of population statistics, e.g. unemployment levels, type of housing	Investigators' judgements and knowledge of confounding factors is used	The result is not a population sample, so there are problems of representativeness Practical applications of data may be less Needs statistical analysis designed for matched populations Overmatching can lead to false conclusions
Analysis: analyse subgroups separately	Compare disease experience of each age group, sex, race, etc. separately (stratified analysis)	Direct control and observation of possible confounding factors	Makes assimilation of results difficult In most studies, there are insufficient subjects to make detailed stratification possible

Table 4.4 Continued

Possible action	Example	Benefit	Cost/disadvantage
Analysis: adjust data statistically	Use techniques to amalgamate results of stratified analysis, e.g. direct or indirect standardization (Chapter 8), Mantel Haensel technique and multiple regression modelling (see also Chapter 9 but consult an introductory statistics or intermediate epidemiology textbook)	Summary measures possible Computers and statistical software make this relatively quick to do	Hard for non-statisticians to understand and do well Actual data are hidden behind summary figures, which are distorted by the process (see Chapter 8) Outputs are not easily used for health-care policy and planning May lead to false sense of complacency that confounders are controlled

constantly varying blood pressure. For that we need long-term recordings of blood pressure at least over several days (ambulatory blood pressure)—a method available in clinical practice but seldom in epidemiology.

Biological variations are not errors but they can cause bias in epidemiology. Imagine two populations with identical blood pressures. If blood pressure measurements on one population were made in the morning and on the other in the evening, the average blood pressure in the two populations would appear different when it is not. The reason is that blood pressure varies across the 24-hour period.

For some variables, the variation in time is so great that making long-term estimates is extremely difficult, for example, in diet, alcohol consumption, and the level of stress.

Measurements of the exposures and confounding factors are often obtained from the subject alone, whereas information on the disease is obtained from the patient's account, the physician's examination, and laboratory tests. Measurement errors in the former, therefore, are more likely to occur than in the latter. Wherever possible, researchers should seek to corroborate their measure by checking more than one source of data.

Measurement errors which occur unequally in the comparison populations are, in line with earlier discussion, considered as epidemiological biases. They can irreversibly destroy a study. For example, in a study where one population is interviewed face-to-face and the comparison population completes a self-completion questionnaire, the results are unlikely to be comparable. The reader may think this example is too obvious to be worth mentioning but this scenario is not unusual, especially in multiethnic, multilingual studies where one or more groups have poor literacy

Box 4.6 Measurement errors in epidemiology

Why are measurement errors in epidemiology likely to be both more common, more difficult to deal with and more important than in other scientific disciplines, say, physics, anatomy, biochemistry, or animal physiology? Consider the effect of measurement error in a study of two populations that are to be compared. There are two possibilities: that errors are equal in both groups or the measurement errors are unequal. What are the consequences of these two possibilities?

and need interviewing. Interviewing is about 10 times more expensive than self-completion questionnaires so, for financial and other practical reasons, this potential bias is sometimes accepted as a necessary compromise. Imagine that the sphygmomanometer in one town is faulty and is underestimating the blood pressure by 10 mmHg. In this town, many people who are hypertensive will be misclassified as not hypertensive, and very few the other way round.

The above two examples illustrate a systematic error, known as a differential misclassification bias. (The degree to which a measure leads to a correct classification can be quantified using the concepts of sensitivity and specificity, and these are discussed in Chapter 6 in relation to screening tests.)

These kinds of differential misclassification errors or biases may be hard to find, but the damage they do is self-evident. If differential errors occur the study may need to be abandoned, unless the extent of the error can be quantified and data corrected. For example, if we find the sphygmomanometer in one town always measured blood pressure 10 mmHg too low, then we could add 10 mmHg to the recorded values. A correction can often be made for measures of physical attributes and for laboratory tests. It is more difficult to correct for differential error in social information collected by questionnaire or interview, and for diagnostic information collected from medical records. Measurement errors which are equal in all comparison populations, known as non-differential errors or biases, are also important, as discussed in the next section on 'Non-differential measurement errors: misclassification'.

Non-differential measurement errors: misclassification

As some error in measurement is inevitable, this problem is universal and for this reason it is often overlooked, but this is why it is so important. Misclassification error occurs when a person is put into the wrong category (or population subgroup), usually because of faulty measurement. For example, in a survey of hypertension in two towns some people who are hypertensive will be misclassified as normal, while others who are normal will be misclassified as hypertensive. Some of this will be due to measurement error. The misclassification may be random, with as many misclassified in one direction as the other. The total number of people with hypertension may be about right. This error is known as a non-differential misclassification bias, in that it affects all subgroups equally (non-differentially). There is a commonly held view that, in epidemiology at least, these errors cancel each other out so they do not matter. This is only true if the purpose of the research is to measure the frequency of disease, but not for studies of associations.

The consequences of non-differential misclassification can be severe in both clinical practice and in epidemiology. Clinically, misclassified persons will be treated wrongly. Information from epidemiological surveys is often sent with the permission of the study subject to the personal physician. Epidemiological mismeasurements can, therefore, trigger unnecessary clinical investigations and treatments (false positive), or, alternatively, convey that there is no problem (false negative misclassification).

The effect of non-differential misclassification error, however, is subtler than for differential error, and therefore more likely to be overlooked, particularly if there is little or no effect on the final prevalence or incidence figure. In measuring the strength of associations between exposures and disease outcomes, however, non-differential misclassification error has an important, and not always predictable, effect. If the misclassification only applies to the exposure or disease outcome then the strength of the association is always reduced, so the main problem is failing to find associations that, in reality, exist. Misclassification, however, affects confounding variables, and the combined effect of the mixture of misclassifications is not so predictable. This is illustrated with a simplified fictitious example. Try the exercise in Box 4.7 before reading on. The imaginary, perfect study is in Table 4.5.

Box 4.7 Misclassification of smoking in a study of cardiovascular disease

Imagine a perfect, error-free study of 20 000 women, 10 000 are cigarette smokers, and the rest are not. Our interest is in the occurrence of new cases of cardiovascular disease (CVD) over 10 years (cumulative incidence of disease). Say that over 10 years, 20 per cent of cigarette smokers develop a CVD compared with 10 per cent of those not smoking. The rate of disease in the smoking group is doubled (relative risk is 20%/10% = 2). Table 4.5 shows the true results, given no mismeasurement hence no misclassification (which is not possible in practice).

Let us assume that misclassification in exposure occurred 20 per cent of the time, so that 20 per cent of women actually smoking cigarettes were classified as not smoking, and that 20 per cent who were not cigarette smokers were classified as smoking cigarettes. Assume that there is no misclassification of disease outcome, and the disease incidence remains the same. Before reading on, you should modify the figures in Table 4.5 and recalculate the relative risk of disease (you may use percentages) given this misclassification. (There is a second exercise in appendix 4.1 where the steps are given in more detail. That exercise also includes outcome misclassification.)

Tables 4.6 and (with reorganization) 4.7 give the results. Table 4.6 shows the effects of misclassification. The investigator does not, however, usually know how much misclassification there is. For the investigator the data look like Table 4.8. The reason for this is shown by the reorganization of the data in Table 4.6 into 4.7, and then into Table 4.8.

The risk of cardiovascular disease (CVD) in the as-observed apparently 'smoking group' with 20 per cent misclassification is 1800/10 000. In the as-observed apparently 'not cigarette smokers group' it is 1200/10 000. Recalculating the relative risk using the data in Table 4.7:

$$\frac{\text{Incidence rate in those apparently on the pill } 1800/10\ 000}{\text{Incidence rate in those apparently not on the pill } 1200/10\ 000} = \frac{0.18}{0.12} = 1.5.$$

Therefore, the relative risk is 1.5 (with misclassification), rather than 2 (without misclassification) as shown in Table 4.8. That is a big difference.

This example illustrates the principle that when the misclassification is of the exposure then the measure of the association (here the relative risk) is reduced. Misclassification will, inevitably, also arise in measurement of the disease outcome.

Table 4.5 Imaginary, perfect, and therefore impossible study of cardiovascular outcome and cigarette smoking: no misclassification

True classification of cigarette smoking status	Cardiovascular disease		Total
	Yes	No	
Yes	2000 (20%)	8000	10 000
No	1000 (10%)	9000	10 000
Total	3000	17 000	20 000

Table 4.6 Smoking and cardiovascular disease: 20 per cent misclassification of cigarette smoking—the figures are those that would result given this degree of misclassification

Observed classification of smoking with 20% error	Cardiovascular disease		Total
	Yes	No	
Yes smoker, classified right (incidence 20%)—smoker	1600	6400	8000
Yes smoker, classified wrong (incidence 20%)—'non-smoker'	400	1600	2000
Subtotal	**2000**	**8000**	**10 000**
No, classified right (incidence 10%)—non-smoker	800	7200	8000
No, classified wrong (incidence 10%)—'smoker'	200	1800	2000
Subtotal	**1000**	**9000**	**10 000**
Total of subtotals	**3000**	**17 000**	**20 000**

In reality, there will be misclassification simultaneously in both measurement of exposure and in disease outcome, and this will distort the results even more. Generally, non-differential misclassification error weakens the association and so lowers the relative risk. This principle may break down when misclassification occurs in confounding variables, with unpredictable results. The association may be strengthened or reduced. The demonstration of this is beyond this book, but there is a reference to a paper by Greenland (1980) giving access to the literature.

Table 4.7 Smoking and cardiovascular disease: 20 per cent misclassification of cigarette smoking. The rows shown in bold show the data as the investigator sees it

Observed classification of cigarette smoking status	Cardiovascular disease		Total
	Yes	No	
Yes, classified right (smoking cigarettes) so incidence rate is 20%	1600	6400	8000
Yes, classified wrong (actually not cigarette smokers) so incidence rate is 10%	200	1800	2000
Subtotal—results as seen by investigator	**1800**	**8200**	**10 000**
No, classified right (not cigarette smokers) so incidence rate is 10%	800	7200	8000
No, classified wrong (actually smoking cigarettes) so incidence rate is 20%	400	1600	2000
Subtotal—results as seen by investigator	**1200**	**8800**	**10 000**
Total	**3000**	**17 000**	**20 000**

Table 4.8 Smoking and cardiovascular disease: 20 per cent misclassification of cigarette smoking—as the investigator sees it in summary (the lines in bold in Table 4.7)

Apparent classification of cigarette smoking	Cardiovascular disease		Total
	Yes	No	
Yes	1800 (18%)	8200	10 000
No	1200 (12%)	8800	10 000
Total	3000	17 000	20 000

Other than awareness, what can investigators do about non-differential measurement error misclassification bias? The answer is to do studies to measure its extent and then adjust the data accordingly. To do this requires validity studies that assess to what extent measures are accurate (i.e. valid). The concepts here are discussed again in Chapter 6 within the context of screening and screening tests, and in particular sensitivity and specificity of tests.

4.2.6 Regression to the mean

A closely related problem, and one that combines selection and measurement biases is regression to the mean, a phrase coined by Francis Galton (1822–1911), where regression means 'to revert to' to or 'return to'. (This is not regression analysis.) This bias has come to light from the observation that measurements that initially lie at the extremes tend to move nearer the average on subsequent measurements. Wherever appropriate or possible, the population across the range of measures should be studied rather than taking a sample from one end of the spectrum. Of course, this may not be appropriate where the focus of interest is in those at the extremes rather than those at the average.

The phenomenon of regression to the mean can also be observed across generations, the classic example being that the offspring of very tall (or very clever, obese, short, energetic, sporting, beautiful, etc.) people tend to be less so than their parents, rather than equally or even more so. Offspring of parents who are short on these qualities tend to have more of them than their parents. Such a general phenomenon must have a general cause. Before reading on, reflect on some possible explanations and try the exercise in the next paragraph. The clue is that regression to the mean relates to the issue of chance and measurement.

Imagine that we have used waistline measurement to find overweight people for a study to prevent obesity. Let us say that we set a value of 90 cm (36 inches) as the cut-off of interest. We measure the waist using a tape measure. We follow instructions on how best to do this surprisingly complex task. In 1000 people, we find 200 who exceed this cut-off. We call these 200 back for a repeat measure in four hours. Why might there be fewer than 200 people exceeding the cut-off? Leave aside the possibility that they lost weight in the interim, that they had been fasting prior to measurement or even that the measurements have been made with a different protocol (all good explanations, but even if they did not occur, regression to the mean would still be there).

In essence, the cause is random error or random variation. The answer is that some of the 200 people had been mismeasured because of random error. Those who had been mismeasured with too low a waist (i.e. truly over 90 cm but mismeasured as less so) are not in our group of 200 who have returned, but those mismeasured too high are back, that is, they were not truly over 90 cm originally. When they return for the second measurement, some of these 200 will be measured too low because of mismeasurement error. Some of those previously measured too high will now be measured correctly, that is, less than 90 cm. Our group of 200 people may dwindle to 180 people or even less.

If, rather than calling back the 200 subsample, we had re-measured all 1000 people, some of the 800 who had a waist of less than 90 cm (36 inches) would now have one above the cut-off for the same reasons. Then, the total number of people with a waist of more than 90 cm may well still have been about 200, but they would not have been exactly the same group as the original 200 people.

In the second example of offspring having less extreme characteristics than their parents, the explanation is that those characteristics arise partly from chance events that are unlikely to be repeated. The reasons why a person is extremely clever are complex—numerous genes, nutritional factors, and environmental and social stimuli among many other factors will be important. Some of these will be chance effects. Their repetition across the generations is unlikely. Sometimes the phenomenon will have occurred as a result of an unlikely combination of such events. So, when the circumstances giving rise to the phenomenon are repeated, a more likely combination of events is likely to result. As explained in section 3.3.1, the DNA of the parents is combined and reshuffled in a process called meiosis. If both parents had gene variants with high potential for extreme intelligence it is possible, indeed, likely that the offspring will not inherit such a favourable collection of gene variants (just because your parents won the lottery does not mean you will). The same reasoning can be applied to environmental factors leading to extreme intelligence.

Regression to the mean is of particular importance in epidemiology when subsamples of the population are followed over time, either to examine the effects of interventions (when the apparent effect may be misleading), or when the association between risk factors and outcomes is to be studied (the effects are underestimated, just as for non-differential mismeasurement). The solution here, in addition to awareness, is to assess the extent of the bias through repeat measurements, usually in a subsample of the study population, and then to adjust the results for the whole of the study population.

In these examples, the strength of the association is generally reduced or diluted—hence this phenomenon is also known as regression dilution bias. You have collected the data as well as possible and now turn to analysis. What errors/biases still await us?

4.2.7 **Analysis and interpretation of data**

In virtually every project, the potential for data analysis is far greater than that actually performed. The choice of which data to analyse, the way to analyse them, and how to present the findings are usually left to the investigators. Clearly, the choices will be informed by their prior interests (and biases, meaning preferences and even prejudices) and expertise of the researchers. These choices will usually be good ones. Sometimes their choices will be poor, misleading, negligent, malicious, and even fraudulent.

There is no easy solution to the potential problem of biased or shoddy analysis. External scrutiny by objective advisers of the research protocol, including the plan for data analysis and interpretation, is one important safeguard. This is done increasingly, especially for clinical trials. Since the second edition of this book was published, there has been a simmering but unresolved controversy on whether the analysis of all studies should follow the approach of randomized trials with predefined analysis. This seems like a good idea but critics of the proposal warn that this could curtail creativity and discovery through more spontaneous analysis based on following interesting paths that result from ongoing analysis. I will return to this in Chapter 9, but for the moment let us note that, as a minimum, all analyses should be recorded and reported. This is the only way for readers to see whether the researchers might have biased the interpretation by selecting their favoured results (called cherry picking), while hiding or ignoring other results. It is also the best way of evaluating the effect of making multiple comparisons. Another step, and one more difficult to achieve, would be the inclusion of objective, uninvolved people in the research team at the data analysis and interpretation stage. Before reading on, you may wish to reflect on what else investigators might do to help avoid potential problems like these.

As a minimum, investigators should ensure that their analysis is driven by prior stated, preferably written and published in a public place, hypotheses, research questions, and analysis strategies. One controversial proposal, being implemented slowly, is that investigators should make public both their data and data collection proforma; for example, questionnaires, data, analysis strategy, and other information required to replicate the analysis. Then anyone could check the work or analyse the data differently. Some scientific journals require that authors of manuscripts reporting original research make the data available on request. In practice, this requirement is rarely imposed, and is unlikely to be except in the case of suspected fraud. Researchers' resistance to these requests and increasing demands, imposed by funders and journals, is easy to understand. In addition to issues of data ownership and intellectual property, there are also concerns about data privacy, given it is often impossible to ensure complex data sets are truly anonymous. There is, however, another danger and that is of external researchers who are not familiar with the limitations and content of data making errors and misinterpretations in their secondary analyses. Even worse, there is a possibility that an analysis might be constructed to serve vested and biased interests; for example, reanalysis by the tobacco companies might be designed to counter already published work.

Given these safeguards, statistical analysis of data can proceed. There are numerous pitfalls in the process, so readers will need to turn to specialist courses and books. A brief overview is, however, given in Chapter 9. After analysis comes write-up and publication.

4.2.8 **Publication**

In discussing publication, I focus on the peer-reviewed journals providing a semi-permanent globally available record and not theses, internal reports, or even internet articles. There is an adage that sums up the world of modern academic research—publish or perish. The pressure to publish, to do it fast (before the competitors), and to go for the prestigious, high 'impact' factor, and competitive peer-reviewed journals has intensified. The same culture is spilling over into the work of service-based epidemiologists. The reasons are not important here, but knowledge of this culture is essential for the interpretation of the published record of science.

The first consequence is that the research team will be motivated to write the work in a format and language (almost invariably now English is the first choice) suitable for such journals and they will target international journals. The work may never reach, or be readable by, the population studied, the professionals who helped in the study or those who might implement it, the policymakers and media.

The second consequence is the publication is likely to be short, although some exceptions are emerging with internet-based journals, as I consider later. The pressure to make choices on what to report is intensified at the publication stage, particularly in scientific journals. The article will usually be written in 1500–6000 words (the most prestigious journals are usually at the shorter end of the spectrum). Research submitted as a short report may be 800–1400 words, and if as a research letter to the editor, even shorter. Choices on the data to be presented will be combined with choices on emphasis and interpretation. In most circumstances, only a part of the analyses can be published.

Convention dictates that the authors indicate their preferred interpretation, and that data are never published without discussion (the latter being the ultimate but impractical solution to the problem of bias in interpretation). Editorial guidelines usually indicate that novelty, originality, interest, and readability will be key criteria for publication. Researchers write accordingly, by highlighting the points of interest to themselves, and equally to editors and readers. Exaggeration of the novelty or interest of the work is probably the norm rather than the exception, because without it the chance of publication, especially in prestigious journals, is diminished.

In epidemiology the usual point of interest in publication, determined by the dominant paradigm, is the difference in the pattern of disease between compared populations, the potential to understand disease causation, and the effects of interventions. Other perspectives and interpretations are usually secondary. Similarities between populations are too seldom commented on, even though they may be even more important.

Manuscripts showing interesting findings (positive results in intervention trials, differences in disease patterns or risk factors in most other epidemiology) are most likely to be published in widely read journals. Other findings are often unpublished, or published in specialist journals or as reports to the funding agency, which may be confidential or difficult to get. There is, nonetheless, a good case for research to be written as a full report with fewer constraints on the word limits from which papers are later published, especially if both report and papers were available to the reader on the internet.

The result of these problems with publication is a biased understanding of the differences and similarities in the disease patterns of populations and an exaggerated view of the importance of associations between risk factors and disease outcomes. For intervention studies, where no, or no important impact has been found, the results may never be published, especially if publication would undermine a commercial interest, for example, the effectiveness of drugs and medical technologies. This has huge importance for systematic reviews and meta-analyses (see Chapters 5 and 10).

This is known as publication bias and it has been recognized as a matter of immense importance. Many solutions have been generated, including open access journals that accept all papers that are methodologically sound, irrespective of novelty, originality, or perceptions of interest. Trial and protocol registration in advance, and detailed reports to funders that are published sometimes in in-house journals, are other solutions.

Methods have been developed to assess whether publication bias is likely in a systematic review. Search techniques have been refined to unearth unpublished work—and some journals welcome long forgotten unpublished work, especially on trials.

The impact of these and many other actions remains unclear at this point, especially as the incentives and pressures on academic researchers remain as described in the opening paragraph of this section. The culture seems to incentivize and embed publication bias, and at the extreme, scientific fraud, perhaps the worst form of error and bias in science (see also sections 10.10.2 and 10.12). It is from this imperfect and biased record that law, policy and strategy are developed, as discussed below.

4.2.9 Judgement and action

The summary results and interpretation of important epidemiology will, at some point, probably be examined by decision-makers, whether the public, politicians, industrialists, policy-makers, or other researchers. It is likely that controversial interpretations, especially those proposing changes that threaten others interests, will be contested. Interpretation of data is a matter of judgement, which depends not only on scientific methods but also on the prior values, beliefs, and interests of the observer.

Epidemiologists expend much effort to teach epidemiology widely to students and practitioners of the health sciences and statistics, especially in the public health fields, so that

---

Box 4.8 Exercise

Using the list of potential causes of bias in column 1 of Table 4.1, analyse the information in Exemplar 4.1.

---

their work can be more widely interpreted (and, hopefully, used). The interpretation is often contested. A pattern seen by one observer as clear evidence of the detrimental effect of smoking on respiratory health may be seen by another observer as due to error, bias, confounding, or another cause such as air pollution. Epidemiological factors are under close scrutiny at present—for example, include those relating to sugar, salt, carbohydrates, fats, and alcohol—and this small list relates only to dietary constituents.

According to Thomas Kuhn (1996), a key characteristic of science is that the scientist and the peer group are the sole arbiters of the meaning and validity of the theory and data (see also section 10.5). Epidemiology differs from other physical and biomedical sciences in that the data are usually of direct interest to a wide range of people and, moreover, are much more amenable to interpretation by non-epidemiologists. Epidemiologists are not the sole arbiters of the theory and data. Epidemiologists have, therefore, the dual responsibilities of minimizing the impact of their own biases and preventing the misinterpretation of data and misleading recommendations by others, and especially those with vested interests. Sound data interpretation rests on sharp critical appraisal skills (see Chapter 10).

4.3 **A practical application of the research chronology schema of bias and error**

The above 'research cycle'-based discussion of error and bias in epidemiology is now illustrated by a study of the possible impact of industrial air pollution in Teesside on the health of populations living close by. Exemplar 4.1 gives the title and abstract of the study together with some background and comments.

Do the exercise in Box 4.8 and examine exemplar 4.1 before reading on. Unusually, this study was followed by a formal examination of the impact of the research on the populations studied; again, interested readers may wish to read how the study report was perceived (Moffatt *et al.* 2000). Table 4.9 provides my answers to the exercise for comparison with yours.

Table 4.9 The research cycle framework for bias in epidemiology and the Teesside study of health and the environment

Bias	Examples of source of bias
Research question	The question focused on industrial air pollution, the interest of the investigating team and the people of Teesside, especially in area A but not of the local industry and local authority, which would have preferred a focus on road traffic pollution, or a focus on all forms of pollution. From their perspective, this particular focus could have been seen as a bias.
Choice of populations	The study questions focused on one population living closest to industry (the population of interest living in Zone A). Another population was included because of the interests of the local authority, but investigators chose certain parts of the area in which this second population lived, to maximize comparability with the population living closest to industry (Zone B). Other populations were chosen on their comparability to the population of interest (living in Zones C and S). These choices were necessarily both selective and exclusionary.

(continued)

Table 4.9 Continued

Bias	Examples of source of bias
Participation in a study	Unequal interest in the issue of industrial air pollution was reflected in unequal response rates with higher response in the three Teesside areas than in the comparison area in Sunderland (Zone S).
Comparing populations which differ	While the populations were very similar on a wide range of relevant indicators, it would be impossible to show they were comparable on all potentially important exposures, say living near an asbestos plant 30 years before the study. There is no solution to this limitation. We have to do our best—just as the palaeontologist needs to use fossil evidence and cannot decry her inability to travel into the past. The study used both sampling and analytic methods to alleviate this problem.
Assessment of disease	The comparison rests on the assumptions that the (i) diagnostic effort, skill, and facilities were equal in the areas studied (a reasonable assumption in this case), and (ii) that subjects close to industry do not report health problems with more diligence (an assumption which cannot be accepted without testing).
	In view of funding and time constraints, general practice records were not studied in the Sunderland area.
Assessment of factors which could cause disease	The assumptions and limitations were similar to those for assessment of disease.
	Misinformation is a potential problem for, arguably, the populations living close to the industry have a vested interest in showing an association between pollution and ill health while the local industries had the opposite interest.
Follow-up	Not applicable.
Outcome	Not an issue affecting the interpretation of the study.
Analysis and interpretation of data	Many potential alternative analyses of the huge data set were avoided despite extreme pressures to veer away from the central hypotheses. A focus on the study questions was maintained by referring to the study proposal. While the investigators were trying to keep an open mind, for some people the expectation and preferred outcome was an association between industrial air pollution and health, while for others it was the opposite. The analysis was searching, with detailed subgroup analysis going beyond the stated hypotheses, to seek such associations.
Interpretation by readers and listeners	The complex findings were interpreted by industry as showing no causal association. Health and local authorities preferred to focus on the issue of poverty rather than on air pollution. Most of the researchers interpreted the data as showing that air pollution from industry was important to respiratory health and that more research was warranted.

Box 4.9 Exercise on assessing the impact of repeating the study, removing errors and biases, and removing confounding factors

What happens to an association when the following actions are taken?

◆ Where the association was thought to be a chance result, repeating the study on a larger population

◆ Removal of errors and biases

◆ Repeating the study in a population where the confounding factor is absent

Table 4.10 Effects of some actions to test role of chance, error, bias, and confounding in assessing associations

Action	Effect on association
Repeat the study	Association usually disappears if it was chance
Remove error and bias	Association usually disappears if it arose from error or bias but will become clearer and stronger if not
Repeat study in a place where confounding factor is absent	Association usually disappears

4.4 **Conclusion**

Error is inevitable in all sciences, but is particularly important and likely in those studying humans. Scientists need to be especially careful about errors that may be applied in health settings, and hence damage health or waste resources. Bias is a subtle error and both more likely to be overlooked or, even when sought, remain undetected. In this chapter, I have utilized the central epidemiological strategy—research studies of the comparison of populations—to discuss bias. Bias, in an epidemiological context, is especially important when errors affect comparison groups unequally. Since this is often, perhaps always, the case, bias is a central issue in epidemiology.

Confounding is a special and difficult matter. It remains one of the critical issues for all aspects of epidemiology. Currently, confounding is not viewed as a bias. Confounding has traditionally been considered and discussed in the context of bias.

As Chapter 9 on study design discusses, most epidemiological studies have similar problems in controlling error, bias, and confounding, and mostly these are inherent in the survey and disease registration methods that underlie epidemiology. Before reading on, do the exercise in Box 4.9, and then look at the answers in Table 4.10.

Exemplar 4.1: **Abstract of an environment and health study for analysis based on the research cycle approach to bias**

This study is a classic example of how epidemiologists get involved in complex public health problems. In addition to helping with the problem, most epidemiologists would hope to use the opportunity to advance methods and produce generalizable knowledge that will be useful elsewhere. This work was on an issue that causes controversy around the world—does living near heavy industry damage local residents' health?

Title

Does living close to a constellation of industries impair health? A study of health, illness, and the environment in north-east England.

Study objective

To assess whether public and professional concerns that industrial air pollution from petrochemical and steel industries in Teesside, north-east England, contributed to poor health, particularly high mortality rates.

Design

Populations which were similar on a broad range of census indicators of social and economic circumstances, but which varied in the distance of the home from major industries were compared on a broad range of health indicators including mortality, morbidity, self-reported health, health-related lifestyles, occupational histories, social circumstances, and attitudes to industry. The underlying hypothesis was that respiratory health, in particular, would show gradients with the worst health in those populations living closest to industry.

Setting

Twenty-seven housing estates, nineteen in Teesside and eight in Sunderland, two conurbations in the north-east of England, were the focus of the study. The estates were aggregated, on the basis of distance and direction from industry, into zones (designated as A, B, and C in Teesside where A is closest to industry, and S in Sunderland).

Main measures

Census data (1981 and 1991), and mortality (1981–1991), cancer registration (1983–1994), birthweight and stillbirth (1981–1991) and fetal abnormality (1986–1993) statistics were compiled for all 27 areas. General practitioner consultation data (1989–1994) were studied in 2201 subjects in 12 Teesside estates. A population-based sample survey in 1993 based on self-completion questionnaires of 9115 subjects provided data on social circumstances, lifestyle, occupation, and health status. Current pollution levels were estimated by air quality measures and computer modelling of emissions from industrial, road traffic, and other sources; estimates of past exposure were made from a twentieth-century land-use survey and historical pollution data.

Main results

The estates chosen for study were extremely economically deprived and comparable on a broad range of indicators including residential histories and unemployment, especially when grouped into zones. Mortality rates were high but there were no consistent and statistically and epidemiologically significant differences in all cause, or all age mortality, or for most specific causes. Lung cancer in women was, however, highest closest to industry: Zone A SMR (standardized mortality ratio) = 393, Zone B = 251, Zone C = 242, Zone S = 185; where the standard population had a value of 100 (see Chapter 8 for details on the SMR). A less striking gradient was observed for respiratory disorders. Lung cancer registration ratios were consistent with mortality data.

There were no associations between proximity to industry and birthweights, stillbirths, fetal abnormality, and general practice consultation rates. For the self-completion questionnaire, data response rates were higher in Teesside areas compared to Sunderland areas. However, in these data, on a broad range of measures of both respiratory and non-respiratory health, including asthma, there were no important variations across the study zones. Smoking habits across the populations compared were similar.

Land-use data showed prominent heavy industry in the Teesside area, and that the contemporary proximity of the housing estates to industry was echoed in the past. Air quality data indicated major improvements in air quality in the preceding 20 years. Levels of major pollutants were generally below guide values.

Conclusions

Living close to a constellation of major petrochemical and steel industries was not associated with most health indicators, whether mortality or morbidity, including disorders such as asthma which had been a cause of concern to health professionals. Lung cancer in women was an important exception. In the absence of plausible explanations based on differences in social and lifestyle factors, exposure to past industrial pollution is the prime explanation. Further research and monitoring of lung cancer rates is warranted.

Note: This abstract is similar to that in Bhopal *et al.* 1998, *Occupational and Environmental Medicine*, 55, pp. 812–22, published with permission from the BMJ Publishing Group.

Concluding remarks (2015)

I will return to this study in section 10.4.2 when I discuss theory in epidemiology. From a practical point of view this detailed work made progress on a controversy that had persisted in Teesside for over 100 years. This said, probably no one was satisfied! Public pressure groups thought their problems had been minimized, the big industries that the findings potentially tarnished their reputation unfairly, and local government (in the middle) that the issue of poverty was more important than industrial pollution. Many people commented that the closure of industry threatened health. From my perspective, more than 20 years after the study, I was surprised at how on so many outcomes we found no association between outcomes and proximity to industry. I drove from Newcastle Upon Tyne, itself an industrial city, to Teesside on many occasions. The pall of air pollution that hung over the City of Middlesbrough was striking. My bias, though kept private, was that we would find extensive evidence of possible adverse effects of proximity to industry. This was another reminder that expectations are often overturned by research data.

When epidemiological data are applied to provide health advice to individuals and to shape clinical or public health policy, error, bias, and confounding are especially important. The reasons are threefold. First, these kinds of data problems may well be anticipated by those checking the evidence who are likely to read papers with a critical perspective but they may be missed. Second, by the time the work is ready for clinical or public health application, the research field is likely to be mature, so there will be a lower anticipation of these kinds of problems. Third, health states, even lives, are at stake at this stage. The implication of this is that the rudiments of critical appraisal (see Chapter 10) are essential for those doing applied epidemiological research. Equally, knowing that there may be health-care implications, and that health professionals and policymakers may be using their work, epidemiologists need to make explicit the potential limitations of their work. This action may, however, undermine the prospects of publication (see section 4.2.8).

Epidemiology has identified many types of errors and biases, and hundreds have been listed. The epidemiological approach to tackling them has been pragmatic rather than theoretical, such that problems have been identified and solutions developed. I am not aware of an epidemiological theory on why error and bias occur. To develop such a theoretically based understanding, one might start with statistical and social science perspectives on these topics.

Statistical theory is, largely, about random (chance) variations. The theory is used most commonly in epidemiology to calculate the probability that a finding of difference, or one more extreme than that *actually found*, occurred by chance alone (i.e. in truth there is no difference). The result is usually given as a P-value, the letter P standing for probability, often but misleadingly said to be a 'significance level'. The probability value is no more than these words imply. The number signifies no clinical, public health, or epidemiological significance. The assessment of real significance is a matter of judgement. Bias cannot be studied in this kind of statistical way. Nonetheless, approaches to the possible quantification of biases are available (see Chapter 9).

One of the most fundamental observations of social sciences on the nature of science is that the scientific endeavour is not objective but open to the influence of society and context. This view helps to explain many scientific actions that lead to error and bias, for example, the Tuskegee Study already mentioned in this chapter and also discussed in Chapter 10. In light of this insight, social scientists may include within their writings their personal background and values so the reader can see how their perspective may have influenced their work and especially data interpretation. This is a possible conflict of interest. This is not the practice in epidemiology or closely related disciplines, though it may be worth considering. The conflict of interest that epidemiologists focus on is mainly financial. In studying and classifying bias, I have promoted the framework provided by the chronology and structure of a research project—this is an atheoretical approach.

The main principles relating to this chapter and which apply to all studies include:

+ develop research questions and hypotheses in ways which help to benefit all the population or at least those studied, will minimize harm, and will maximize the public health goals of epidemiology;

+ study representative populations, whenever possible, especially in studies of the frequency of risk factors and diseases;

+ where a representative population is unnecessary; for example, for proof of concept studies of causal relationships, consider whether the results are likely to generalize and check by replicating the findings in other populations;

+ measure accurately and with equal care across comparison groups;

+ compare like-with-like or, in practice, approximately like-with-like;

+ check for the main findings in subgroups before assuming that inferences and generalizations apply across all groups;

+ for findings from unplanned exploratory analyses, prioritize corroboration with other data sets;

+ check for and take into account confounding, bearing in mind confounding factors might not be measured, or measured imprecisely;

+ a single study should only exceptionally be accepted as accurate enough for application;

+ in interpreting associations, first consider artefact, and when this is set aside, apply causal frameworks (Chapter 5);

+ publish in a way to avoid publication bias;

+ maintain a critical stance at all times, including post-publication, whether of single studies or meta-analyses (Chapters 9 and 10).

Summary

Epidemiological studies are prone to error, because they usually study complex matters in human populations in natural settings and not in laboratory conditions. The large size of many epidemiological studies imposes time and cost constraints, which may promote errors. Bias is a kind of error that is sometimes subtle, and one that is differentiated from random error (hence, sometimes called systematic error). Bias in epidemiology may be thought of as error which affects comparison groups unequally or leads to inappropriate inferences about one group compared with another. Error and bias may be inherent in the research question and the hypothesis, but this is a relatively neglected matter that needs attention.

Three great and broad problems confront epidemiologists: selection of study populations; quality of information; and confounding. Selection and imperfect information cause biases. Confounding is not an error or bias as normally understood but it leads to errors of data interpretation. Confounding causes an error in the assessment of the meaning of an association between a disease and risk factor. It results from comparing groups, which differ in characteristics that are associated both with the disease and the risk factor under study, without fully accounting for such differences.

The different epidemiological research designs have similar problems with error and bias, which are mostly inherent in the survey and disease registration methods. Principles which apply to all studies and help to minimize these errors include: construct research questions and hypotheses carefully; study representative populations when possible; when representative populations are not needed, in concept of causality studies, consider generalizability at the interpretation stage; measure accurately and with equal care across groups; compare like-with-like; take into account confounding; and check before assuming that inferences and generalizations apply across groups. Epidemiologists should present and publish the data with impartiality and integrity. The chronology and structure of a research project offers a pragmatic framework for the systematic analysis of error, bias and confounding.

Sample questions

Many of the questions at the end of Chapter 9 are highly relevant to this chapter.

Question 1 What is misclassification bias (or error), and why is it important in measuring risk factor–disease outcome relationships?

Answer Misclassification bias occurs when we categorize a person wrongly, for example, a smoker is classified as a non-smoker, or a person with rheumatoid arthritis is classified as having osteoarthritis.

Misclassification can occur in both risk factors and outcome variables. Where risk factor–outcome relations are under study, we are usually interested in the relative risk of the outcome in those with and without the risk factor. If misclassification is greater in one of these two groups, the relative risk will be exaggerated. The study may be irreversibly destroyed.

Where classification occurs equally in those with and without the risk factors or in those with and without the disease, the relative risk is usually diminished. The study may reach a wrong conclusion, but the damage is sometimes repairable by adjusting for the degree of misclassification. When there is misclassification in confounding variables, the result is not predictable—the association may even be stronger.

Question 2 How can we control confounding in epidemiology?

Answer We can control for confounding by, above all, awareness, foresight, and planning. This will alert us to compare like-with-like wherever possible. Strategies to do this include restriction of who is recruited to the study, and matching (but beware matching has its own problems, including overmatching). In trials, random allocation of people into intervention and control groups is of great help. Further control of confounding is achievable by stratified analysis, standardization methods, and multivariable analysis where confounding factors are entered as covariates.

Question 3 Why might bias occur in the wording of an epidemiological research question? What can you do to minimize such a bias? Illustrate your answer with at least one example.

Answer Bias in epidemiology can be thought of as errors that are not equal in the compared populations. Errors can arise from prejudices (conscious or subconscious), stereotypes, or lack of awareness and they can affect the research question. For example, imagine we are interested in the question of hygiene and its relationship to gastrointestinal infections in children of unemployed families. The question could be posed as:

- (a) Are the higher rates of gastrointestinal infections in children of unemployed parents related to their poorer hygiene?

    Or

- (b) Are there any differences in the hygiene practices of children that are associated with the employment status of their parents and that might be associated with gastrointestinal infections?

An issue such as this is open to bias. While bias in the minds of investigators is not easily set aside, the second question, written in a neutral way, reduces the potential for bias. The first question is posed in a way that points to the expected answer.

Question 4 What biases may arise in a cohort study assessing a possible association between a risk factor and disease, for example, dietary salt intake and the development of hypertension?

Answer Bias can be thought of as a type of error that affects comparison groups unequally so that the risk factor or intervention effect under study tends to be systematically over or underestimated and hence erroneous conclusions may be drawn.
Biases can be categorized according to the chronology of a research project:

- Question bias. Processed food industry funded studies might aim to discredit the importance of dietary salt in blood pressure control.

- Selection bias. Restricting study participants by gender, age group, ethnicity, or volunteer status.

- Participation bias. Differential non-response/participation rates or loss to follow-up.

- Information bias. Diet and blood pressure are both difficult to measure accurately. This would be a great problem especially if measured more inaccurately in some subgroups.

- Intervention bias. Although cohort studies do not impose an intervention as such, differential treatment of risk factor and control groups (e.g. in frequency or intensity of follow-up), may bias results.

- Interpretation bias. Unintentional or intentional misinterpretation of results to reflect researchers' preferred outcome.

- Publication bias. Only putting forward preferred results for publication leads to biased availability of evidence.

  - Confounding (while not bias, it is relevant to the question). The risk factor and control groups may be dissimilar in other factors that influence the development of hypertension. Diet is linked to a range of other health behaviours, for example, alcohol intake, which may influence blood pressure.

Question 5 What is publication bias? Why is it important in epidemiology?

Answer The pressures and difficulties of publication, particularly in scientific journals, can generate biases. The article will usually need to be short. Choices on the data to be presented will be combined with choices on emphasis and interpretation. Editorial guidelines usually indicate that originality, interest, and readability will be key criteria for publication. Researchers write accordingly, by highlighting the points of interest to themselves, editors, and readers. Manuscripts showing interesting findings (positive results in trials, differences in disease patterns in most epidemiology) are most likely to be submitted, and to be accepted, for publication in widely read journals, while others are often left unpublished or published in specialist journals, or as reports to the funding agency. The result is a biased understanding of the differences and similarities in the disease patterns of populations, an exaggerated view of the importance of associations between risk factors and disease outcomes, and an exaggerated view on the effectiveness of interventions.

References

Bhopal, R.S., Moffatt, S., Pless-Mulloli, T., *et al.* (1998) Does living near a constellation of petrochemical, steel, and other industries impair health? *Occupational and Environmental Medicine*, **55**, 812–22.

Greenland, S. (1980) The effect of misclassification in the presence of covariates. *American Journal of Epidemiology*, **112**, 564–9.

Jones, J.H. (1993) *Bad Blood: The Tuskegee Syphilis Experiment*, 2nd edn. New York, NY: Free Press.

Kuhn, T.S. (1996) *The Structure of Scientific Revolutions*, 3rd edn. Chicago, IL: The University of Chicago Press.

Lillie-Blanton, M., Anthony, J.C., and Schuster, C.R. (1993) Probing the meaning of racial/ethnic group comparisons in crack smoking. *Journal of the American Medical Association*, **269**, 993–7.

Moffatt, S., Phillimore, P., Hudson, E., and Downey, D. (2000) 'Impact? What impact?' Epidemiological research findings in the public domain: a case study from north-east England. *Social Science and Medicine*, **51**, 1755–69.

Popper, K.R. (1989) *Conjectures and Refutations: The Growth of Scientific Knowledge*, 5th edn. London, UK: Routledge.

Porta, M. (2014) *A Dictionary of Epidemiology*, 6th edn. New York, NY: Oxford University Press.

Appendix 4.1

Further exercises on misclassification

For simplicity, we will use cumulative incidence with the denominator fixed as at the beginning of the study.

Imagine a study of 20 000 women, 10 000 are on the contraceptive pill and the rest are not. Our interest is in the occurrence of new cases of cardiovascular disease (CVD) over 10 years (cumulative incidence of disease). Say that over 10 years, 20 per cent of those on the pill develop a CVD compared with 10 per cent of those not on the pill. The rate of disease in the oral contraceptive group is doubled (relative risk = 2). Table A4.1.1 shows the true results, given no misclassification. This is not realistic.

Let us assume that misclassification in exposure occurred 10 per cent of the time, so that 10 per cent of women actually on the pill were classified as not on the pill, and that 10 per cent who were not on the pill were classified as on the pill. This level of misclassification seems realistic for studies that are based only on self-reported data.

Assume that there is no misclassification of disease outcome, and the disease incidence remains the same. Before reading on, you should modify the figures in Table A4.1 and recalculate relative

Table A4.1 Imaginary and perfect but impossible study of cardiovascular outcome and pill use: no misclassification

True classification of pill use status	Cardiovascular disease		Total
	Yes	No	
Yes	2000	8000	10 000
No	1000	9000	10 000
Total	3000	17 000	20 000

risk of disease given this misclassification. Tables A4.2 and A4.3 give the results. The following steps and questions, and if necessary dummy Table A4.8, should help you with this exercise (the textual answers are also given on pages 127–129):

(1) For the group of women taking the pill (from Table A4.1), calculate the number of women correctly classified as on the pill and the number of women on the pill who are misclassified, that is, wrongly classified as not being on the pill.

(2) For the group of women not taking the pill (Table A4.1), calculate the number of women correctly classified as not on the pill and the number of women misclassified, that is, wrongly classified as on the pill.

(3) Create two rows of data, that is, the numbers of women correctly classified as on the pill (from step 1) and numbers incorrectly classified as on the pill (from step 2). For these

Table A4.2 Pill and cardiovascular disease with an imperfect but possible study: 10 per cent misclassification of pill use

True classification	Cardiovascular disease		Total
	Yes	No	
Yes, classified right (incidence 20%)	1800	7200	9000
Yes, classified wrong (incidence 20%)	200	800	1000
Subtotal	2000	8000	10 000
No, classified right (incidence of 10%)	900	8100	9000
No, classified wrong (incidence 10%)	100	900	1000
Subtotal	1000	9000	10 000
Total of subtotals	3000	17 000	20 000

Table A4.2 shows the reality of the effects of misclassification. The investigator does not, however, know how much misclassification there is. For the investigator the data look like Table A4.4. The reason for this is shown by the reorganization of the data in Tables A4.2 and A4.3, and then into A4.4.

Table A4.3 Pill and cardiovascular disease: 10 per cent misclassification of pill use, bold rows as seen by the investigator

Classification of pill use status in this imperfect study	Cardiovascular disease		Total
	Yes	No	
Yes, classified right (on the pill so incidence rate is 20%)	1800	7200	9000
Yes, classified wrong (actually not on the pill so incidence rate is 10%)	100	900	1000
Subtotal	**1900**	**8100**	**10 000**
No, classified right (not on the pill so incidence rate is 10%)	900	8100	9000
No, classified wrong (actually on the pill so incidence rate is 20%)	200	800	1000
Subtotal	**1100**	**8900**	**10 000**
Total	3000	17 000	20 000

women, calculate the number of CVD cases and non-cases in each subgroup, that is, for women correctly classified as on the pill and for women misclassified as on the pill. *Remember: women truly taking the pill have a 20 per cent chance of developing CVD whereas women truly not on the pill, even though misclassified as such, have a 10 per cent chance of developing CVD.*

(4) Create two rows of data, that is, for women correctly classified as not taking the pill (from step 2) and for those misclassified as not on the pill (from step 1). Calculate the number of CVD cases in each subgroup. *Remember: women truly taking the pill have a 20 per cent chance of developing CVD, whether they are classified correctly or not, whereas women truly not on the pill have a 10 per cent chance of developing CVD, again, irrespective of the classification.*

(5) Add up the number of women and cases in your work in step 3 above to create a single row of data. (If you have difficulties, Table A4.3 should be helpful, but try to do this yourself.)

(6) Add up the number of women and cases in your work in step 4 above to create a single row of data. (If you have difficulties, Table A4.3 should be helpful, but try to do this yourself).

(7) Create a new (blank) 2 × 2 table. Now add the number of CVD cases and non-cases for women apparently on the pill (whether correctly classified or misclassified) and women apparently not on the pill (whether correctly or incorrectly classified). *Remember: in each case, combine CVD cases and non-cases from the correctly classified and misclassified subgroups of women.* Calculate the subtotals and totals and then the proportion with CVD in each group. Lastly, calculate the percentages of women with CVD in these groups, divide the percentages, and interpret the relative risk.

Table A4.4 Pill and cardiovascular disease: 10 per cent misclassification of pill use and as the investigator sees it

Apparent classification of pill use	Cardiovascular disease		Total
	Yes	No	
Yes	1900	8100	10 000
No	1100	8900	10 000
Total	3000	17 000	20 000

(8) Compare the results (relative risk) obtained in step 7 above to the risk estimate calculated earlier in step 1. How many times more common is the disease in pill users now? Is the extra risk in pill users as high as before? What has happened?

The risk of CVD in the cigarette smoking group with 10 per cent misclassification is 1900/10 000. In the 'not on the pill group' it is 1100/10 000. Therefore, the relative risk is

$$\frac{1900/10\ 000}{1100/10\ 000} = \frac{0.19}{0.11} = 1.7$$

Misclassification will, inevitably, arise in measurement of the disease outcome also. Let us now assume that there is 10 per cent misclassification there. For simplicity, assume there is no misclassification of pill status (so use Table A4.1 as the starting point). Before reading on, try to work out the result. Table A4.1 shows the data as observed by the investigator. Tables A4.5, A4.6, and A4.7 give the results.

Before reading on calculate the effects of 10 per cent misclassification of outcome—see Table A4.5 for the results, which are simplified in tables A4.6 and A4.7.

Table A4.5 Pill and cardiovascular disease. Ten per cent misclassification in measurement of disease outcome: reorganization of Table 4.5

True classification of pill status	Cardiovascular disease						Subtotal	Total of subtotals
	Yes			No				
	Classified right	Classified wrong	Subtotal	Classified right	Classified wrong	Subtotal		
Yes	1800	200[†]	2000	7200	800[*]	8000	10 000	
No	900	100[§]	1000	8100	900[‡]	9000	10 000	
	2700	300	3000	15 300	1700	17 000	20 000	

[*]10% of 8000 (row 1, column 3, Table A4.1); [†]10% of 2000 (row 1, column 2, Table A4.1);
[‡]10% of 9000 (row 2, column 3, Table A4.1); [§]10% of 1000 (row 2, column 2, Table A4.1).

Table A4.6 Pill and cardiovascular disease: 10 per cent misclassification in measurement of disease outcome: reorganization of Table A4.5

Oral contraceptive	Cardiovascular disease				Total
	Yes		No		
	Yes correctly classified as CVD	Misclassified as CVD	CVD, but misclassified as no	No CVD, correctly classified	
Yes	1800	800*	200†	7200	10 000
No	900	900‡	100§	8100	10 000
	2700	1700	300	15 300	20 000

*10% of 8000 (row 1, column 3, Table A4.1); †10% of 2000 (row 1, column 2, Table A4.1); ‡10% of 9000 (row 2, column 3, Table A4.1); §10% of 1000 (row 2, column 2, Table A4.1).

Now the relative risk (from Table A4.7) is

$$\frac{2600/10\ 000}{1800/10\ 000} = \frac{0.26}{0.18} = 1.44.$$

Answers to the questions posed above on the misclassification of exposure (pill status):

(1) For the group of women taking the pill (Table A4.1), calculate the total number of women correctly classified as on the pill and also the number of women misclassified as not on the pill. Group of women on the pill (n = 10 000):

  90 per cent or 9000 women are correctly classified as on the pill
  10 per cent or 1000 women are misclassified as not taking the pill

(2) For the group of women not taking the pill (Table A4.1), calculate the total number of women correctly classified as not on the pill and also the number of women misclassified as not being on the pill. Group of women not on the pill (n = 10 000):

  90 per cent or 9000 women are correctly classified as not on the pill
  10 per cent or 1000 women are misclassified as on the pill

Table A4.7 Pill and cardiovascular disease. Ten per cent misclassification in measurement of disease outcome: reorganization of Table A4.6 to show results as investigator perceives them

Oral contraceptive	Cardiovascular disease		Total
	Yes	No	
Yes	2600	7400	10 000
No	1800	8200	10 000
Total	4400	15 600	20 000

Table A4.8 Dummy table for reorganizing misclassified data

Classification of pill use status	Cardiovascular disease		Total
	Yes	No	
On the pill, and classified right (so incidence rate is truly 20%)			
Wrongly said to be on the pill (so incidence rate is truly 10%)			
Subtotal			
Classified right (not on the pill so incidence rate is truly 10%)			
Classified wrong (actually on the pill so incidence rate is truly 20%)			
Subtotal			
TOTAL			

(3) For the group of women said to be taking the pill, calculate the number of CVD cases in each subgroup, that is, women correctly classified as on the pill and those misclassified as on the pill.

Among the 9000 women correctly classified as on the pill, there are 1800 cases of CVD—20 per cent chance of developing CVD

Among the 1000 women misclassified as on the pill, there are 100 cases of CVD—10 per cent chance of developing CVD

(4) For the group of women said not to be taking the pill, calculate the number of CVD cases in each subgroup, that is, women correctly classified as not on the pill and those misclassified as not on the pill.

Among the 9000 women correctly classified as not on the pill, there are 900 cases of CVD—10 per cent chance of developing CVD

Among the 1000 women misclassified as not on the pill, there are 200 cases of CVD—20 per cent chance of developing CVD

Table A4.9 The proportion of participants with CVD in each group

Exposure/Outcome	CVD	No CVD	Total
On the pill	1800 + 100 = 1900	7200 + 900 = 8100	10 000
Not on the pill	900 + 200 = 1100	8100 + 800 = 8900	10 000
Total	3000	17 000	20 000

On the pill: the proportion with CVD is 1900/10 000 = 0.19 (or 19%).

Not on the pill: the proportion with CVD is 1100/10 000 = 0.11 (or 11%).

Relative risk = 0.19/0.11 = 1.73.

(5) Now add the number of CVD cases and non-cases for women as in step 3, and this number is 1900. Since the total number of women is 10 000, the remainder of non-cases is 8100.

(6) Now add up the number of CVD cases and non-cases for women as in step 4 and this number is 1100. The number of non-cases is 8900.

(7) As before, create a new (blank) 2 × 2 table. This is Table A4.4 as above and in more detail below in Table A4.9.
Calculate the subtotals and then the proportion with CVD in each group. Lastly, calculate and interpret the relative risk (text above - RR = 1.73).

(8) Compare the results (relative risks) obtained in steps 7 (above) and from Table A4.1.
The calculation from Table A4.1 shows the relative risk when there is no misclassification that is 'ideal world' scenario; the relative risk in step 7 shows the effects of 10 per cent misclassification in the exposure, which has biased the risk estimate towards the null.
(These step-by-step answers are not given for the misclassification of outcome but are similar.)

Chapter 5

Cause and effect: The epidemiological approach

Objectives

On completion of the chapter you should understand:

- that the purpose of studying cause and effect in epidemiology is to generate knowledge to prevent, cure, treat, and control disease;

- that cause and effect understanding is particularly difficult to achieve in epidemiology because of the complex development of diseases over long timescales and because of ethical restraints on human experimentation;

- how causal thinking in epidemiology depends on and contributes to other domains of knowledge, both scientific and non-scientific;

- the importance of setting out a causal framework in advance of designing a study;

- the potential role of causal graphs in both concepts (e.g. web of causation) and analytical aids (e.g. directed acyclic graphs);

- the potential contributions of epidemiological study designs for contributing to causal knowledge;

- how to use a systematic approach, which checks for error, chance, bias, and confounding, before reaching judgements on cause and effect;

- the distinction between confounding, moderator, and mediator variables;

- the meaning of interaction and effect modification;

- that epidemiological approaches to, and guidelines for, causality are not a checklist and therefore conclusions must be carefully judged and tentative;

- the value of synthesizing data from epidemiological studies and other disciplines, including laboratory experiments, before reaching conclusions.

5.1 Introduction: causality in science and philosophy and its relevance to epidemiology

Cause and effect understanding is the highest achievement (the jewel in the crown) of scientific knowledge, including epidemiology. Causal knowledge points to actions to break the links between the factors causing disease, and disease itself. As such, it underpins prevention of disease. It also helps to predict the outcome of an intervention and helps to treat disease. To quote Hippocrates writing about 2000 years ago, 'To know the causes of a disease and to understand the use of the various methods by which the disease may be prevented amounts to the same thing as being able to cure the disease' (see Chadwick and Mann 1950). This is both a modest exaggeration and an understatement. Sometimes we know the exact cause of a disease but we can neither prevent it nor cure it (e.g. serious genetic disorders); but where we can prevent it, the result is far superior to curing the disease (e.g. it is better to prevent lung cancer than cure it through surgery, chemotherapy, and radiotherapy).

Epidemiology enjoys the status of a science. As in all sciences including physics and chemistry, epidemiological understanding of cause and effect does not have to be 100 per cent complete or accurate to permit useful application. After all, gravity is still a mystery but scientists have learned enough about it to land a rocket on a comet. Arguably, more so than in other sciences, in epidemiology even partial understanding must be applied as quickly as possible, for it may be a life and death matter. There is, therefore, an ethical responsibility to apply knowledge even when, from a scientific point of view, further research is advised. Yet, this ethical imperative may be perilous.

Early application of knowledge sometimes has devastating effects and sometimes beneficial effects. Sylvia Tesh (1988) gives two examples of this. The public health endeavours of the nineteenth century, including the building of sewers, the delivery of clean water, and the improvement of the sanitary conditions of the home and workplace, were driven by the 'miasma' theory of health and disease. This theory presumed that noxious air carrying 'miasma' released from filth in the environment was the cause of most of the prevalent diseases, including cholera. Though wrong, the miasma theory worked and the benefits of the applications of this simplistic theory have been immense and remain the bedrock of public health everywhere. Time has shown the 'filth' allowed microbes (and the insects and other creatures that spread them) to flourish. Many of these diseases were contagious—that is, they spread by contact. There was no 'miasma'.

By contrast, according to Tesh, the contagion theory was both correct and dominant in explaining the occurrence of plague. Jews were, however, incriminated in a poorly understood causal pathway of contagion and thousands were executed in a vain attempt to control plague. Tesh gives a figure of 16 000 Jews killed in Strasbourg alone. (Roy Porter gives a figure of 2000 Jews slaughtered in Strasbourg and 12 000 in Mainz.) The contagion theory was ineffective in this application, which was outrageous, and surely underpinned by the anti-Semitism of those times. Nonetheless, this history has contemporary lessons as some, usually poor or minority, populations are still scapegoated when there are threats of contagious diseases.

The effective application of incomplete knowledge requires art and science. Epidemiology is one of the principle sciences that public health policy draws upon. Recent examples of major public health policy decisions requiring the application of incomplete data include: whether to ban consumption of beef products given the epidemic of bovine spongiform encephalopathy in cattle; what action to take given evidence that living near a nuclear power plant is associated with raised risk of childhood leukaemia; what proportion of daily energy intake should be consumed as fat; what is the recommended daily salt intake; whether we should tax sugar to help reduce obesity; whether we should strive to increase the average birthweight of newborn babies; and whether women should or should not take oestrogen-based hormonal therapy to reduce post-menopausal problems and chronic diseases. These kinds of decisions generate massive controversy that hinges around causality.

To the study of causality, epidemiology has contributed:

◆ a philosophy of health and disease

◆ models that illustrate that philosophy

◆ study designs to produce quantitative evidence

◆ information from quantitative studies on the relationships between numerous factors and diseases

◆ frameworks for interpreting and applying the accumulated evidence.

Box 5.1 Some simple questions in causality in epidemiology

- ◆ What is a cause?
- ◆ What will be the result of a cause in epidemiology?
- ◆ How might we measure the result of a cause in epidemiology?

Epidemiology has absorbed a great deal of causal thinking from other disciplines and the occasionally heard and read proposition that epidemiology is *the* science of causal thinking (whether confined to populations or not) is immodest and false.

Scientific thinking encourages turning empirical observations into theories and hypotheses that permit tests of generalizable cause and effect judgements. Epidemiological reasoning on cause and effect is embedded in observations of disease variation, the discovery of associations between putative causes and the disease, and ways of testing hypotheses so we can use associations to progress towards causation. Epidemiology draws upon the reasoning of other disciplines, including philosophy and microbiology. Epidemiology shares similar problems of disentangling cause and effect relationships with other disciplines (particularly those mainly reliant on observation of naturally occurring events). Solutions to problems are likely to arise from the sharing of ideas among such disciplines.

This background understanding of how science works is necessary to counter the criticism that epidemiological reasoning on cause and effect is merely empirical and atheoretical. On a pragmatic note, epidemiological debates on cause and effect are often in the public eye and, more so than most other sciences—so non-epidemiologists become involved in the interpretation of data and making judgements on their meaning (see also Chapters 4 and 10). This requires that epidemiological approaches to analysis of cause and effect are easy to understand and apply. Before reading on, do the exercise in Box 5.1.

A cause is something which has an effect, that is, it brings about or produces something. In epidemiology, a cause can be considered something that alters the frequency of disease, health status, or associated causal factors in a population. We measure these effects by defining changes in the incidence (preferably), prevalence, and other outcomes due to changes in the presumed causal factors (i.e. exposures or risk factors). We will also measure how other (moderating and mediating) variables alter the relationship between postulated causal factors and outcomes. These are pragmatic definitions, but it is worth knowing more about the broader debates and controversies on cause, and where such simple ideas fit. This is important so that epidemiologists can converse about cause and effect in multidisciplinary settings, where pragmatic definitions may be questioned, or even derided.

5.1.1 Some philosophy

Philosophers have grappled with the nature of causality for thousands of years (Cottingham 1996). Aristotle, for example, held a broad view that there were four elements to cause, which have been reconsidered in the context of a house by John Dreker, as extracted in Cottingham. The causes of a house are the material (the stone, brick, or wood), the formal (the plan), the efficient (the thing which puts it into effect, here the builder), and the final (the purpose, being to create a comfortable home). Aristotle foresaw one effect could have several causes. The cause of Legionnaires' disease is, at its simplest, exposure to the causal bacteria. From an Aristotelian point of view, the four causes would be: the existence of living bacteria (material); the essence of the nature of the relationship between bacteria and humans (the formal); the delivery of an infective dose by some mechanism, such as a cooling tower (the efficient); and the quest for processes to increase human comfort that leads to complex water systems such as cooling towers (final).

David Hume's philosophy has also been influential (Cottingham 1996). Hume's view that a cause cannot be deduced logically from the fact that two events are linked, but needs to be experienced or perceived at a deep level, is crucially important to epidemiology. Just because thunder follows lightning does not mean thunder is caused by lightning (indeed, it is not as we discuss later). When we flick a light switch the light may go on, but this does not prove that the one act causes the other. To stretch your imagination, can you think of alternative explanations, no matter how absurd they seem?

One explanation is that there is someone observing and as soon as you flick the switch, he or she puts the light on. This is, indeed, absurd, but it is possible. To someone who had no understanding of electrical circuits it might seem more plausible than the truth. When we understand the mechanism of electrical circuits, however, we accept that there is cause and effect.

This perspective is echoed in the axiom, 'association is not causation'. Cause and effect deductions need more than linkage; they need understanding. Hume's thoughts are relevant to the debate on black box epidemiology. The black box metaphor comes from the increasing availability of technology as a closed unit, not amenable to easy opening and exploration, for example, a DVD player, modem, or mobile telephone. The unit works, or if it does not it is discarded and replaced, without regard to what the problem is. This has become an apt metaphor for epidemiological research based on the study of associations (risk factor epidemiology) and the evaluation of complex interventions. The late Petr Skrabanek (1994) described it as epidemiology where the causal mechanism behind an association remained unknown but hidden (black), but with the inference that the causal mechanism was within the association (box). Skrabanek argued that the purpose of science is to open and understand the black box, which epidemiology too often failed to do. While failing to understand the association (or the effective components of a complex intervention) is a limitation, the greater problem occurs when the true causes lie outside the putative association (i.e. outside the black box)—and that happens.

The contribution of another philosopher, John Stuart Mill, captured in his 'canons', is so similar to the modern ideas of epidemiology that it is discussed in the section on guidelines for causality (section 5.6.1). Philosophical discussion on the nature of causality, questioning whether causes can be stated definitively or only as a matter of probability is of importance to epidemiology. Epidemiology tends to work closely with statistics, which deals with probability, and tends to side with this approach.

5.2 Epidemiological causal strategy and reasoning: the example of Semmelweis

The epidemiological strategy is simple but its successful execution is not. To reiterate, at the population level diseases form patterns, which are ever-changing. Over short time periods the changes are largely, but not exclusively, caused by environmental changes. The exception is that genetic changes in microbes can be rapid and hence the pattern of human microbial diseases can change fast. Over long time periods, that is, over many generations, genetic variation also changes the population pattern of human disease. Clues to the causes of disease are inherent within these patterns. These patterns, therefore, can be studied both to generate and test ideas on causation and to test out ideas developed in other fields of enquiry. The combination of epidemiological and other types of observation is particularly valuable.

The epidemiological mode of reasoning combined with other observations is illustrated by the discovery by Ignaz Semmelweis of the general cause of puerperal fever. Semmelweis (1818–1865)

Table 5.1 Births, deaths, and mortality rates (%) for all patients at the two clinics of the Vienna maternity hospital from 1841 to 1846

First clinic (doctors)			Second clinic (midwives)		
Births	Deaths	Rate (%)	Births	Deaths	Rate (%)
20 042	1989	9.92	17 791	691	3.38

Source: data from Semmelweis I. The etiology, concept and prophylaxis of childbed fever, 1983 [excerpts] In: Buck C, Llopis A, Najera E, Terris M (eds.). *The challenge of epidemiology–issues and selected readings.* Washington: Pan American Health Organization (PAHO) Scientific Publication, Copyright © 1988 PAHO. pp. 46–59.

was training in obstetrics in Vienna when he observed that the mortality from childbed fever (now known as puerperal fever) was lower in women attending clinic 2, run by midwives, than in those attending clinic 1, run by doctors. He also noted that women who gave birth in the street, or prematurely, had a lower mortality than those in clinic 1. The statistics he collected are given in Table 5.1. Do the exercise in Box 5.2 before reading on.

Semmelweis also noted that while the cases in clinic 2 were sporadic, in clinic 1 a whole row of patients might be sick at the same time. Semmelweis was perplexed but saw that the pattern he observed meant an endemic cause, that is, the cause lay within the clinic itself. He tried, unsuccessfully, to solve the problem by delivering the mothers by laying them on their sides rather than on their backs. At this stage, based on a case series study (see Chapter 9 for details on this design) Semmelweis has observed a pattern, come to a general conclusion (internal, not external cause), developed a hypothesis, and tested an intervention which was unsuccessful (delivery position). It could be said that he has observed an association but the explanation remains hidden. This makes unravelling the mystery even more, not less, important. At the time there was no developed suite of methods in epidemiology—if there had been a case–control study would have been the next step (see Chapter 9 for this study design). Equally importantly, there was no field of medical microbiology either.

A year or so later, in 1847, his colleague and friend Professor Kolletschka died following a fingerprick with a knife used at an autopsy. Kolletschka's own autopsy showed inflammation to be widespread in his corpse, with peritonitis and meningitis. Semmelweis's mind was alert and he connected the childbed fever disease in women with that of his friend. He wrote:

> Day and night I was haunted by the image of Kolletschka's disease and was forced to recognize, ever more decisively that the disease from which Kolletschka died was identical to that from which so many maternity patients died.

> Semmelweis (reprinted 1988, p. 52)

Semmelweis was 'compelled to ask' whether cadaverous particles, that is, the substance passed from the cadaver (corpse) Kolletschka dissected, had been introduced into the vascular systems of maternity patients, as seemed to have happened in the case of his friend.

Box 5.2 Causal question from statistics presented in Table 5.1

Do these figures spark off any ideas of causation in your mind? What explanations can you generate? Reflect on this question before reading on.

Semmelweis's inspired idea was that particles had been transferred from the scalpel to the vascular system of his friend and that the same kind of particles were killing maternity patients. He foresaw that the particles could be transferred from the hands of medical students and doctors to the women during pelvic examinations. If so, something stronger than ordinary soap was needed for handwashing. He introduced chlorina liquida, and then for economy, chlorinated lime. These substances, unlike ordinary soap, have antiseptic properties. The maternal mortality rate plummeted, reaching the level of the midwives' clinic.

Although Semmelweis was not the first to link puerperal fever to lack of hygiene, his contribution was huge; particularly because of the systematic, epidemiological evidence he accumulated and the way he tested his ideas (hypotheses). The epidemiological observations outlined the problem and prepared the mind to seek a solution, itself inspired by clinical and autopsy observation, and tested by experimentation and epidemiological monitoring of outcomes.

Two great principles are illustrated by this work. First, deep and generalizable knowledge lies in the explanation of disease patterns, rather than in their description, which is just the first step. The questioning (and persistent) mind may solve the riddle inherent in the pattern. Second, inspiration is needed, and may come from unexpected sources, as here from Kolletschka's autopsy. Such inspiration needs to be converted into a scientific hypothesis so it can be tested by scientific observation or experiment, as by Semmelweis's interventions, first in the way labour was conducted (unsuccessful), and then of handwashing with chlorinated lime (successful).

Most disease patterns remain unexplained despite lengthy study and others are never explored fully (so-called cul-de-sac epidemiology). Those that are explained usually lead to profound insights. Epidemiology does not, however, have the tools to demonstrate biological disease mechanisms. Whether the cause is biochemical—as in scurvy, or social, as in the rise of suicide in populations hit by unemployment—epidemiologists are reliant on other sciences to be equal partners in pursuit of the mechanisms. Action cannot always, however, await understanding of the mechanism. A contemporary example of this is the use of epidemiological data showing that laying an infant on its front (prone position) to sleep raises the risk of 'cot death', or in medical terms sudden infant death syndrome. Yet, the prone position was long and wrongly advocated as a means of avoiding the potential danger of infants inhaling their own vomit. A campaign to persuade parents to lay their infants on their backs has halved the incidence of cot death. In countries where the evidence has not been implemented, we have seen no such change. The mechanism is yet to be fully explained but the association is agreed as causal.

It would be several decades after Semmelweis that, among others, Louis Pasteur firmly established an old idea—the germ theory of diseases—to be true and the bacterial nature of the cadaverous particles was established. Then Semmelweis' discovery could be understood. Even in this straightforward disease we see complex layers of causation: the organization of health care; the behaviour of doctors in relation to autopsies; hygiene practices; cadaverous materials; and transfer of bacteria from doctors to mothers in labour. This complexity is the topic we cover next, where we consider models of causation.

5.3 Models of cause in epidemiology

5.3.1 Interplay of host, agent, and environment

The idea that disease is *virtually always* a result of the interplay of the environment, the genetic and physical make-up of the individual, and the agent of disease, is one of the most important of the cause and effect ideas underpinned by epidemiology. This theory applies both to diseases said

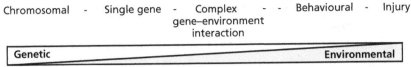

Fig. 5.1 Line of causation—a simple model for considering genetic and environmental factors.

to be multifactorial (e.g. cancers or heart disease) and to diseases which are by their definition a result of a single cause, such as tuberculosis, a drug side effect, or an overdose. This way of thinking, shared with social scientists, contrasts with the strong focus on very specific and narrowly defined causes (reductionist approaches) of most sciences, including medical sciences.

Diseases attributed to single causes are invariably so by definition. For example, tuberculosis is a disease that has many manifestations. It is characterized by a multiplicity of diffuse signs and symptoms, which affect nearly every part of the body. Some diseases, for example, sarcoidosis, are often indistinguishable from tuberculosis clinically, while the microscopic findings in Crohn's disease look very similar to tuberculosis. In some ways tuberculosis is a number of diseases (e.g. pulmonary tuberculosis, cutaneous tuberculosis, tuberculous meningitis), some of which are indistinguishable from other diseases. The fact that tuberculosis is caused by the tubercle bacillus is a matter of redefinition following Koch's discovery of the causal bacterium in 1882. Another perspective is that the causes of tuberculosis are many, including malnutrition and overcrowding.

This idea is captured by several well-known disease causation models such as the line, the triangle, the wheel, the web, and the pie. These models help to organize ideas about causes and strategies to prevent and control disease. In analysing causes, it is advisable to move from simple to complex models.

Figure 5.1 illustrates the idea of the line of causation. First, an arbitrary division is made between genetic and all other causes, categorized by convention as the environment. The line conceptualizes causes as lying on a spectrum from being wholly caused by genetic factors, or by environmental ones. Although the interaction of the genome and the environment is the key to understanding causation, the gene–environment division, though artificial, is widely used as a simple first step in analysing causes. At one extreme lie disorders which are almost entirely genetic, such as Down's syndrome (trisomy 21). At the other extreme lies injury arising from a road traffic accident. Most disorders lie in between. One of the early judgements required on diseases of unknown cause is the likely relative importance of genetic and environmental factors, for the preventive or control strategy will be fundamentally different. Try the exercise in Box 5.3 before reading on.

Figure 5.2 shows how epidemiology can help to make judgements on the question in Box 5.2. Diseases where the incidence varies rapidly over time or is different in genetically similar groups are clearly strongly influenced by environmental factors, while diseases which have a stable

Box 5.3 Exercise on gene and environment in causation

Think about the causes of three or four health problems or diseases that you or your friends or relatives have had. Place them on the line of causation. (Use these diseases for the following exercises too.)

Think through the cause of disease X using this model (Box 1.7, Chapter 1). What is your judgement? Is disease X likely to be genetic or environmental? Why? What makes you favour genetic factors over environmental ones?

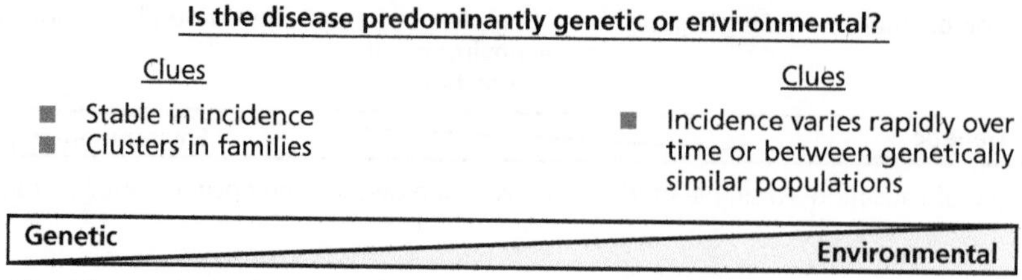

Is the disease predominantly genetic or environmental?

Clues	Clues
■ Stable in incidence ■ Clusters in families	■ Incidence varies rapidly over time or between genetically similar populations

Genetic   Environmental

Fig. 5.2 Line of causation: epidemiological clues to environment or genetic causation.

incidence or are clustered in blood relatives are more likely to have strong genetic influences. Figure 5.3 places some diseases on this spectrum.

The triangle, wheel, and the web are more complex versions of the same concept as the epidemiological line. Each model has its strengths and limitations for helping to clarify causal thinking. Each model is, however, a simplification—that is the value of a model. The categories of host, agent, and environment (Fig. 5.4) are arbitrary. While the meaning of the words host and agent of disease are self-evident, or can be illustrated with simple examples (Boxes 5.4 and 5.5), this is not the case for the environment, which has an immensely broad meaning (Box 5.6). The host and agent are, of course, both part of the environment. The environment, in this context, is arbitrarily defined to mean factors other than the host and the agent of disease. The environment, in particular, can be split to some benefit into several categories, such as the social, chemical, or physical environment.

Boxes 5.4, 5.5, and 5.6, list some of the many host, agent, and environmental factors which are generally important causes of population level variations in human disease. Of the factors listed in Table 5.2, age is the most powerful, and for many diseases, particularly of the reproductive tract, sex equally or even more so. Obviously, neither age nor sex are direct causes of disease outcomes, but they are on the causal pathway. Age is a measure of time, and all causes need time to have their effects, some needing many decades. Paradoxically, however, these two factors are seldom studied as causal factors but as confounders. Before reading on, reflect on why this might be so.

In using epidemiological comparisons to spark *new* understanding of disease causation, it is essential that the populations compared are alike in *known* causal factors, of which age and sex are the most important. Hence, we see the almost routine use of age and sex matching or adjustment techniques in causal epidemiology (Chapters 4 and 8). This said, even for variables such as age and sex, the causal effects and mechanisms are complex and cannot usually be

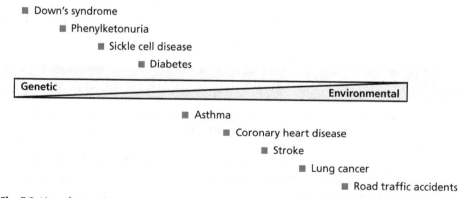

■ Down's syndrome

    ■ Phenylketonuria

        ■ Sickle cell disease

           ■ Diabetes

Genetic   Environmental

             ■ Asthma

                ■ Coronary heart disease

               ■ Stroke

                  ■ Lung cancer

                    ■ Road traffic accidents

Fig. 5.3 Line of causation: some examples of where disease/health problems lie.

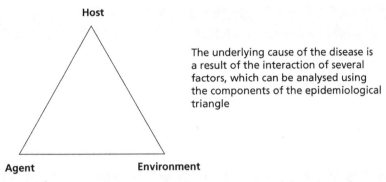

The underlying cause of the disease is a result of the interaction of several factors, which can be analysed using the components of the epidemiological triangle

Fig. 5.4 Triangle of causation.

Reproduced from Centers of Disease Control and Prevention (2012), '*Principles of Epidemiology in Public Health Practice, Third Edition: An Introduction to Applied Epidemiology and Biostatistics*', available from http://www.cdc.gov/ophss/csels/dsepd/ss1978/lesson1/section8.html, 29th Feb. 2016.

specified as biosocial mechanisms. For example, at any age, women have a lower incidence of cardiovascular diseases such as myocardial infarction (heart attack). This sex difference is well characterized, but the mechanisms have not been specified and are likely to involve a mix of genetic, behavioural, and social factors. The human genome project may lead to such mechanistic understanding.

Before reading on, do the exercise in Box 5.7.

The triangle is a useful model for analysing causal relationships and to derive public health strategies, as shown in Figures 5.5 and 5.6, for example, for the control of Legionnaires' disease. In this and other infectious diseases, the concept of the disease agent is central to causation, and usually a specific agent can be identified or assumed.

In explaining population differences in the pattern of disease, agent factors, examples of which are in Box 5.5, receive less attention than they deserve. In infectious disease epidemiology, characterizing the virulence of organisms is difficult and sometimes impossible, and in other diseases conceptualizing the cause as an agent is not easy. The issue of agent virulence is likely to be considered more carefully in future. The reason is that the genome of most pathogenic microorganisms is being mapped and understanding of gene variants associated with virulence is growing fast. The bacterium *Helicobacter pylori*, for example, is associated with severe inflammation and duodenal ulceration in 89 per cent of infections with the VacAsla strains and 20 per cent of infections with the vac s2 strain. Virulence genes can be identified and potentially can be removed to create organisms that are less pathogenic to humans.

Box 5.4 Causes of diseases: examples of host factors

Genetic inheritance
Age
Sex
Previous disability
Behaviours (such as smoking)
Height and weight
Cholesterol in blood

Box 5.5 Causes of diseases: examples of agent factors

Virulence of a microorganism
Serotype of microorganism
Antibiotic resistance of microorganism
Cigarette—tar content
Type of glass in motor car windscreen

Box 5.6 Causes of diseases: examples of environmental factors

Home overcrowding
Air composition
Workplace hygiene
Weather
Water composition
Food contamination
Animal/human contact
Cooling tower use
Radiation

Table 5.2 Control of Legionnaires' disease: triangle and levels of prevention

	Agent	**Host**	**Environment**
Primary	Design and hygiene of water systems to prevent growth of bacteria	Smoking cessation and general health improvement	Use and location of cooling towers to be regulated
Secondary	Hygiene to keep bacterial growth controlled	Nil—there is no way to pick up cases at the pre-symptom stage	Separate people from source once outbreak has occurred, e.g. if in a hospital ward
Tertiary	Once an outbreak has occurred, decontaminate the water system	Medical therapy	Close damaged cooling towers or water systems; or repair them

Box 5.7 Analysing disease using the triangle of causation

Reconsider your chosen health problems (Box 5.3) using the triangle of causation (Fig. 5.4). Also, think through the cause of disease X (Chapter 1, Box 1.7) using this model. Finally, think through how these problems could be controlled by actions targeted at the host, agent, and environment.

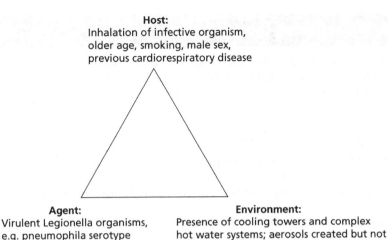

Fig. 5.5 Analysis of the causes of Legionnaires' disease: triangle of causation.

The concept of the disease agent also works with many non-infectious agents, for example, cigarettes, motor cars, and alcohol can be considered as the agents of disease and injury. A reduction of the tar content of cigarettes, and hence their virulence (in the literal sense of being toxic or hostile to health) could be responsible for some of the recent reduction of lung cancer incidence.

The interaction of the host, agent, and environment is rarely understood. For example, the effect of cigarette smoking is substantially greater in poor people than in rich people. The reason is unclear. It may be that there is an interaction between the agent (cigarettes), host factors such as nutritional status, and environmental factors such as air quality. These ideas are illustrated as follows in the simpler context of Legionnaires' disease.

Legionnaires' disease is a pneumonia (an inflammation of the lungs) that presents with some atypical features. It results from the inhalation, by susceptible people, of virulent organisms belonging to the genus *Legionellaceae* (legionellas for short). The organisms that cause Legionnaires'

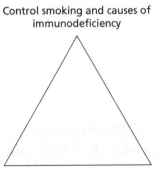

Fig. 5.6 Analysis of the control of Legionnaires' disease: triangle of causation.

Box 5.8 Reflection on the value of models

Consider how your thinking on the cause of Legionnaires' disease has changed because of the analysis in Figures 5.5 and 5.6, and the analysis you conducted on the diseases you chose in Box 5.3. What has been the additional value of employing this kind of model?

---

disease are environmentally acquired. The causal microorganism is found in most natural waters and is usually harmless. It is, therefore, a simplification to say that this normally harmless bacterium is *the* cause of Legionnaires' disease. Such a view could lead to erroneous, costly, and ineffective action to control this disease through futile attempts to eliminate this widely distributed organism from water.

The underlying cause of Legionnaires' disease lies in the creation by humans of water systems which permit the organism to thrive and be aerosolized at sufficient concentration to cause human disease. The ageing of the population, the presence of immunocompromized people, and people who impair their lung's defence mechanisms by smoking are also important causal factors. The bacterium, which is not normally a human pathogen, finds itself interacting with humans in this environment. The triangle of causality provides a framework for this type of reasoning, as illustrated in Figure 5.5. An understanding of the range of causes permits the development of a rational preventive strategy as shown in Figure 5.6. Before reading on, do the exercise in Box 5.8.

In a systematic analysis based on a model, as shown in Figures 5.5 and 5.6, attention is deflected from the microorganism as a specific cause, to the environment, host, and agent as interacting causes. This thinking broadens the control strategy. On current thinking the most effective approaches are to design better complex water systems, and to use hygiene and chemical measures to inhibit bacterial growth.

Table 5.2 shows how the epidemiological triangle can be combined with the schema of the levels of prevention to devise a comprehensive framework for thinking about possible preventive actions. Primary prevention is action to prevent the disease or problem from actually arising; secondary prevention is the early detection of the problem to prevent its damaging effects; and tertiary prevention is to contain, and if possible reverse, the damage already done. (As an aside, most clinicians and policy-makers working in clinical settings combine tertiary prevention with the secondary prevention category, calling it all secondary prevention. Epidemiologists and public health practitioners, in this context, usually conform to this simpler schema.) It is worth re-emphasizing that these frameworks aid systematic thinking by simplifying the problem into logical constituent parts. Before reading on, do the exercise in Box 5.9.

Figure 5.7 shows the wheel of causation. The principles behind this model are as for the triangle, but it emphasizes the unity of the interacting factors. The genetic make-up of the individual and its expression in the body (called the phenotype) is shown as the hub of the wheel, but enveloped

---

Box 5.9 Combining causal models and the levels of prevention

Think about the control of the three or four health problems you picked and disease X (Chapter 1, Box 1.7) using the triangle and the levels of prevention. Create a table from the information in Box 5.4 and a figure like Figure 5.6.

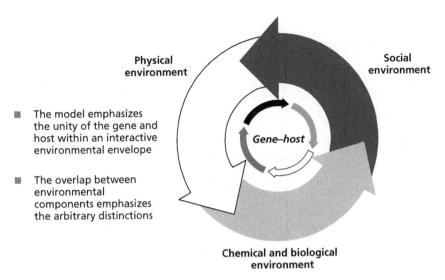

Physical environment

Social environment

- The model emphasizes the unity of the gene and host within an interactive environmental envelope

- The overlap between environmental components emphasizes the arbitrary distinctions

Gene–host

Chemical and biological environment

Fig. 5.7 Wheel of causation.

Reprinted, with minor adaptation, from *Epidemiology: An Introductory Text*, 2nd edition, Mausner JS and Kramer S, Philadelphia, PA: WB Saunders, Copyright © 1985, with permission from Elsevier.

within an interacting environment. This version of the model emphasizes the fact that the division of the environment into components is somewhat arbitrary.

In Figure 5.8 the wheel model is applied to phenylketonuria, the classic genetic disorder. Phenylketonuria is an autosomal single gene disease (autosomal means it is not on the sex chromosomes). As a result, an enzyme required to metabolize the dietary amino acid phenylalanine and turn it into tyrosine is deficient, and so phenylalanine accumulates in the blood, causing brain damage. Early diagnosis, usually through screening, and then following a diet low in phenylalanine can prevent the disease. The cause of this disease could be said to be a faulty gene. The cause

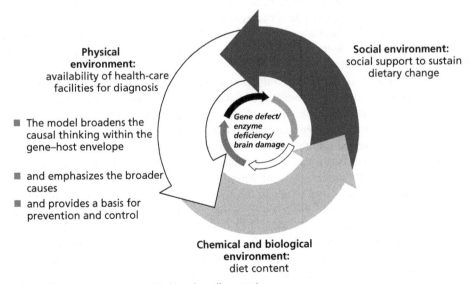

Physical environment: availability of health-care facilities for diagnosis

Social environment: social support to sustain dietary change

- The model broadens the causal thinking within the gene–host envelope

- and emphasizes the broader causes
- and provides a basis for prevention and control

Gene defect/ enzyme deficiency/ brain damage

Chemical and biological environment: diet content

Fig. 5.8 Wheel of causation applied to phenylketonuria.

- There is no single cause

- Causes of disease are interacting

- Disentangling causes is almost impossible

- Causality may be two way

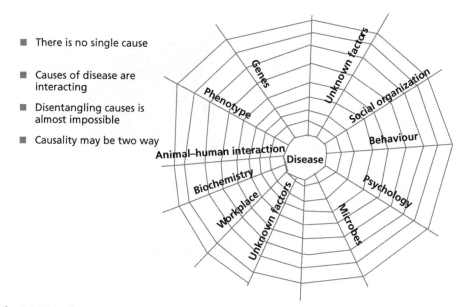

Fig. 5.9 Web of causation.

of the disease is, in reality, a combination of a faulty gene, exposure to a diet containing a high amount of phenylalanine (about 15% of the protein of most natural foods), and in the case of failure of diagnosis and dietary advice, a social environment unable to protect the child.

For many disorders such as coronary heart disease, and many cancers, our understanding of the causes is highly complex. Either the causes are truly complex, or equally likely, our understanding is too poor to permit clarity. These disorders are referred to as multifactorial or polyfactorial disorders. As discussed earlier, all disorders have several causes and where that is not the case, it is simply a matter of our definition. In disorders with multifactorial causation often no specific causes are known, many factors appear to be important, and mechanisms of causation are not apparent. (Usually, greater knowledge of causes brings simplification. For example, until recently gastric ulcer was thought of as a complex, multifactorial problem associated with stress. Now, we know the bacterium *Helicobacter pylori* lies at the heart of causation. Gastric ulcers are no longer thought of as multifactorial disorders.)

The complexity of these multifactorial diseases is not captured by the line, wheel, and triangle concepts (which remain useful nonetheless) and is better portrayed by the metaphor of the spider's web. In some portrayals, the web is shown as a highly schematized diagram, more like an electronic circuit or an underground transport map. Such portrayals tend to underestimate the complexity and overestimate the state of understanding. The web, as shown in Figure 5.9, emphasizes the interconnections among the postulated causes. This model, more than the others, indicates the potential for the disease to influence the causes and not just the other way around. For example, lack of exercise may be one of the causes of heart disease but the disease can also cause people to stop exercising (called reverse causality). The metaphor of the web permits the still broader causal question: where is the spider that spun the web? (after Krieger 1994). The question can be answered at a number of levels, for example, evolutionary biology, social structures, economics, and role of industries. This question chimes with Rose's concept of the causes of the causes (Chapter 2). The analysis of heart disease causation using the web of causation begins to illustrate the great complexity of this disease (see Fig. 5.10).

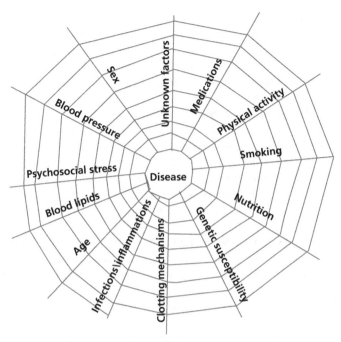

Fig. 5.10 Web of causation and coronary heart disease.

The purpose of models is to simplify reality and promote understanding. The web permits us to grasp the complexity of multifactorial diseases but the line, triangle, and the wheel help us to focus on their essentials and think through practical actions. Before reading on, do the exercise in Box 5.10.

Models provide a means of analysing causal pathways and a foundation for the application of epidemiological knowledge to public health action. Narrow causal thinking based on single causes, in contrast, can mislead epidemiologists into prematurely believing that a problem has been resolved and can seriously distort public health action. Models also help to lay out what is, and what is not, known. Causal models also help us to understand the ideas of necessary or sufficient causes, ideas that have been formalized in the interacting causal components model (causal pies) considered below.

5.3.2 Necessary and sufficient cause, proximal and distal cause, and the interacting component causes, models: individuals and populations

Epidemiological thinking on causality has been influenced by the concepts of necessary and sufficient cause. Mostly, this thinking relates to causation at the individual level (I will consider the

Box 5.10 Analysing disease using the wheel and web models

Review the health problems or diseases that you picked and disease X (Chapter 1, Box 1.7) using the wheel and web models.

implications for populations at the end of this section). *A Dictionary of Epidemiology* tells us that a necessary cause is a factor whose presence is required for the occurrence of the effect. It defines sufficient cause as a set of conditions, factors, or events sufficient to produce a given outcome. A factor, or a group of factors, whose presence leads to an effect is a sufficient cause, so some causes of diseases are said to be sufficient in themselves to induce disease while others are said to be necessary components in a larger jigsaw of causes. For example, the tubercle bacillus is required to cause tuberculosis but, alone, does not always cause it, so it is a necessary, not a sufficient, cause. In other words, a single factor does not cause this disease. This is, of course, the key message of the causal models discussed here.

The problem in practice is that a cause on its own rarely induces a disease in an individual except for extremely serious genetic defects. The necessary and sufficient causes model has theoretical value for analysing causes, but in epidemiology, as Susser (1977) points out, most causal factors are neither necessary nor sufficient, but contributory. Try the exercise in Box 5.11 before reading on.

Down's syndrome is the name given to a disorder where a person has a highly characteristic appearance (leading to the previous name, mongolism), and who will inevitably be mentally retarded because they have three chromosomes at the position of chromosome 21 instead of the normal two (trisomy 21). This genetic feature is a sufficient cause of Down's syndrome. In other words, this chromosome abnormality alone will lead to the characteristics that define Down's syndrome.

Sickle cell disease (two sickle cell gene alleles per cell) is a genetically inherited condition. The position is not quite the same as for Down's syndrome because the word disease leads to an expectation that the person has, or will develop, a health problem. The presence of sickle cell genes is a necessary cause of sickle cell disease. In milder cases especially, external stimuli such as infections are required to cause clinical disease. Here we have another example (phenylketonuria was discussed earlier) of genes being necessary, but not always sufficient causes of genetic diseases.

Scurvy occurs when there is insufficient vitamin C in the diet to maintain health, usually due to lack of fruit and vegetables. This does not occur in natural circumstances, but does when a restricted diet is taken, as in the past by sailors on long voyages in sailing ships, and nowadays by food-related problems or in the mentally disturbed. Vitamin C insufficiency is both a necessary and sufficient cause of scurvy. By definition, other diseases, several of which look like scurvy, are not scurvy unless there is a lack of vitamin C. Yet, dietary insufficiency of vitamin C is unnatural, so other factors, in practice, come into play.

For tuberculosis, exposure to the bacillus is necessary but not sufficient in most people, and in many people the organism is controlled in the host. For both tuberculosis and scurvy, contributory causes include poor socio-economic conditions. These increase both the risk of exposure to the necessary cause and, for tuberculosis, the likelihood of the organism establishing a clinically important infection.

Box 5.11 Necessary and sufficient causes for some disorders

Consider the causes of one or all of Down's syndrome (trisomy 21), sickle cell disease, tuberculosis, scurvy, phenylketonuria, and lung cancer. If the cause is sufficient, its presence alone would induce the disease and if it is necessary, the disease would not occur in its absence. What do you think: are the causes sufficient and are they necessary?

For phenylketonuria, the necessary cause is a genetic defect and that together with a diet containing normal amounts of phenylalanine is sufficient (Fig. 5.8).

For lung cancer tobacco smoke, by far and away the most important causal factor is neither necessary nor sufficient, for there are many other causes. Some smokers do not develop the disease and some non-smokers do.

This analysis shows the strengths and weaknesses of the necessary/sufficient cause concept. When a specific cause of disease is known it can be incorporated into its definition. The specific cause becomes necessary by definition. For multifactorial diseases, at least at present, there are no known necessary causes. The example of lung cancer illustrates this well. In practice, except for unusual or unhelpful scenarios (e.g. a bolt of lightning, or falling off a cliff), there are no single sufficient factors that inevitably lead to chronic diseases or death. Ageing (and birth!) is probably the only sufficient cause of death. The concept of sufficient causes has, therefore, veered from single causes to groups of causes.

Rothman's interacting component causes model (Fig. 5.11) has emphasized that the causes of disease comprise a constellation of factors. It has broadened the sufficient cause concept to be a minimal set of conditions which together inevitably produce the disease. Different combinations of these factors may cause the disease. Figure 5.11 is a simplified version of Rothman's ideas. Three combinations of factors (ABC, BED, AEC) are shown here as sufficient causes of the disease. Each of the constituents of the causal 'pie' is necessary, and hence contributes to 100 per cent of the risk of disease attributed to that particular combination of causes. The factors are conceived to act in a biological sequence, which determines the period between the beginning of causal action and the initiation of disease. It follows that control of the disease could be achieved by removing one of the components in each 'pie'. If there were a factor common to all 'pies', the disease would be eliminated by removing that factor alone. In this case removing factor A would remove all the disease caused by the first and third constellation of causes. This mode of reasoning, and model, is hard to apply to specific diseases but has considerable theoretical value.

A sequence of causes can be considered in terms of time, and also in terms of space. Causes that are close to the individual—in terms of time or space—are sometimes referred to as proximal causes, in the sense of 'near to'. Those that are distant are called distal causes in the sense of 'away from'. To give an example, proximal causes of lung cancer would be smoking cigarettes and exposure to radiation. Distal causes would be poor diet, poverty, or tobacco farming. Distal causes are sometimes referred to as upstream.

Each of the three components of the interacting constellations of causes (ABC, BED, AEC) are in themselves sufficient and each is necessary

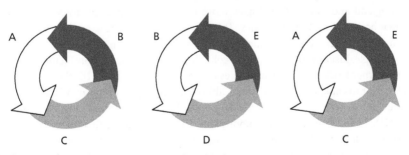

Fig. 5.11 Interacting component causes.

The problem with these complex models, in practice, is that we do not have the knowledge to define even a sufficient constellation of causes, that is, we cannot define the 'pies' in Figure 5.11. The components of the pies, as sufficient causes, must be acting differently than if they were separate (when they do not cause disease). There is, therefore, a modification of the biological effect (i.e. biological interaction that leads to disease). The model is, therefore, useful in thinking about the issues discussed in section 5.4.

The model is also pertinent to thinking about the strength of the association (section 5.6.2) and relative and attributable risk (sections 8.4 and 8.6). Interested readers should consult Rothman's writings.

Epidemiology is a population science but the work has to have meaning and applications for individuals, otherwise it would be of little or no use to clinicians and others, including health promoters, when dealing with patients. Clinicians apply probabilities in the management of the individual. It is true that sufficient causes can rarely be defined at the individual level. This is not true, though it is seldom discussed, at the population level. We know many single causes are sufficient to alter the incidence of disease at the population level and we can predict the consequence with great certainty. So, at the individual level smoking cigarettes is not a necessary or sufficient cause of lung cancer. At the population level, it is not a necessary cause of a rise in lung cancer, but alone, it is a sufficient cause of a rise in the incidence of lung cancer. Therefore, the mostly theoretical concepts of necessary and sufficient causes can find practical and firmly grounded applications at the population level.

5.4 Susceptibility, risk/effect modification, and interaction

We have already considered, briefly, the idea of disease susceptibility, for example, in the extreme case where some diseases rarely, or never, occur because humans have no susceptibility to them. Even for human diseases, exposure to the causes is often common but the disease is rare. The fact that some people who are exposed to the known causes get disease, and others do not, implies there are other factors that determine the outcome, as emphasized by all the models we discussed.

Whether we consider trivial problems such as the common cold, or serious diseases such as coronary heart disease (CHD), it is clear that some individuals are more susceptible than others. Epidemiology cannot help with understanding such individual differences. The same variable susceptibility, however, applies to populations, where epidemiology can shed light. In the case of the common cold the reasons tend to be fairly obvious: poor populations living in overcrowded conditions are more susceptible to being exposed to the common cold virus, may get a larger dose, and may have lower resistance and therefore are more likely to get ill.

For CHD it is not at all clear why, to take one of many potential comparisons, Indian-born women in England and Wales should have more CHD than predominantly White European-origin women born in England and Wales. This observation seems real, and not a data artefact. In fact, on first principles we would expect the opposite because of less smoking in Indian-born women for example. Just as with the common cold, there must be one or more factors that increase Indian-born women's risk. Typically, in studies of ethnic variations in CHD, the known risk factors do not appear to explain such differences, although at least part of this may be due to difficulties in measuring risk factors precisely. There may be unknown factors that cause these differences in risk of CHD. Such factors may even modify the risk of CHD through known risk factors; for example, hypertension may be a more potent cause of CHD in one ethnic group than in another. If that were true, the question of why this is remains. At this point, speculation is usually required, for example, unknown genetic variations, or life-course effects, possibly related to fetal development that alter susceptibility to the effects of high blood pressure.

The factor that influences susceptibility is known as a risk modifier or effect modifier, and there is said to be an interaction between the study exposure and the effect modifier on outcome. Strictly speaking, it is an association modifier but the word *effect* is now embedded. Interaction is a word from statistics and is used, mostly, loosely and synonymously with effect modification, but care is needed in the use of these terms as will be considered later. Risk and effect is best judged in epidemiology by how the incidence of disease is changed by exposure to the risk factor (Chapter 7), and it is quantified using either absolute or relative measures of risk (Chapters 7 and 8).

Risk or effect modification is different from confounding. It occurs when two factors reduce or increase risk. Before reading on, do the exercise in Box 5.12.

The possible combined effects are that the coexistence of these factors can lead to the addition of the individual cumulative incidence or relative risks, less than the addition of the two (antagonism, or negative interaction), or more than the addition of the two (synergy, or positive interaction). Our default situation, and expectation on first principles, is that at least the two risks will be combined. We call this the additive model of effect modification. There are good reasons for basing biomedical and public health research and practice on this model (readers should consult Kenneth Rothman (2012) for the arguments but be aware that this is still a controversial area). In this case, if there is no effect modification or interaction, the cumulative incidence in this population is 100 (baseline) plus 200 (excess from smoking), plus 200 (excess from alcohol)—that is, 500 per 10 000. This gives a relative risk of five. If our research shows a different result—say 800 per 10 000 or 300 per 10 000, and it is not a result of chance, error, or bias (including confounding), then we have risk modification on the additive scale. The two risk factors, smoking and alcohol, are then combining to give a result other than that expected on the additive effect. We can say that the presence of one factor has modified the effect of the other.

A simple definition of effect modification is this: the association between a risk factor and an outcome differs in subgroups of the population. In this example, the association between smoking and cancer X has been altered by the presence of alcohol, and vice versa, and this alteration occurs on the additive scale in a subgroup of the population, where both risk factors are present.

Box 5.12 Potential effects of smoking cigarettes and drinking alcohol on a hypothetical cancer X

When two (or more) causal risk factors coexist, what is the likely effect on the outcome? For example, say that smoking cigarettes triples the risk of cancer X, and drinking alcohol also triples the risk. What is the risk of cancer X in a population where people both smoke cigarettes and drink alcohol? Let us say that the cumulative incidence of disease in people who do not drink or smoke is 100 per 10 000 people. In those that smoke, the risk is 300 per 10 000 people, 200 extra cases per 10 000 people being contributed by smoking (relative risk 3, excess relative risk 2, where excess relative risk is relative risk minus the baseline risk, which is by definition 1), and similarly for those that drink alcohol (200 extra cases per 10 000 people, relative risk 3, excess relative risk 2). Assume the four groups of people—those who do not smoke or drink, those who smoke, those who drink, and those who both smoke and drink—are identical in every other respect, that is, there is no confounding. Now imagine we have 10 000 people who all drink alcohol and smoke cigarettes. What are the possible combined effects in this group? You may wish to prepare an appropriate table including the cumulative incidences and relative risks to test your thinking, before looking at Table 5.3(a), which summarizes the text that follows.

The two risks might have large modifying effects, perhaps even so much that the effects are multiplicative or more; that is, the two factors of smoking and alcohol together increase relative risk by ninefold ($1 \cdot 3 \cdot 3$; the 1 signifying baseline risk, in the absence of the two risk factors) and not by fivefold ($1 + 2 + 2$). If a third factor (say a gene variant) also tripled relative risk, people with the three factors would have a 27-fold risk ($1 \cdot 3 \cdot 3 \cdot 3$) and not a sevenfold risk as for the addition of baseline and excess risks ($1 + 2 + 2 + 2$).

In fact, this multiplication effect is often seen. As a result, sometimes statistical interaction is defined as a departure from the expectation of multiplication of risks. Investigators can conclude, sometimes without meaning to because as we will see the claim is not tenable, that there is no effect modification, because there is no departure from multiplication of risks. Logically, if there is no interaction on the additive scale then there must be interaction on the multiplicative scale (negative interaction), and if there is positive interaction on the multiplicative scale, then there must be interaction on the additive scale also.

The combined effects might be even bigger than 27. Then we would have effect modification demonstrable even using statistical methods that are based on the multiplication of risks. It is, however, exceptional to demonstrate such large interactive effects in epidemiology.

These additive and multiplicative considerations in relation to risk are important to the development of research questions, study design, analysis of data, the choice of statistical methods and analysis programmes, and interpretation of data. Statistical models sometimes assume a multiplicative model of risks. They may use logarithms, where addition is equal to multiplication, for example, for logarithms on base 10, where 0 is 1 in ordinary numbers, and 1 is 10 in ordinary numbers, the addition of the logarithms 1 plus 1 is equivalent to 100 in ordinary numbers. (The multiple logistic regression model and the Poisson regression model are examples. The multiple logistic regression model uses natural not decimal, logarithms.) Other models, for example, multiple linear regression, do not use logarithms.

In epidemiology and statistics, the concept of effect modification is increasingly discussed as interaction. Interaction is often demonstrable on the additive scale (relating to the biological and public health concept of interaction) but rarely on the multiplicative scale.

In the classic and most commonly cited example of effect modification (interaction) between smoking (tenfold increased risk) and asbestos (fivefold increased risk), the combined effect on lung cancer is multiplicative with a combined greater than 50-fold increased relative risk (compared with 15.1, i.e. 1 plus 9.9 plus 4.2, on the additive model). This result, summarized in Table 5.3 (b), has been shown by Hammond *et al.* (1979). If this interaction had been tested out using statistical analysis based on the multiplication of risks as the standard approach, investigators could have concluded that there was no effect modification. Such a general conclusion would be wrong because there is interaction on the additive model. If the combined effect had been substantially more than 50, there would also have been interaction on a multiplicative scale. The important point is that the risk of lung cancer in smokers who are exposed to asbestos is much higher than in those not so exposed.

One difference between confounding and effect modification is that the exposure–outcome association would be similar in all levels (strata) of a confounder but that the exposure–outcome association differs in different levels (strata) of an effect modifier. Confounding is an obstacle to proper interpretation that should be controlled for but effect modification is of causal and public health interest and should not be controlled. (A variable can act as both a confounder and an effect modifier in different circumstances, e.g. age.)

Table 5.3 Effect modification for (a) cancer X (imaginary) and (b) lung cancer (real)

Exposure	Cancer X cumulative incidence/10000		Relative risk	
(a) Imaginary data	Actual	Excess*	Actual	Excess
No smoking, no alcohol**	100	0	1	0
Smoking, no alcohol	300	200	3	2
Alcohol, no smoking	300	200	3	2
Smoking and alcohol				
No effect modification on the additive model	500	400	5	4
Effect modification on the additive model (example)	800	700	8	7
(b) Based on classic example (Hammond *et al.*)	Lung cancer Death rates/100 000		Relative risk	
	Actual	Excess	Actual	Excess
No smoking or asbestos	11.3	0	1	0
Smoking, no asbestos	58.4	47.1	5.2	4.2
Asbestos, no smoking	122.6	111.3	10.9	9.9
Asbestos and smoking				
- no effect modification (as expected) if no additive model interaction	169.7***	158.4	15.1	14.1
- with effect modification on additive model (as found)	601.6	590.3	53.2	52.2

*Over baseline

**Baseline

*** 169.7 = 11.3 + 47.1 + 111.3

As we will discuss in Chapter 8, there are two main ways of presenting risk data—by absolute/actual risk, and relative/comparative risk. In discussing interactions, we should clarify which approach and analysis we intend to pursue, our prior definition of interaction, and the causal model we are assuming. In the classic example discussed just now involving smoking and asbestos in lung cancer, the interaction is clear if the causal model is an additive one. If, however, the chosen causal model presumes a multiplication of risks, then there is no important departure from that. The latter is an awkward interpretation, as this is the prime example of interaction, in the sense of effect modification, in epidemiology.

The surprising conclusion of this is there is always interaction from a statistical perspective. It is vital, therefore, for researchers to tell us how they examined interaction, why they did so, and on what scale there was interaction. Unfortunately, this essential and simple information is only exceptionally provided (this can sometimes be inferred from the kind of statistical analysis done). My recommendation to readers is to think of interaction as a departure from additive risks (following Rothman's advice (Rothman, 2012)): Rothman recommends stratified analysis to spot effect modification, prior to statistical analysis of interactions. That way examination of effect modification is not just a by-product of analysis.

Interaction can also occur when the outcome is a continuous variable, for example, blood pressure or cholesterol levels. The current trend is for very large studies and this is driven by the large samples required for studying gene–environment interactions.

The promise of the new genetics is to clarify the nature of individual and group-level susceptibility to diseases, and the variable response to treatments. Gene variants can act as effect modifiers/interactive factors of the relationship between an environmental exposure and an outcome. The problem is that studies that can accurately assess interaction need to be very large, especially when effects are small (as with most gene variants). Mostly, studies that report there is no interaction are too small to reach such a conclusion, and many others have applied the wrong conceptual approach. If there is heterogeneity in the effects of a risk factor within populations, as is highly likely, there must be effect modification/interaction and vice versa. Failure to seek or notice risk modification can lead to a false measure of population risk and the possibility of missing an important finding, at least for population subgroups. The importance, in practice, of effect modification/interactions is under debate.

Causal graph methods that are helpful in data gathering, analysis, and interpretation have become available in epidemiology (mainly developed and advanced in other disciplines), and these are considered next. At present, these methods do not incorporate effect modification, and are being developed for this.

5.5 Causal graphs: introducing the directed acyclic graph

A diagram (or graph) that makes explicit the postulated relations between variables is recommended. Producing such a diagram is difficult because it requires considerable understanding, including of the biology, of the topic under study. This step is a component of a disciplined approach to research that includes prior statement of a fully articulated scientific hypothesis (not merely the statistical null hypothesis) and a detailed analysis plan prepared in advance. With a hypothesis, causal diagram, and an analysis plan, we can assess whether the results of the research fit with our prior presumed causal understanding. If yes, that increases confidence that our prior understanding was correct. If not, then it motivates us to alter and improve our hypothesis and causal diagram. This can then be checked with new research. The field of causal diagrams in epidemiology is large, complex, and is developing fast. One important and increasingly used form of causal diagram is called the directed acyclic graph (DAG). The field has been advanced by, among others, Judea Pearl, who is a professor of computing sciences and statistics. Pearl has claimed in his book *Causality* (second edition) that causality has been mathematized. While this claim is not (yet) true for epidemiology and related population health and medical sciences, it merits examination.

The DAG is based on graph theory in mathematics and can be written as an algebraic equation (in a form known as a structural equation model). Equally, algebraic equations can be expressed as DAGs. This property allows DAGs to be used both for expressing potential causal pathways, and for guiding and interpreting data analysis. The field of DAGs has vocabulary that is different but related to that of epidemiology. Some of this vocabulary is in Table 5.4, which also re-expresses it in similar epidemiological terms. The DAG uses lines and arrows (Table 5.5) that follow formal rules.

Assume we have a relationship between two variables (A and B) that we believe is potentially causal. Before examining the DAG approach, we will look at this relationship in general terms. To make this less abstract let us name A as the variable physical inactivity (PI) and the outcome B as coronary heart disease (CHD). It is known that physical inactivity can cause CHD, but also that CHD can cause inactivity. This complex relationship can be designated as circular:

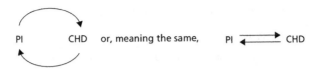

Epidemiology simplifies this kind of problem by examining the possibilities separately. Probably the best way to do this is by studying young people long before they get the outcome, here CHD, which occurs in later life. Therefore, we could, for example, consider the relationship between physical inactivity in early life, childhood, adolescence, and early adulthood and the outcome

Table 5.4 Terminology commonly used in DAGs in relation to similar or related terminology in epidemiology

DAG terminology	Epidemiology terminology for similar ideas
Ancestors	Distal causes
Back door pathway	Confounding variable(s) creating the association
Block/blocking	Eliminating an association through, for example, adjusting, stratifying, etc.
Blocked path	An association that has been eliminated as it has been controlled for, e.g. by adjusting for confounders
Blocking	Presence of confounding or selection bias
Child	Effect, outcome
Collapsibility	The measure of the association is not affected whether examining stratified or overall, actual (crude) rates
Collider	A variable that is caused by both the exposure and outcome under study
Collider stratification bias	See M-bias
Conditioning	General term to include stratification, standardization, and adjustment in a model (conditioning means holding a variable constant)
Descendants	Effects on potential causal path including mediators
D-connected	The postulated causal path is open (see open path and path)
D-separation or D-unconnected (directional separation)	The postulated causal path is closed
Endogenous selection	See M-bias
Identification	Analysis of associations to separate error/bias/confounding from causal effects
M-bias	Berkson's bias/selection bias. It arises from, for example, adjusting for a collider
Nodes	Variables
Open path	Potential causal relationship, i.e. association
Parent	Proximal cause
Path	The route to potential causality, i.e. from A to B
Vertices	Variables

Table 5.5 Symbols used in the construction of directed acyclic graphs (DAGs)

Symbol	Name of symbol
————	Edge. This edge is undirected, i.e. there is no arrow to give the direction
>	The direction indicator for an edge
⟶	Directed edge (arrow) indicating association (arrow can be thickened to denote stronger association)
X	Variable or in some notations variables conditioned on X (the practice of putting variables in a box is not always followed in epidemiology)
. . . .	Association induced by collider bias
< · · · · · >	Bidirected edge, denoting an association induced by confounding (the line can be solid)

CHD in middle age and beyond. In this case we postulate and study that physical activity leads to CHD i.e. PI → CHD. It is not plausible that CHD in middle age leads to inactivity earlier. So in doing this, we have simplified our research.

In contrast to this example from a chronic disease, nearly all infectious diseases have the simple A → B relationship where A is the infectious agent and B is the outcome; for example, A is the measles virus and B is the illness. It is not plausible that measles illness causes the acquisition of the measles virus.

So, for causal analysis we usually start by simplifying the matter under study. Simplifying means the construction of models (in the same way that an architect may create a model building). The DAG is a model. The equation describing the DAG is also a model. The DAG needs specification of exposure (A) and outcome (B) and, ideally, on the ancestors and descendants (see Table 5.4) of A and B.

A relationship between A and B can be expressed as A – B, so A and B are connected by a line that we call an edge. The variables are called nodes. Does A cause B or does B cause A (the problem of reverse causation)? As it is designed to help causal analysis, the DAG method does not permit two-headed (bidirectional) arrows. The word acyclic means there are no cycles in the graph. When complex cyclical relationships are to be studied, other types of causal graphs need to be used (theory is available). Of course, we could create two DAGs, one for A → B and the other for A ← B. We could plan and run the analyses separately. Let us assume that our interest is in A causes B, then we can express that as

$$A \rightarrow B$$

If A → B, it could either increase B (positive association) or decrease B (negative association). The DAG can be used to show this, for example, by having one colour for positive relationships and another for negative ones or plus/minus signs. Clearly, the researchers need a high level of knowledge to set out these kinds of decisions in advance.

Let us assume that our understanding of the relationship between physical inactivity and CHD is not based on our reading of fabricated, seriously biased, or chance research results (i.e. that it is a reasonable proposition).

What else do we need to consider in this DAG to make it informative? First, we must consider the possibility that a third variable (C) is creating the relationship A → B, that is, there is confounding (known as a backdoor path in DAG terms). The confounding factor could be age, sex, socio-economic status, or similar variables.

This can be expressed as

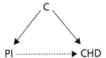

Here the dashed line denotes the possibility of a confounded relationship. As we already know if we adjust for C, and C is a confounding factor creating this relationship, then the association between A and B will greatly reduce or even disappear. The dashed line will disappear. This is described as closing the backdoor path.

If we control for a confounding variable and the association between A and B disappears, we can redraw the DAG either without an arrow between A and B, or with a dotted line between A and B to signify that relationship is confounded.

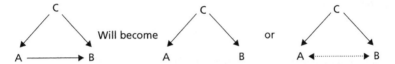

When both our variables of interest are associated with a third variable, presumed causally in that direction, this variable is called a collider. If there is a collider D, then we have

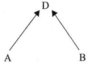

If we control for collider D, we induce a spurious association between A and B, which is denoted as

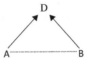

The dotted line has no arrows, which distinguishes it from confounding.

It is possible that both physical inactivity and CHD cause an effect that is important in the relationship, for example, social isolation (I)

So

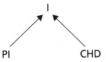

I (social isolation) is called a collider. The collider blocks the path from P1 to CHD but adjusting for it opens it up, the opposite of adjusting for confounding (closing the back door path). Here a biased association may be created between PI and CHD because of adjustment for social isolation. This is not at all an unfamiliar concept (even though it is still an unfamiliar term) in epidemiology, but the use of DAGs has made it clearer. We have already discussed this in Chapter 4 with the example of Berkson's bias. In this example, let us assume that, in fact, there is no association between PI and CHD as in the above diagram (no line connecting the two). If we condition on the collider I, we would hold it constant. One of several ways of doing that is to study only socially isolated people, that is, stratify. In this group, there will be an association between PI and CHD, if these two variables are among the causes of social isolation, which seems plausible. The term *collider stratification bias* includes a range of biases that have varying names in epidemiology (e.g. Berkson's bias).

In analysis, our aim is to help separate non-causal and causal associations so we can see we must not control for colliders (or their descendants or ancestors) and mediators (or their ancestors or descendants), but we should control for confounders. If the study is free of error/bias, and all confounding factors are included, then the DAG reflects a causal structure and the resulting analysis reflects a causal relationship between A and B. Of course, this ideal state is not actually achieved.

We may ask how physical inactivity causes CHD. One possibility, among others, is that it does so through obesity (O).

$$PI \rightarrow O \rightarrow CHD$$

Obesity might, for example, work through raised cholesterol (CH).

$$PI \rightarrow O \rightarrow CH \rightarrow CHD$$

Obesity and cholesterol would, therefore, be postulated to be intermediate variables (synonym, mediators). If, however, we adjust statistically for the intermediate variable O and the relationship between PI and CHD remains completely unaltered then it is not, actually, acting as an intermediate variable. If the association weakens or disappears, then the case for O being a mediator is strengthened. However, this interpretation requires that the outcome, here CHD, does not cause the intermediate (i.e. obesity), which common sense tells us is plausible but we make the assumption this in not true. (In our DAG we may either use different colours for the lines/arrows for different kinds of variables, or use different line widths or use broken lines.)

Therefore, our revised causal proposition might be that after adjusting for potential confounding factors, we think physical inactivity leads to CHD through obesity and cholesterol.

So, this DAG will be

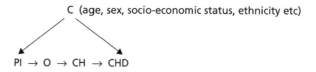

We can see the DAG has helped to think through and clearly express, in a way that everyone can understand, complex relationships between confounders (C), the exposure/risk factor (PI), intermediate variables (O, CH) and the outcome (CHD). Our knowledge and data sets both tend to be incomplete, so this is a provisional model. The model should also include uncertainties. Uncertainties can be added, for example, as U for unmeasured variables and error terms.

If we know of variables that are potentially important in the relationship but have not been measured, they should be added to the DAG so we can immediately see the limitations of the study. So, for example, it may not be physical inactivity that is important but the fact that physically inactive persons may spend less time outdoors, thereby being less exposed to sunshine or to the social benefits of meeting neighbours and people on the street. These could be unmeasured confounders or mediators. Our study may well have no data, either because these variables were forgotten, omitted deliberately, or most probably it was not feasible to collect the data, possibly for reasons of time and cost. The DAG helps by being explicit on the limitations of the causal analysis.

Again, these unmeasured variables could be picked out using a different colour or different kind of line. Here, these are shown as unmeasured confounders in *light grey*. These unmeasured factors are treated here as confounders, but they may actually be on the causal path. Investigators need knowledge and judgement to decide where the variables belong.

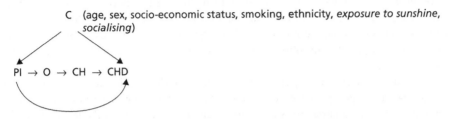

C (age, sex, socio-economic status, smoking, ethnicity, *exposure to sunshine, socialising*)

PI → O → CH → CHD

Of course, physical inactivity may have effects on CHD either directly (without mediators as shown by the direct arrow) or through a completely different pathway than obesity (e.g. through endothelial dysfunction). The effect of the direct and indirect paths can be quantified. This extra, endothelial pathway, could be added (but this is beyond our purposes here). There may be confounding in the relationships between the intermediate variables and both exposure and outcome, which needs to be considered. Ideally, the DAG (and statistical model) should include confounders not only between PI and CHD, but also between other variables on the path.

The DAG is also telling us an important story about the variables that are not shown. The DAG is telling us that the investigators do not think these are important in this particular causal path. For example, diet is not mentioned. If that is not an oversight, then we can deduce the investigators think that diet has no relevance here. If so, excluding diet is the correct decision. Variables that do not connect to causal and confounding variables on the DAG should be excluded, even if they connect to the outcome through some other causal path, for example, smoking cigarettes and CHD. Ideally, investigators would explain why variables like this were not included. DAGs do not include statistical interaction, although this area is being developed.

A variable may be a moderator, mediator, and a confounder variable (e.g. socio-economic position). The elements of such a variable that are thought to be moderators or mediators need to be separated from those thought to be confounders, and should be labelled differently, for example, SEP1, (income), SEP2 (education), SEP3 (housing tenure), etc.

Software is available for drawing DAGs, for example, DAGitty (www.dagitty.net). This software uses colour coding with confounders in red, mediators in green, and no effect in grey. Currently, a variable can only have one status in this software. The DAG software shows which variables are, and which are not, essential for measuring the association between A and B.

Exemplar 5.1 illustrates a study that shows how the process works.

Exemplar 5.1: Factors associated with prediabetes (Bardenheier *et al.* 2013)

Bardenheier *et al.* used the cross-sectional United States National Health and Nutrition Examination Surveys (NHANES) 2001–2006 to test a hypothetical causal model for prediabetes in people aged 50 years or more. NHANES had data on 2230 eligible people without diabetes. The study was motivated by observing that while many risk factors for prediabetes had been identified, they had not been examined simultaneously as a coherent system or model. They identified a statistical method called structural equation modelling (see glossary) as a way of testing a hypothetical model. Their hypothetical models before and after analysis can be examined in their original coloured format at this URL: http://care.diabetesjournals.org/content/36/9/2655.full.pdf

The variables that were measured were shown in rectangles, and those that were not measured but reflected in or derived from observed variables were shown in ovals and are known as latent variables. The arrows indicated the postulated direction of association.

Based on the investigators' knowledge, itself reflecting prior research, 10 major variables were identified as either direct or indirect predictors on the causal path to prediabetes. Arrows showed 27 paths from these variables to the outcome. Some of the variables were composite ones based on several measured variables, for example, socio-economic position (a latent variable; SEP), while others were single (and therefore measured); for example, high blood pressure.

The model was assessed using structural equation modelling with factor and path analysis. Factor analysis can group interrelated variables (factors are the lowest common denominators for a number). Path analysis assesses the direct and indirect effects of the factors identified. The factor analysis approach reduced the number of individual variables, which has statistical advantages, as well as easing examination of the model.

In the model, there were variables that had no number (i.e. age, race/ethnicity, and sex). These were identified as potential confounding variables. They were not entered as potential direct effects, while family history was. The authors justified this as follows: 'Because age, sex, and race/ethnicity are strong, non-modifiable confounders related to most of the other factors in the model, their direct effects, while included, are not shown in the graphic of the final model. Although family history is non-modifiable, it is specific to diabetes risk and therefore is examined as a factor of interest.'

The analysis used advanced statistics that is both beyond the scope of the book and unnecessary to understand the key points.

The structural equation model indicated that in the SEP factor (group of variables) the number of family members did not contribute. In the poor diet factor, saturated fats and processed meats did not contribute. The latent constructs were shown to be correlated with each other. To create a model fitting the data better, total cholesterol and BMI were removed. Then the direct effect of diet on high-density lipoprotein (HDL) cholesterol was dropped. Age, sex, and ethnicity were shown to have direct effects on most factors.

The model was reconstructed with the 10 postulated directly causal variables.

Concluding remarks

The outcome of prediabetes is not a complex one compared to many chronic diseases or syndromes such as CHD or asthma. The paper shows, however, how complex the putative causal relationships are. Yet, the authors have also taken a pragmatic decision to treat three major variables (age, sex, ethnicity) as confounding variables, rather than as direct effects or intermediate variables. This simplifies the thinking greatly. The great merit of this paper is the immense effort the authors have expended in creating a credible, theory-based causal diagram. They have then used data to assess the model. The data suggested a slightly different model that provided the best fit between the postulated model and the calculated model. The authors have, after this mammoth effort, made no claims to having produced a definitive model. Rather, recognizing the limitations of their data, in particular the cross-sectional design, they have urged further examination of the model, but with cohort data. They have also showed in what respect this model aligns with the published literature. This paper exemplifies how causal epidemiology might be done.

In my view, all papers working with associations aiming to contribute to the causal basis of a subject should provide the causal diagram based on current evidence (in the introduction) and the refined version following their research (in the discussion), as Bardenheier and colleagues did.

Source: data from Bardenheier *et al.* (2013) A novel use of structural equation models to examine factors associated with prediabetes among adults aged 50 years and older: National Health and Nutrition Examination Survey 2001–2006. *Diabetes Care*, Volume 36, Issue 9, pp. 2655–62.

DAGs and related diagrams help to design studies and to analyse data. By pointing to data which are needed, they can make research more efficient. Using DAGs is also changing basic concepts in epidemiology, an example being the realization that adjusting for a collider can cause bias, that is, a spurious association. If a variable is both a collider and a confounder then adjustment for it removes confounding, but can induce bias. Obviously, stratifying a sample into separate groups is a selection bias, but so is selecting a sample (except perfectly randomly), or non-response, missing data, subgroup analysis, or adjusting for a variable in regression analysis. So, selection bias (and hence colliders) are unavoidable in the practice of epidemiology.

The strength of the DAG approach is that it openly presents the assumptions guiding the analysis and interpretation of the data. The DAG, unlike the statistical analysis, is a causal model, albeit a postulated one.

DAGs can be very complicated so variables can be grouped, for example, as demographic variables, or as behaviour-related ones to help simplify the diagram.

The output is not a causal truth, but an opportunity for the investigators to assess whether the data fit the model. If there is a close match with most of the variances explained, then it would be reasonable to infer that the DAG is reflecting a causal structure, at least as portrayed in these data. The ultimate goal is to strip out bias and error, so what is left must be causal. This process is called identification.

The field of causal diagrams is enriching epidemiology and we are seeing these diagrams increasingly, though mostly in specialist journals. They have not, however, 'mathematized causality' (a claim by Judea Pearl) in epidemiology, which is still based on judgement as discussed in section 5.6. DAGs have the potential to contribute substantially to the formation of such judgements.

An even more complex approach is the logic diagram, which tries to produce a model that shows the full complexity of reality including non-causal, non-linear relationships. One of the best known of these diagrams is that produced by the Foresight Report on obesity (see http:// www.noo.org.uk/NOO_about_obesity/causes). (Government Office for Science 2007).

5.6 Guidelines (sometimes erroneously called criteria) for epidemiological reasoning on cause and effect

5.6.1 Comparison of epidemiological and other guidelines for causal reasoning

Turning epidemiological data into an understanding of cause and effect is challenging and perhaps the most difficult aspect of the subject. Unfortunately, there is a widespread tendency to reach easy, but often premature or wrong conclusions. The commonest problem is either to declare, or interpret, an association as causal when it quite possibly a result of confounding or reverse causality. This problem may be becoming more common, partly because of media involvement. It is not easy to present the nuances of data interpretation in a news sound bite or even press release.

Conclusions with strong caveats are not newsworthy, and, indeed, may not attract the attention of the top journals either.

To convince colleagues and the public, epidemiologists need an explicit mode of reasoning. Scientists, like all other human beings, rely on intuition in evaluating evidence and making judgements. Einstein intuitively understood the theory of relativity years before he published it and before there was empirical evidence to support his findings. The theorems of the mathematical genius Srinivasan Ramanujan were intuitive and many have yet to be resolved, although they are generally accepted as correct based on precedent. These are only two of many examples. The lesson for epidemiology is that subjective judgements on cause and effect should not be dismissed but tested empirically. Epidemiologists place much emphasis on the evaluation of empirical data, and have devised (and adopted from other disciplines) so-called criteria for causality. *Criteria* is an inappropriate word, as it encourages a checklist approach; *guidelines* is better.

The use of such guidelines for reaching causal judgements in epidemiology is controversial. They are not, and must not be used as, a checklist or algorithm for causality. There is no causality score. Rothman and Greenland (1998) provide a vigorous critique of the limitations of causal guidelines as stated so clearly by Bradford Hill (1965). A set of guidelines has been so closely linked to this exposition that they are commonly known as the Bradford Hill criteria, although he called them considerations. Similar principles had already been developed, indeed published, long before their inclusion in the 1964 United States Surgeon General's report on smoking and health, so their close association to one person is not appropriate. These kinds of guidelines are only sporadically used and it is evident that new scholarship and research is needed to update them. Some work has been published examining the meaning of such guidelines in the context of genetic epidemiology. The guideline-free approach—simply relying on measures of the association alone, has not been sufficient. The existing principles are valuable and I have distilled them here, together with some additional thoughts. Clearly, such guidelines should be seen as a framework for thought about the totality of evidence including from non-epidemiological studies.

Epidemiological causal reasoning comes under frequent attack, particularly from people and organizations that do not agree with particular research findings. It is a cliché, but one with barbs, that epidemiological results on cause and effect which are making headlines one week will be replaced by results reporting the opposite the next. One such result making headlines as I write is that dairy fats are good for cardiovascular health, overturning some 30–40 years of epidemiologically based views to the contrary. All sciences refine, re-adjust, and sometimes reverse their conclusions but unlike epidemiology, their debates do not usually make headline news internationally. Exemplar 5.2 considers this.

Exemplar 5.2: Headline: 'Toasties get you laid, fat prevents dementia and I'm a sex god' (*The Sunday Times*, 12 April 2015, p. 19)

Epidemiologically based health stories are common, often making headlines in newspapers, television, and social media. This article in *The Sunday Times*, one of the United Kingdom's important and serious newspapers, exemplified the mixture of amusement, bemusement, and humorous derision that journalists, including specialist health journalists, subject epidemiology to. The journalist Rod Liddle writes a funny article, but one with serious points to make.

A survey associating eating cheese toast (toasties) with a good sex life is not taken seriously by Liddle, but it does show that people like to collect, publish, and discuss these kinds of statistics. Seventy-three per cent (73%) of those eating toasted cheese sandwiches reported enjoying sex at least once a month, but only 63 per cent of those preferring other snacks did so. This report came from a dating website. This lighthearted discourse is then followed by a serious one.

Liddle then moves on to a study published in a prestigious journal of two million people showing that being overweight was associated with lower risk of dementia. To quote: 'This is an awful thing for our state sponsored health fascists to contemplate.' The result of our efforts to curb obesity, he says, may well lead to a nation of agreeably thin people who have no idea of what they are doing. He then lambasts conflicting advice: 'One day eggs are bad, the next day they are good. One day Lurpak* is an agent of Satan, the next you are advised to spread it thickly and maybe put some bacon on it.' He says you end up trusting nothing as it is all disproved next week.

Concluding remarks

If there were not so much truth in this amusing and lighthearted derision, it would be funny. However, it rings so true that we epidemiologists need to take it seriously. The reporting of lighthearted statistics and serious epidemiology is unfortunate because the general reading public might not appreciate the difference.

(*a brand of butter).

The more serious criticisms are that epidemiologists' reasoning lacks a theoretical basis and it falls short of the more rigorous thinking in the experimental sciences. These criticisms are unhelpful and unjustified. Causal thinking in epidemiology draws upon the theories and principles of other disciplines including philosophy, the laboratory sciences, and the social sciences and is theoretically grounded, though this may not be obvious. Epidemiology is predominantly an observational and not experimental science, as are demography, astronomy, geology, evolutionary biology, palaeontology, and archaeology. Epidemiology is far more complex than most sciences, and experimentation in epidemiology is strictly limited by ethical constraints on human research. Epidemiology has, moreover, contributed new ways of thinking about causality when experiment is not possible. Epidemiological guidelines are, furthermore, designed for thinking about the causes of disease in populations and not in individuals. When applied to the individual, as in the courtroom, they are wanting but that is a criticism of those who misapply them rather than of the discipline.

Table 5.6 summarizes some of the cause and effect thinking in microbiology, health economics, philosophy, and epidemiology. There are commonalities of reasoning. The approach to establishing causality in the experimental medical sciences is illustrated by the Henle–Koch postulates, as discussed in detail by Susser (1977) (Table 5.6, column 1). These postulates also have limitations. First, consider the postulate the organism must be present in every case. This is impossible to show for many bacterial diseases including tuberculosis. (In clinical practice, a trial of anti-tuberculosis therapy is sometimes required when the patient has a clinical picture of tuberculosis but the organism cannot be grown in the laboratory.) Second, the organism must be grown in pure culture. Viral organisms are particularly hard to grow, and so are some bacteria such as the mycobacterium causing leprosy. Third, when inoculated into a susceptible animal (or human) the specific disease should occur. Animal models are sometimes not available, and even when they are the induced disease may be different from the human version. Fourth, the organism must be recovered from the animal (or human), but this is often not achieved.

The Henle–Koch postulates are a counsel of perfection and too stringent. Evans (1978) points out that even when they were developed, it was recognized that they were not to be applied rigidly, and that Koch believed that the cholera bacillus caused cholera even though the postulates were not achieved. According to Evans, leprosy, typhoid fever, syphilis, malaria, mycoplasma pneumonia, and *Chlamydia trachomatis* infection are among the microbial diseases which have causes

Table 5.6 A comparison of four modes of thinking about causality

Microbiology: Henle–Koch's postulates	Philosophy: Mill's canons	Economics	Epidemiology: some related modes of reasoning for causality[1]
The microorganism causing the disease can be demonstrated in every case of the disease	Method of concomitant variation: the phenomenon which varies when another phenomenon varies in a specific way is either a cause, an effect, or connected through some fact of causation	The future cannot predict the present	The cause precedes the effect (temporality)
The organism can be isolated and grown in pure culture	Method of agreement: if there is only one circumstance in common in instances of the phenomenon, then the common circumstance is the cause of effect	The effect (y) can be predicted more accurately by using values of the cause (x) than by not using them	The disease is commoner in those exposed to the cause (strength)
Animals (or humans) exposed to the cultured organism develop the disease	Method of difference: if there is only one difference in the circumstances when a phenomenon occurs compared with when it does not occur, that difference is part of the cause or effect	Instantaneous causation does not exist, since there is a time difference between independent actions. If A, itself, causes B, and A did not exist, B would not have occurred	The amount of exposure relates to the amount of disease (dose–response)
The organism can be grown from the experimentally exposed animal (or human)	The method of residues: remove from the phenomenon any part known to be the effect of known antecedents (causes), and the remainder is the effect of the remaining antecedents	One cause can have many effects and one effect many causes. The putative cause A may have an effect by itself or be a part of the cause	The causes are linked to diseases in specific and relevant ways (specificity). Altering the amount of exposure to the cause leads to change in the disease pattern (experiment or natural experiment). Different types of studies reach similar conclusions (consistency)

[1]The guidelines for causality have been reduced to six by the author for simplicity. Biological plausibility is discussed in the text and is, strictly, not an epidemiological concept.

Source: data from Susser M. *Causal thinking in the health sciences*, Second Edition. New York: Oxford University Press, Copyright © 1977, pp. 70–71; Charemza WW and Deadman DF. *New directions in econometric practice: general to specific modelling, cointegration, and vector autoregression* Second Edition, Cheltenham: Elgar, Copyright © Elgar; Hicks J. *Causality in economics*. Blackwell, Oxford, Copyright © 1979 John Wiley and Sons.

that do not meet the criteria. Furthermore, with new technologies such as antibody tests and DNA sequencing available, the postulates are being superseded. Epidemiologists need to be aware of such criteria, both as a standard to incorporate into their own work, and so they can discuss causality in the context of infectious disease epidemiology.

Some philosophers' ideas were considered in section 5.1. John Stuart Mill (1806–1873) was a British philosopher and economist who succinctly offered a practical interpretation of causal thinking in philosophy, the nub of which is now known as Mill's canons (Table 5.6, column 2). Susser (1977) has discussed these in the epidemiological context. The principles are of importance to epidemiology and are essentially incorporated into its own guidelines. The method of concomitant variation corresponds to current ideas on correlation and association (see section 8.15); the method of agreement to the search for a factor in common (e.g. in an outbreak of Legionnaires' disease, all those sick may have been to a particular air-conditioned hotel); the method of difference is at the core of epidemiological thinking (e.g. why do some people get heart disease and others of the same age and sex do not?); and the method of residues echoes modern ideas of experiments of preventive action, to establish what proportion of disease can be prevented, or where this is not possible, calculations of attributable risk (see Chapter 8). (Readers should note that the order in which the canons are presented in Table 5.3 does not correspond to Mills's numbering of his canons, e.g. the method of concomitant variation is the fifth in his list.)

Economics also evaluates associations in similar ways (Table 5.6, column 3). Even more than epidemiology, health economics relies on observation and modelling, with the scope for experiment being extremely limited. According to Charemza and Deadman (1997), the operational meaning of causality in economics is more on the lines of 'to predict' than 'to produce' (an effect). A scan of the third and fourth columns shows the similarity in concept, if not detail, between economics and epidemiology.

The nub of epidemiological reasoning (Table 5.3, column 4) is that the cause:

◆ must precede the effect

◆ should raise the incidence of the disease in a population

◆ should have a greater effect in greater quantity

◆ be associated with specific and relevant effects

◆ should show consistent effects across a number of studies.

These epidemiological ideas are similar to Mill's canons and to thinking in health economics.

Evidence from experimentation, natural or by design, on humans or animals, may show that manipulating exposures changes the disease. Experimentation may also elucidate the mechanisms by which this happens. The cause–effect relationship should make biological sense. These latter ideas, now integral to epidemiology, are those of the other biological sciences. The epidemiological guidelines for causality are not an idiosyncratic epidemiological invention. Their validity, as a collective, needs to be assessed empirically.

In the modern era an amalgam of epidemiological and basic science guidelines are adopted as the standard for causal thinking, as shown in the example in Box 5.13 and in the ensuing examples. Before reading on, try the exercise in Box 5.13.

In Kaposi's sarcoma (Box 5.13), the first and second items of evidence match the ideas underpinning the Henle–Koch postulates. The third and fourth match epidemiological concepts (strength of association) and the data could be converted to a measure of strength, such as relative risk (see Chapter 8). The fifth item is a mixture of microbiology (distribution in tissues) and epidemiology (transmission). The sixth item is, again, epidemiology, as is the seventh (temporality).

The principle is this: causation is established by judgement based on evidence from all disciplines. Failure to meet some guidelines (with the exception that the cause must precede the effect, which is not easy to establish conclusively) does not dismiss causality and achievement

Box 5.13 An exercise on causal thinking in medical science and causal guidelines

Can you see the links between the evidence listed below and the causal guidelines in Table 5.3? Which of these pieces of evidence match the guidelines for causality?

Aetiology of Kaposi's sarcoma: Evidence cited for a herpesvirus as the cause;

1. Viral sequences (DNA) can be detected in sarcoma tissues in most cases.

2. Such sequences are rarely detected in other tissues.

3. Virus is detected in blood cells in 50 per cent of cases but not in controls.

4. HIV positive patients who had the virus in blood cells had a greater risk of developing sarcoma than comparable patients without the virus.

5. The virus is probably sexually transmitted and is found in semen and other genital tissues of healthy adults.

6. Antibody levels in blood correlate with presence of sarcoma.

7. Antibody levels rise before Kaposi's sarcoma appears.

Conclusion: Kaposi's sarcoma is caused by a herpesvirus (Beiser 1997, p. 581).

Source: data from Berisera C. Recent advances: HIV infection-II. *British Medical Journal*, Volume 314, Issue 7080, pp. 579–582, Copyright © 1997 BMJ Publishing Group Ltd.

of some guidelines does not ensure it. The currently popular 'hierarchy of evidence' places the systematic review and the human experiment (trial) at the apex of the evidence pyramid. This is understandable for studying the effectiveness of interventions on humans. In doing this in causal epidemiology, one side effect is to dismiss too readily other kinds of evidence. This matters for causal thinking, especially where the question is difficult to resolve using epidemiology alone (e.g. alcohol and heart disease). Just as we would expect laboratory scientists to examine the evidence from human population studies in reaching their conclusions, it is important that population scientists consider the findings of laboratory work.

Epidemiology often establishes cause in populations unequivocally, but this information only applies to individuals in a probabilistic way, which does not prove cause and effect at the individual level. Try the exercise in Box 5.14 before reading on.

The answer is that we do not know the cause at the individual level. If the person is a non-smoker, the cancer may have arisen from passive exposure to tobacco but perhaps is more likely to be due to other factors. If the person is a smoker, the cause is most likely smoking, but may result from other factors such as exposure to radiation or asbestos. There is no way, at present, to distinguish a lung cancer (or heart attack) resulting from smoking from a lung cancer (or heart attack) arising from another cause.

Box 5.14 Causes of lung cancer in populations and in individuals

If 90 per cent of all lung cancer in a population is due to smoking, and assuming that is correct, what is the likelihood that in an individual with lung cancer the cause was smoking?

A drug or public health intervention may be effective in a population but harmful to an individual. For example, exercise may be good generally but lead to collapse and death in some individuals. Some people are harmed by alcohol while others benefit, and the net effect on the health of the population as a whole is unclear. In contrast to alcohol, the net health effect of tobacco consumption is overwhelmingly negative.

These kinds of counterintuitive observations on causality lie at the heart of disputes between population scientists and those whose work is based on individuals. Immunization may or may not harm individuals as is sometimes claimed (e.g. MMR and autism, and whooping cough vaccine and neurological disorders), but the benefits far outweigh these harms at population level epidemiological studies show. To prove harm in these particular circumstances, that is, to the individual, is beyond the scope of epidemiology and requires other kinds of sciences. Equally, to prove there is no harm to individuals is also impossible for epidemiology. We can, however, show there is no sizeable harm to the population. The problem is that sciences based on individuals are also unable to predict well at the individual level. As a result, epidemiology is used in a setting and context for which it is not designed, in the absence of better alternatives. A great deal of the criticism of epidemiology arises from failing to separate what it can and cannot do.

Epidemiological data are, therefore, difficult (possibly impossible) to apply in legal cases about individuals. To quote Evans discussing the issue in the United States of America:

> Legal requirements are concerned with the risk in the *individual*, the plaintiff, and whether the preponderance of evidence supports the conclusion that *that* exposure 'more likely than not' resulted in *that* illness or injury in *that* person.
>
> (1978, p. 194)

Evans contests that a higher order of proof and specificity is required in legal proof than in epidemiological proof, concluding that epidemiological evidence is often inapplicable in this context. Epidemiology is a science based on studies of groups and cannot be directly applicable to individuals, and this is an inherent limitation. Equally, a factor demonstrated to cause a disease in an individual, by a science of individuals, say toxicology or pathology, may not be demonstrable as harmful in the population, possibly because harmful effects are balanced by beneficial ones. This is an inherent limitation of a science of individuals. The problem lies not with epidemiology itself, but with those who apply epidemiology in these circumstances. The law also extrapolates from population data to the individual. The standard of proof in epidemiology is not of a lower order than in law, but it is of a different order and for a different purpose. The problem is that so often the best we can offer the individual is average risk derived from the study of groups similar to that individual. That is a limitation of medical sciences collectively. We now consider how epidemiological guidelines for causality help to analyse the causal basis of associations observed at the population level.

5.6.2 **Application of guidelines to associations**

The association (or link or relationship) between disease and postulated causal factors lies at the core of epidemiological thinking. Mostly, such associations are found by observing that disease varies with time, place, or characteristics of persons in observational data. An association rarely reflects a causal relationship, but it may. The preceding chapters on variation and error showed how to separate the probably not causal association from the possibly causal one. Having accounted for chance, error and bias, and confounding, logically, what remains is a causal relationship. The problem is that accounting for these factors is not a foolproof process. That is why we need to go to the next step of synthesizing the evidence to strengthen our conclusions. Once we learn how to conduct perfect studies and data analysis, this step will become unnecessary. For the foreseeable future, however, it is essential. We have a further problem, however, and that is that there is no foolproof, or even consensual, process of synthesizing the evidence. The approach described here is a distillation of now-standard concepts developed over the last 50–70 years. These and other approaches need more work.

Table 5.7 begins the questioning and reasoning process often used in epidemiology to make the difficult judgement on whether an association may be causal. These six guidelines are a distillation of, and echo, the 10 Alfred Evans postulates in *A Dictionary of Epidemiology*, the reasoning in the United States Surgeon General's report on smoking and health, and the nine Bradford Hill considerations. The causal challenge is illustrated by the pyramid of associations and causes in Figure 5.12. The pyramid displays the axiom 'association is not causation' with my qualification, '... but rarely it may be'. Try the exercise in Box 5.15 before reading on.

We shall now look at these guidelines in more detail. A visual summary is in Figure 5.13.

i. Temporality

Did the supposed cause precede the effect? In Figure 5.13, the first panel shows the relative risk (RR) of disease rising over time following exposure. In this image, a lag period is shown with the risk increasing over time and then stabilizing. We would not expect the effect to be immediate. Some causes (e.g. carcinogens) take many decades to have an effect. If the effect is simultaneous with or precedes the proposed cause, the association is definitely not causal in the direction postulated. There may be reverse causality, that is, the outcome actually affects the supposed cause; for example, early undetected cancer leads to low weight, not low weight leads to cancer. If there is no clear answer the judgement will be tentative, irrespective of other data, no matter how convincing these are. If the effect follows the action of a proposed cause, the association may be a causal one and the analysis can proceed. This matter of timing is referred to as temporality. Demonstrating that this guideline is satisfied does not usually establish causality. Why might this be so? Reflect on this question before reading on.

The supposed cause under study may not be the only exposure that changed. There may have been many changes, and the temporal relation under study may be coincidental. If a perfect experiment (trial) only changed one exposure and the outcome is altered, this evidence alone would, usually, be accepted as causal. Before reading on, do the exercise in Box 5.16.

Thunder follows lightning, at least as perceived by humans, but is not caused by it. Both are generated simultaneously by an electrical discharge in clouds. The later arrival of the thunder is simply a result of the slower speed of sound than of light. Without an understanding of the nature of thunder and lightning, erroneous conclusions about cause and effect are likely. Empirical observation seduces us to err. Generating alternative explanations is an essential discipline in epidemiology. The epidemiological imagination needs to be cultivated for this. Our alternative explanations can be put to the test. It would be hard to test the lightning and thunder association. Earlier, when discussing Hume (section 5.1.1) we considered the association between flicking a switch and a light going on. If the act of flicking similar switches in other settings turns on a light, we are likely to accept a cause and effect relation on empirical grounds. The empirical observation has no explanatory power for exceptions, for example, when the light does not go on because of a break in the wiring, or when it goes on even without the switch being flicked, by water penetration. When there is a deeper understanding of the nature and action of electrical circuits, the association may be agreed as causal, especially if it explains exceptions. Just because B follows A does not, of itself, prove a causal relation. Deeper understanding, opening and understanding the black box, is essential.

Table 5.7 Questions underlying the guidelines for causality and implications of answers for interpretation of associations in populations

Question underlying guideline	Label for guideline	Evidence		
		Unsure	No	Yes
Does the supposed cause precede the disease (or other effect)?	Temporality	Judgement premature	Not causal	Causal relation possible
Does exposure to the supposed cause raise the incidence of disease?	Strength of association	Judgement premature	Not causal in the population context but does not rule out causal effects in individuals	Causal relation in populations possible
Does varying exposure to the supposed cause lead to varying amounts of disease?	Dose–response	Not critical	Causal relation still possible if there is a threshold effect	Strengthens case for a causal judgement
Is the association between supposed cause and disease(s) limited in range	Specificity	Not critical	Not critical but extra caution—a sign of artefact	Strengthens causal claim
Is the association between supposed cause and outcome consistent across different studies and across populations and subgroups?	Consistency	Defer decision, and await further research unless an immediate judgement is essential	Judgement will require explanation for inconsistent results	Strengthens causal claim
Does manipulating the level of exposure to the supposed cause change disease experience?	Experimental confirmation	Not always possible, so not critical	Caution needed for a causal claim	Strong confirmation of a causal relation
Is the way that the supposed cause exerts its effect on disease understood?	Biological plausibility	Not critical	Not critical but great caution needed for causal claim	Causal judgement strengthened

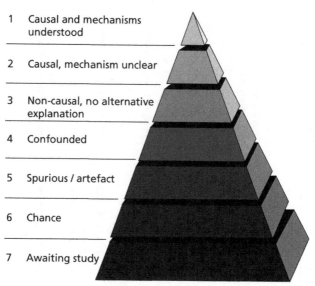

Fig. 5.12 Pyramid of associations and causes.

1   Causal and mechanisms understood

2   Causal, mechanism unclear

3   Non-causal, no alternative explanation

4   Confounded

5   Spurious / artefact

6   Chance

7   Awaiting study

Box 5.15 Linking associations and causality in risk factors/outcome relationships

Can you think of an exposure/risk factor variable with an association that fits with each category in the pyramid? Once you have attempted this, have a look at Table 5.8.

Table 5.8 Examples of associations fitting each level of the pyramid of associations

Level	Example
1. Causal, understood	Common in infectious and toxic disease but still quite rare in chronic diseases with examples being tobacco, asbestos, radiation, and lung cancer
2. Causal, unclear	Posture when sleeping and sudden infant death syndrome
3. Non-causal, no alternative explanation	Suicide and smoking
4. Confounded	Alcohol and lung cancer
5 Artefact	Numerous
6. Chance	Numerous
7. Awaiting study	By definition, no examples but most associations are yet to be discovered

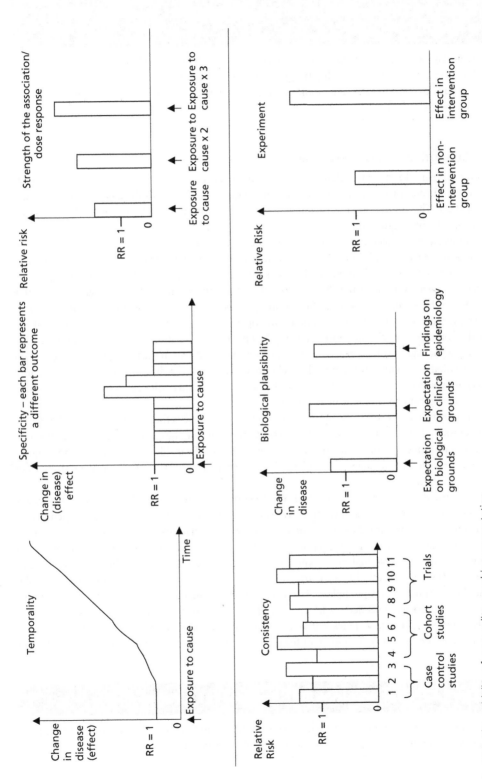

Fig. 5.13 The guidelines for causality: graphic representation.

Box 5.16 The deduction of cause and effect from the linkage of events

Reflect on whether the linkage of two events provides convincing evidence on cause and effect. For example, thunder follows lightning. Does lightning cause thunder?

    If you observe this once or a thousand times, does it make a difference? What other explanations might there be?

ii. Strength and dose–response

Does exposure to the cause change disease incidence, and if so, what is the shape of this relationship? If not, or we are unsure, there is no epidemiological basis for a conclusion on cause and effect. The failure to demonstrate this does not, however, disprove a causal role. Reflect on Box 5.17 before reading on.

    The cause or its effect may be so rare that there are insufficient cases available to reach a conclusion. Alternatively, or additionally, the effect may be very small. Epidemiology is not good at demonstrating causal links when the rise in disease incidence is low, for example, less than 10 per cent excess. Alternatively, there may be some people in the population in whom the cause is operative while in others it has an opposite effect, leading to the view that there is no association. It might be reasonable to say that the cause studied was operative in causing disease in individuals but not at the population level. The cause may only be operative in the presence of a cofactor, that is, as part of a package of sufficient causes. The cofactor may be absent in the time, place, or population you studied. The same study somewhere else may have reached a different conclusion. The cause may be operative on everyone. If oxygen is the cause of, say, pancreatic cancer we cannot show this epidemiologically (or possibly in any way).

    The most usual way of assessing strength and dose–response is the relative risk (see Chapter 8). Other ways of measurement include the correlation coefficient, the regression coefficient, absolute rates, odds ratios, and other measures of associations and effects. (Some of these and other measures are considered in Chapters 7 and 8.) The greater the relative risk, the greater the strength of the association.

    Does the disease incidence vary with the level of exposure? If yes, this is a dose dependent effect and the case for a causal relation is advanced, but if not, the effects may be independent of the amount of exposure. Allergy is one example where trivial doses of substances such as peanuts can cause life-threatening reactions. For most exposures, the relationship with disease is not linear, but the principle that more exposure leads to more disease tends to hold. For high blood pressure there is a threshold above and below which adverse effects arise. Above the threshold, the dose–response concept applies. Below the threshold, the effects are unclear but some minimal blood pressure is needed for life. For weight and alcohol consumption, there is an apparent adverse effect at both low values and high values (called a J-shaped distribution). Dose–response can be considered as a development of the concept of the strength of the association; that is, does

Box 5.17 Epidemiology fails to uncover a cause

Can you think of circumstances when exposure to a causal factor does not change, or cannot be demonstrated to change disease incidence, yet the exposure is a cause?

Box 5.18 Strength of association in a perfect, counterfactual study

Imagine that we had the perfect study. In an imaginary world, we can even have the counterfactual data, that is, what the risk would be in the same population if that population did not have the risk factor. Would these data alone—that tell us the strength of the association—suffice for a cause and effect judgement? What about in the real world?

the strength of the association vary with the level of exposure? The second panel in Figure 5.13 shows the risk of the disease increasing in people exposed to the cause (the unexposed group has an RR of 1 by definition), with the risk increasing with greater exposure. It is generally accepted that the size of the relative risk matters in causal interpretation. In a well-designed study, if the relative risk is 5 or more we veer towards causal explanations, whereas if it is 1.5 we worry more about non-causal effects. There is no single metric to describe the strength of the association but by custom and practice, the following is a rough guide: weak associations imply RR <2; moderate associations imply RRs of 2 to 3.9; strong associations imply RRs of 4 or more. Before reading on, try the exercise in Box 5.18.

Assuming temporality was established, from a population perspective this evidence from the perfect study in Box 5.18 would be causal. The closest we come to this, in reality, is the well-designed experiment, in epidemiology the trial (Chapter 9). If a trial were free of all errors and biases, the strength of the association would, together with temporality, reflect causality. As yet, all epidemiological trials are imperfect and on selected populations. If trials were perfect, we would need only one on any topic and we would not need any systematic reviews or meta-analyses. In our imperfect but real epidemiological world, the other guidelines are, therefore, of importance.

iii. Specificity

Is the association of the supposed cause limited to relevant diseases and are diseases associated with a limited number of supposed causes? If so, we would say the association is specific. This idea is called specificity. Imagine a factor which was linked to all health effects. Why would that be? It is hard to explain (except through some error). Unless the links to a broad range of diseases can be explained, the case for causality is weakened. Non-specificity is characteristic of spurious associations (e.g. underestimating the size of the population denominator; Chapter 7). Some factors do have broad effects, for example, poverty and cigarette smoking. However, even these are not associated with more of every health problem. In the United Kingdom, poverty is associated with less malignant melanoma, a skin cancer that includes within its sufficient causes, sunburn and excess exposure to sunlight. This observation makes sense because these causes are often a result of holidays in hot climates. Those in poverty are less able to afford to expose themselves to these causes than richer people. Panel 3 in Figure 5.13 shows that following exposure to a possible cause, the RR was increased for two adjacent disease outcomes of 11 studied. This is indicating reasonable specificity. While specificity is not a critically important guideline, epidemiologists should take advantage of the reasoning power it offers.

iv. Consistency

Is the evidence within and between studies consistent? It is wise to be tentative if it is not. Unless the inconsistency can be explained, the case for causality is weakened. Consistency is linked to generalizability of findings. Experience tells us that causal effects tend to be widely applicable, while spurious associations are often local. The systematic review and meta-analysis are ways of assessing consistency in a rigorous way and are considered briefly in Chapter 9.

Panel 4 in Figure 5.13 shows 11 studies using three kinds of design. While the relative risk varies, in every case it is above the reference value of 1. This is compelling evidence. It is possible, however, that all 11 studies are making the same kind of error, although given a few are trials it is hard to imagine a non-causal explanation. Trials are experiments, the next guideline to be considered.

v. Experiment

Does changing the exposure to the supposed cause change disease incidence? If yes, this is experimental confirmation. Sometimes there have been natural experiments, with changes over time in exposure to risk factors. For example, a spill of a pollutant into a water supply, the closure of a factory, the availability of a new product, redundancy in a factory, economic collapse of a society, or a change of policy (e.g. putting fluoride into a water supply). Perhaps the greatest of these experiments is the mixing of the genes in Mendelian randomization (see Chapter 3 section 3.3.1 and Chapter 9). These natural experiments can be vitally important. Often there is no such evidence, and some form of deliberate experimentation will be necessary.

The problem is that human experiments or trials are sometimes impossible on ethical grounds and are always difficult and expensive to organize. Ethically, the individual involved must have the potential to benefit and yet there must be uncertainty on the question posed. For risk factors, as opposed to protective factors, there may be no such benefit. Then the experimental approach requires a valid *in vitro* or animal model. Causal understanding can be greatly advanced by laboratory and experimental observations. Such data must be integrated with epidemiological observations, to ensure that the theoretically predicted effects do occur in free-living human populations. Experimental methods are introduced in section 9.7 on trials. The ethics of epidemiology are particularly important to these studies (section 10.10). Panel 5 in Figure 5.13 shows an experiment with an intervention. The non-intervention group by definition is assigned a relative risk of one. We see the risk is increased in the intervention group. There is an effect, but it is an adverse one. If the trial were perfect, this would be causal evidence at least in the type of population studied.

vi. Biological plausibility

Is there a biological mechanism by which the supposed cause can induce the effect? This is the guideline of biological plausibility. If there is plausibility, the case for a causal effect will be easier to advance. For truly novel advances, however, the biological plausibility may not be apparent. For example, it is biologically plausible that laying an infant on its back to sleep may lead to it inhaling its own vomit. This biologically plausible theory, which informed parenting behaviour for decades, has been overturned by the biologically implausible observation that laying a child on its back halves the risk of cot death compared to the side or front. The mechanisms are still being worked out. That said, biological plausibility remains important, particularly in confirming causality. The analogy is with the light switch; when there is understanding of the electrical circuit, the causal basis of flicking the light switch is confirmed. An understanding of electrical discharges in clouds explains the association between thunder and lightning (see i. Temporality). Ultimately, biological processes govern all diseases and adverse health outcomes, without exception. This applies to social and physiological processes alike—so the ill effects of economic deprivation on health must, ultimately, occur through biology. Understanding these processes is important. Clinical and other scientists are not easily persuaded by epidemiological evidence that does not fit into biological understanding.

Demonstrating biological plausibility is not part of epidemiological methods. This does not, however, mean epidemiologists can forget about it. Epidemiologists need to understand the biology of the diseases they study, explain their hypotheses in biological terms, and propose and promote (sometimes even lead) biological research to test hypotheses. The precedent and inspiration for such work is abundant, as we saw in Chapters 1 and 2 with syndrome X (pellagra) and the work of Joseph Goldberger (and his colleague Edwin Syderstricker).

Panel 6 in Figure 5.13 shows a situation where on biological and clinical grounds we might expect an increased risk of disease. If epidemiology demonstrates this prior expectation, that is powerful. It is less powerful, but still useful, when in retrospect, biological and clinical ideas are invoked to explain an epidemiological finding. An example of the latter is my four-stage model synthesizing the published evidence to try and explain a well-established epidemiological observation that South Asians have about four times the risk of type 2 diabetes mellitus compared to White Europeans in the same context (Bhopal, 2013). The model can be tested by further epidemiological studies.

5.6.3 Judging the causal basis of the association

The investigator can now proceed to a conclusion, but the interpretation ought to be tentative as judgements on cause and effect are not necessarily universal. An association which meets many or even all of the causal guidelines may, at least theoretically, be non-causal. George Davey Smith, Andrew N. Phillips, and James D. Neaton (1992) have shown, for example, that the association between cigarette smoking and suicide meets many (but not all) of the guidelines for causality including temporality, strength, and dose–response. Yet, they argue, the association is not causal.

The guidelines are particularly valuable in exposing the lack of, or contradictory nature of, evidence for causality, for indicating the need for further research and for avoiding premature conclusions. This said, sometimes firm judgements are possible, and at other times are forced upon us, even in the face of limited evidence. A judgement may be essential when policy is to be made. Using a causal framework makes the judgement explicit. Table 5.9 indicates how the questions implicit in causal guidelines can be applied to weigh up evidence.

Three examples of the case for causality (illustrating the need for a systematic mode of analysis) are shown in Table 5.9: diethylstilboestrol as a cause of adenocarcinoma of the vagina (Herbst *et al.* 1971); smoking as a cause of lung cancer (Doll and Bradford Hill 1956); and residential proximity to a coking works as a cause of ill health (Bhopal *et al.* 1994). Before reading on, reflect on the exercise in Box 5.19. Readers are invited to read the original studies (listed in References).

At the time that the key studies referred to in Table 5.6 were published, the authors claimed that the smoking–lung cancer association was causal (true, but many remained unconvinced), that diethylstilboestrol had caused adenocarcinoma of the vagina (this was accepted), and that residential proximity to a coking works had caused respiratory morbidity, but not mortality. The latter case was not, however, accepted as solid, though it was the best that was achievable.

5.6.4 Interpretation of data, paradigms, study design, and causal guidelines

Causal knowledge is born in the investigator's imagination and understanding. Scientific data do not, in themselves, offer knowledge. Indeed, the same data can be interpreted in quite different ways, depending on the investigator's way of thought. For example, data that one scientist, Samuel Morton, interpreted as showing clear differences by race in cranial capacity and hence brain size and ultimately intelligence, was interpreted by another, Stephen Gould (1984), as showing no noteworthy differences. This arose because of differences in the way they saw the world—including the research world. This way of seeing the world is often referred to as the paradigm.

Table 5.9 Three examples of applying the guidelines for causality

Question	Smoking and lung cancer	Diethylstilboestrol and adenocarcinoma of the vagina	Living near a coking works and ill health
Does the supposed cause precede the disease (effect) (temporality)	Yes, clearly so	Yes, maternal exposure to diethylstilboestrol preceded the disease in the offspring	Yes, the coking works was functioning before most people in the study were born
By how much does exposure to the cause raise the incidence of disease? (strength)	Greatly and as much as 20 to 30-fold in smokers of 20 or more cigarettes per day	Greatly, as estimated from the first case–control study	The excess of disease is modest, varying for each specific cause but is rarely more than 30–50% greater than expected
Does varying exposure lead to varying disease? (dose–response)	Yes, there is a clear relationship and more smoking causes more disease	No clear evidence from the study	The evidence is suggestive that the closer the residence to the coking works, the greater the effect on health
Does the cause lead to a rise in a few relevant diseases? (specificity)	No, numerous diseases show an association with smoking	Only one outcome was studied	Yes, the association is restricted mainly to some respiratory diseases
Is the association consistent across different studies and between groups?	Yes, the association is demonstrable in men and women, and across social groups internationally	Decisions had to be taken on the one study	There are no directly comparable studies, but it fits with understanding of the role of industrial air pollution
Is the way that the cause exerts its effect on disease understood? (biological plausibility)	Only partly. The tar in cigarettes contains important carcinogens	At the time of the discovery, no	Generally, yes, specifically no. Coking works produce complex mixtures of emissions. Most knowledge is on single components of air pollution, not mixtures
Does manipulating the level of exposure to the cause change disease experience? (experimental confirmation)	Yes. Reducing consumption of cigarettes reduces risk. Persuading people to smoke more would be unethical. Tobacco is carcinogenic to animals	At the time this was unknown	Not known. An experiment is not possible, but the plant closed during the research, producing a natural experiment. Closure of the coking plant was not linked to changes in consultation with a general practitioner, but on days when pollution levels were high, the consultation rates were also high

Box 5.19 Reaching a judgement on cause and effect

Reflect on the evidence in Table 5.9 and deliver a verdict on whether the associations between smoking and lung cancer, diethylstilboestrol and adenocarcinoma of the vagina, and living close to a coking works and ill health are causal.

The paradigm within which epidemiologists work will determine the nature of the causal links they see and emphasize. There is a strong case for researchers to make their guiding research philosophy and paradigm explicit (see also section 10.5).

Causal thinking and study design (Chapter 9) are distinct, though interlinked, issues. No epidemiological design, in practice, confirms causality and no design is incapable of adding important evidence. In all studies, there are limitations and pitfalls. There are differences among the various study designs in both the type of pitfalls and their likelihood (see Chapter 9). While a single observation may spark off causal understanding, it would be wise to exercise great caution until further observations confirm or refute the idea. Exceptionally, however, there may be no time to delay.

Table 5.10 indicates the potential contributions of various study designs to the epidemiological guidelines for causality. Note that with the exception of consistency, to which all designs contribute, and biological plausibility, to which no epidemiological designs contribute directly, all epidemiological studies contribute to some but not all guidelines. This must not be confused with the hierarchy of evidence that has emerged in relation to the effectiveness and cost-effectiveness of interventions, or even of measuring the burden of disease. Each purpose requires its own hierarchy. We have already discussed that the experiment is the pre-eminent causal method, but it can only be applied rarely. Otherwise, there is no hierarchy of causality.

Table 5.10 Potential contributions of study design to causal guidelines

Guideline	Case series	Cross-sectional	Case-control	Cohort	Trial
Temporality	Sometimes	Sometimes	Sometimes	Often	Usually
Strength or dose–response	Sometimes	Sometimes	Often	Always	Always
Specificity	Sometimes for exposure	Sometimes	Sometimes for exposure	Sometimes for outcome	Sometimes for outcome
Consistency	Yes	Yes	Yes	Yes	Yes
Experimental confirmation	Sometimes, in the case of natural experiment	Sometimes, in case of repeated studies, following an intervention	Seldom (but this design is not advised for assessing interventions)	Sometimes, following natural changes	Always
Biological Plausibility	Not directly	Not directly	Not directly	Not directly	Not directly

5.7 **Epidemiological theory illustrated by this chapter**

Several theories underpin epidemiological causal thinking. First, there is the theory that diseases arise from a complex interaction of genetic, social, and environmental factors. This is not the kind of theory that is common in other medical sciences, but it is also fundamental in social sciences applied to health. Second, there is a theory that causes of disease in populations may not necessarily be demonstrable as causes of disease in individuals and vice versa. This theory is very rarely discussed. It is not easy for a science that is applied so much at the individual level to expose such limitations. The third (and pragmatic) epidemiological theory of causation is that reliable cause and effect judgements are achievable through hypothesis generation and testing, with data interpreted using a logical framework of analysis, which draws on multidisciplinary perspectives. This is a theoretical perspective that differs from purely quantitative disciplines. At present, at least, epidemiology does not work with a theory, derived from a mix of mathematics, statistics and computational science, that causality can be inferred from the mathematics, as articulated by Judea Pearl. The ideas underpinning this mathematical theory of causality, however, are being incorporated into epidemiology quite rapidly.

5.8 **Conclusion**

The most important aim of epidemiology is to generate cause and effect theories, to break the links between disease and its causes, and to improve health. The misapplication of such theory may have serious repercussions including deaths on a mass scale, while its proper application can transform the control of disease.

It is difficult to achieve trustworthy causal knowledge because of the complexity of diseases, the long timescales over which many human diseases develop, and ethical restraints on human experimentation. Nonetheless, there is an imperative to act, even when our knowledge is incomplete, for lives depend on our science. In the words of Bradford Hill (1965):

> All scientific work is incomplete—whether it be observational or experimental. That does not confer upon us a freedom to ignore the knowledge we already have, or to postpone the action that it appears to demand at a given time.
>
> Bradford Hill (1965, p. 300)

A rigorous analysis of all the scientific data available is essential, though to quote Bradford Hill again, 'this does not imply crossing every "t", and swords with every critic, before we act'.

Epidemiology engages with health policy-makers and planners who are the users of much of the work. Rothman and colleagues (1998) have helped to open up the prickly question, posed by Lanes, of whether epidemiologists (as scientists) ought to be engaged in choosing between theories of causation, or whether they should simply present the evidence and the theory options to policy-makers and leave the choices to them. Mostly, there are alternative interpretations of data, and it is our theoretical perspective that governs our preference. To take an example, small amounts of alcohol have been shown in many (but not all) kinds of study to be associated with cardiovascular health benefits. Reaching a causal judgement and drawing a policy conclusion is tricky. It may well be that in doing so, the epidemiologist adopts the role of advocate. To refuse to draw a conclusion, however, potentially leaves us paralysed for it is improbable that lay decision-makers would make policy in these circumstances. Generally, epidemiologists tend to draw policy conclusions, and often possibly do so too early. Readers need to ponder on this question and form their own views. The debate continues in the scientific journals. Whatever viewpoint prevails, epidemiology has a responsibility to understand the theories of causation used by other disciplines, and to educate others about the mode of thought in epidemiology.

Notions of epidemiology about causality, for example, that a cause is something which raises the incidence of disease, are not particularly helpful in persuading sceptics who can retort that association is not causation. Demonstrating causation to the sceptics' satisfaction is complex and requires detailed understanding by both parties of causal reasoning in epidemiology. Developing effective actions, a difficult challenge usually achieved in cross-disciplinary partnerships, is also demanding in epidemiological knowledge.

Epidemiology provides a broad perspective on the causes of disease, which contrasts with the narrower one of the physical and most biological sciences. This complementary perspective is a great strength. The causal models reinforce this perspective and provide a framework to organize ideas.

The prevailing attitude in epidemiology, that all judgements of cause and effect are tentative, is both pragmatic and in line with modern thinking about the nature of scientific advances. The increasing understanding that the data do not hold an unequivocal answer, and that the answers derived are dependent on human judgement (symbolized in Fig. 5.14) though apparently common sense, are harder to accept because they give space for subjectivity whereas science prefers objectivity.

Epidemiologists should be alert for the play of chance, error, and bias, reverse causality and confounding; should create causal diagrams and related analysis plans; and should apply guidelines for causality as an aid to thinking and not as a checklist. Only rarely will causal mechanisms be understood, as symbolized by the peak of the pyramid of associations in Figure 5.14. Finally, epidemiology should seek corroboration from other scientific disciplines in terms of both data and scientific frameworks for cause and effect.

Seeking causal associations is like panning for gold, for it usually yields nothing but grit and mud (error and bias). Often we find gold flakes and specks (risk factors, relating to the causal pathway in ways that remain obscure). Sometimes we get a nugget (causal factor). Rarely a gold mine is discovered (a causal theory). Like panning for gold, a great deal of hard work is required to find a gold mine. When it is discovered, panning alone will not be enough, and much sophisticated equipment and skills will be needed to take full advantage of the discovery. In epidemiology, this implies working with other laboratory and population-based scientific disciplines (including social sciences) to gain understanding of the mechanisms by which the cause operates.

In the second edition of this book, I said that epidemiology needs an international council to assess evidence to establish the causal credentials of the multiplicity of associations being generated. Associations would be categorized by this council according to the pyramid of associations and causes, to help guide both future research and public health action, and to plan and deliver

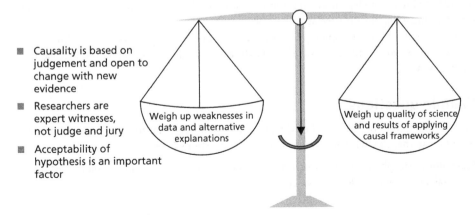

Fig. 5.14 Cause and effect: judgement.

the necessary health interventions. This proposal has been developed and discussed under the interim title of World Council for Epidemiology and Causality (Bhopal 2009) and further discussion is underway. Workshop-based and other discussions have pointed to the difficulties of the task. However, there are precedents. First, the World Council on Epidemiology and Causation (WCEC) would focus on associations in the same way that the Cochrane Collaboration and the UK organization National Institute for Clinical and Public Health Excellence (NICE) do for effectiveness of interventions. Second, this would be an extension of the monographs of the World Health Organization's (WHO) cancer agency, International Agency for Research on Cancer, dealing with the causal effects of carcinogens. However it is done, the task is essential in epidemiology. The vision now is for an independent body working with many partner organizations to spur on concepts, methods in causality, and structured, comprehensive analysis of specific associations, to reach speedier and more robust judgements on whether these might represent cause and effect.

Summary

Cause and effect understanding is the highest form of scientific knowledge, for it permits prediction and generalization, one of the main purposes of science. Understanding of cause and effect has also been a preoccupation of philosophy. A comparison of epidemiological and other forms of causal thinking shows similarity, reflecting the debt which epidemiologists owe to other, older disciplines. Epidemiology is increasingly influencing thought in other sciences.

An association between disease and the postulated causal factors lies at the core of the science of epidemiology. Causal knowledge can be greatly advanced by experimental observations on what happens to disease incidence when the causal factors are manipulated.

In epidemiology, demonstrating causality experimentally is difficult because of the long and complex natural history of many human diseases and because of ethical restraints. Epidemiologists should: hold the attitude that all judgements of cause and effect are tentative; understand that causal thinking demands a judgement; be alert for the play of chance, error, and bias; always consider reverse causality and confounding; utilize the power of causal models that broaden causal perspectives; apply guidelines for causality as an aid to thinking and not as a checklist; and look for corroboration of causality from other scientific frameworks for assessment of cause and effect.

The many guidelines for evaluating the causal basis of associations have here been distilled to six: temporality; strength, and dose–response; specificity; consistency; experimental confirmation; and biological plausibility. Causal models and tools introduced as aids to causal thinking include the line, triangle, wheel, and web of causation; the component cause model and causal diagrams including the directed acyclic graph.

The ultimate aim of epidemiology is to use cause and effect knowledge to break links between disease and its causes, and to improve health. The application of erroneous knowledge has serious repercussions.

Sample questions

Many of the questions at the end of Chapter 9 are highly relevant to this chapter, and you may need to read that chapter before doing some of the questions here.

Question 1 The phrase 'association is not causation' is often used in epidemiology. List five non-causal factors that can lead to association.

Answer Associations that are non-causal can be generated by chance, errors, bias in the selection of study populations, bias in the quality of information, failing to compare like-with-like (confounding), fraud, etc.

Question 2 Which of the guidelines (also erroneously known as criteria) for causal reasoning can clinical trials make a contribution to? Which do they not contribute to?

Answer Trials can contribute to the following causal guidelines:

- Temporality—intervention comes first, outcome is observed
- Strength of the association (dose–response may be possible if varying levels of the intervention are studied)
- Consistency—if they support other studies
- Specificity of the disease outcome, but not exposure (usually only one exposure is changed)
- Experimental confirmation—trials are experiments
- Trials do not contribute, at least directly, to biological plausibility unless specific effort is made to collect data on the biological mechanisms within the trial

Question 3 Which of the guidelines (also erroneously known as criteria) for causal reasoning can cohort studies make a contribution to? Which do they not contribute to?

Answer Cohort studies can contribute to temporality by showing that the exposure precedes disease; to strength of the association by measuring the relative risk; to dose–response by measuring the association as the exposure increases; to consistency either by comparison with other kinds of studies or with other cohort studies; and to specificity, that is, the range of outcomes that exposures lead to. They cannot contribute directly to biological plausibility, although they can test a biologically derived hypothesis. They cannot give experimental confirmation though (a) they can be used to study natural experiments and (b) to find people to do trials (experiments) on.

Question 4 What is the value of the concept of 'consistency' in helping you assess an association?

Answer 'Consistency' of an association is linked to generalizability of findings. The consistent association is similar in different populations and in studies using different kinds of study design. This helps to evaluate an association. For example, causal effects tend to be widely applicable, while spurious associations are often local. Unless the lack of consistency in findings can be explained, the case for an association is weakened.

Question 5 The phrase 'risk factor' is often used in epidemiology. Explain the meaning of this phrase, and discuss how it differs from causal factor.

Answer Risk in epidemiology usually refers to the likelihood (probability) of dying or developing a disease, or its precursors. In epidemiology, our prime interest is in the interaction between the probability of disease, or risk, and those environmental, individual, and social characteristics which influence the risk. Where there is an association with an increased probability of disease in those with such characteristics, the characteristics are called risk factors.

The phrase 'risk factor' does not necessarily imply the characteristic has a causal effect (association is not causation). No causal relationship is presumed, though there is great interest in assessing whether one exists. When a causal relationship is agreed between disease and the risk factor, the phrase causal factor, or simply cause, is used.

References

Bardenheier, B.H., Bullard, K.M., Caspersen, C.J., Cheng, Y.J., Gregg, E.W., and Geiss, L.S. (2013) A novel use of structural equation models to examine factors associated with prediabetes among adults aged 50 years and older: National Health and Nutrition Examination Survey 2001–2006. *Diabetes Care*, **36**, 2655–62.

Beiser, C. (1997) Recent advances: HIV infection–II. *British Medical Journal*, **314**, 579.

Bhopal, R.S., Phillimore, P., Moffatt, S., and Foy, C. (1994) Is living near a coking works harmful to health? A study of industrial air pollution. *Journal of Epidemiology and Community Health*, **48**, 237–47.

Bhopal, R. (2009) Seven mistakes and potential solutions in epidemiology, including a call for a World Council of Epidemiology and Causality. *Emerging Themes in Epidemiololgy*, **6**, 6.

Bhopal, R.S. (2013) A four-stage model explaining the higher risk of Type 2 diabetes mellitus in South Asians compared with European populations. *Diabetic Medicine*, **30**, 35–42.

Bradford Hill, A. (1965) The environment and disease: association or causation? *Occupational Medicine*, **58**, 295–300.

Chadwick, J. and Mann, W.N. (1950) *The Medical Works of Hippocrates*. Oxford, UK: Blackwell Scientific.

Charemza, W.W. and Deadman, D.F. (1997) *New Directions in Econometric Practice: General to Specific Modelling, Cointegration, and Vector Autoregression*, 2nd edn. Cheltenham, UK: Elgar.

Cottingham, J. (1996) *Western Philosophy—An Anthology*. Oxford, UK: Blackwell.

Davey Smith, G. Phillips, A.N. and Neaton J.D. (1992) Confounding in epidemiological studies: why 'independent' effects may not be all they seem. *British Medical Journal*, **305**, 757–9.

Doll, R. and Bradford Hill, A. (1956) Lung cancer and other causes of death in relation to smoking. *British Medical Journal*, **2**, 1071–81.

Evans, A. (1978) Causation and disease: a chronological journey. *American Journal of Epidemiology*, **108**, 249–58.

Gould, S.J. (1984) *The Mismeasure of Man*. London, UK: Pelican.

Government Office for Science. (2007) *Foresight. Tackling Obesities: Future Choices—Project Report*, 2nd edn.

Hammond, E.C., Selikoff, I.J., and Seidman, H. (1979) Asbestos exposure, cigarette smoking and death rates. *Annals of the New York Academy of Science*, **330**, 473–90.

Herbst, A., Ulfelder, H., and Poskanzer, D. (1971) Adenocarcinoma of the vagina: Association of maternal stilbestrol therapy with tumour appearance in young women. *New England Journal of Medicine*, **284**, 878–81. (Reprinted in Buck *et al.* 1988, pp. 446–50.)

Krieger, N. (1994) Epidemiology and the web of causation: has anyone seen the spider? *Social Science and Medicine*, **39**, 887–903.

Liddle, R. (**2015**) Toasties get you laid, fat prevents dementia and I'm a sex god. *The Sunday Times*, 12 April 2015, p. 19.

Mausner, J.S. and Kramer, S. (1985) *Epidemiology*, 2nd edn. Philadelphia, PA: W.B. Saunders.

Pearl, J. (2009) *Causality*, 2nd edn. Cambridge, UK: Cambridge University Press.

Porta, M. (2014) *A Dictionary of Epidemiology*, 6th edn. New York, NY: Oxford University Press.

Porter, R. (1997) *The Greatest Benefit to Mankind: A Medical history of Humanity from Antiquity to the present*. Harper Collins, London.

Rothman, K.J. and Greenland, S. (1998) *Modern Epidemiology*. Philadelphia, PA: Lippincott-Raven.

Rothman, K.J., Adami, H., and Trichopoulos, D. (1998) Should the mission of epidemiology include the eradication of poverty? *Lancet*, **352**, 810–13.

Semmelweis, I. (1983) *The Etiology, Concept and Prophylaxis of Childbed Fever*, translated by Codell Carter, K. University of Wisconsin, Madison. (Excerpted and reprinted in Buck *et al.* 1988, pp. 46–59.)

Skrabanek, P. (1994) The emptiness of the black box. *Epidemiology*, **5**, 553–5.

Smith, G.D., Phillips, A.N., and Neaton, J.D. (1992) Smoking as 'independent' risk factor for suicide: illustration of an artifact from observational epidemiology? *Lancet*, **340**, 709–12.

Susser, M. (1977) *Causal Thinking in the Health Sciences*, 2nd edn. New York, NY: Oxford University Press.

Tesh, S.N. (1988) *Hidden Arguments*. New Brunswick, Canada: Rutgers University Press.

Chapter 6

Interrelated concepts in the epidemiology of disease: Natural history and incubation period, time trends in populations, spectrum, iceberg, and screening

Objectives

On completion of this chapter you should understand:

- that the natural history of disease is the unchecked progression of disease in an individual;

- that natural history ranks alongside causal understanding in importance for the prevention and control of disease;

- that the technical and ethical challenges in describing the natural history of disease are great, particularly where the time between exposure to the causal agents and the onset of disease is long;

- that the incubation period is the time between exposure to a disease cause to the first clinical signs or symptoms of disease;

- that the spectrum of disease is the variety of ways it presents and evolves;

- that time trends in disease in populations describe the progress of disease in populations;

- that the changing pattern of disease in populations over time, and the spectrum of the presentation of disease, are related to natural history;

- that the 'iceberg of disease' is a metaphor emphasizing that the known number of cases (those visible) is outweighed by those not discovered (those invisible);

- how the iceberg of disease phenomenon thwarts assessment of the true burden of disease, the need for services, and the selection of representative cases for epidemiological study;

- that screening is the application of tests to diagnose disease (or its precursors) in an earlier phase of the natural history of disease than is achieved in routine medical practice;

- that the key to screening is a simple test, which can be applied to populations with minimum harm and has a high degree of accuracy in separating those who need more detailed investigation from those who don't;

- that the potential of screening is vast but there are limitations such as the inability to influence the natural history of many diseases, and the need to balance the costs and benefits of earlier diagnosis.

6.1 **Natural history of disease, the incubation period, and acute/chronic diseases**

The natural history of disease is the uninterrupted progression in an individual of the development of disease from the moment that it is initiated by exposure to the causal agents. Do the exercise in Box 6.1 before reading on.

There are four main types of response. First, the exposure may have no evident effect. The exposure may have had no effect because the dose was too low or the recipient was not susceptible. Alternatively, perhaps a cofactor was missing so there was no package of sufficient causes (section 5.3.2). There may, however, have been an effect but one too small to notice. Strictly speaking, then, for such individuals there is no 'history of disease', or even precursors of disease. Nonetheless, from an epidemiological and public health perspective this type of response is important, because we may learn how to protect populations by studying these individuals.

Second, there may be some demonstrable damaging effect of the exposure which may be repaired. Microbiological, immunological, biochemical, genetic, or pathological studies may be able to demonstrate inflammation, biochemical or tissue change, and repair. This type of response is likely to lead to some illness, possibly non-specific symptoms and signs such as tiredness and fever.

Third, the effect may be an illness that is rapidly contained by the body's defence mechanism. In this case, there will usually be a short illness. In the case of tuberculosis, there may be a fever that subsides. The tuberculosis bacilli are controlled, though they may remain alive.

Fourth, the illness may progress until it leads to continuing long-term problems, irreversible damage, or death. This progression may be curtailed by treatment (however, it then no longer represents the natural history of disease, but the prognosis).

The outcome of the exposure will depend on the interactions of host, agent, and environmental factors. For example, an elderly person with cardiorespiratory diseases may die on exposure to smog on a cold wintry day, when similar exposure of a younger person (with the same amount of smog) would have no important adverse effect. The natural history, as outlined in these four responses to exposure, is a biological and clinical concept of great importance to all medical sciences, including epidemiology.

Figure 6.1 provides an idealized view of the concept. The idea is that individuals start life healthy or at least disease-free. As they age, they are exposed to disease-causing agents which, cumulatively, increase their susceptibility to disease, some of it becoming chronic. In the early years, exposure to disease agents causes little lasting harm. This cumulative burden, however, eventually leads to death. With the exception of the period in utero and early infancy, which are perilous times in terms of health risks, this idealized picture is becoming true in the affluent parts of the world, where the pattern of health, ill health, and death generally follows that shown in Figure 6.1. The burden of serious ill health is being 'compressed' into the later part of life. The same concept can be applied to individual diseases.

Box 6.1 **Potential effects of an exposure to a causal agent**

Reflect on the possible outcomes in an individual from exposure to a causal agent. The causal agents to consider include microbes (e.g. those causing Legionnaires' disease or tuberculosis) and inanimate exposures (e.g. particulate air pollution or tobacco smoke).

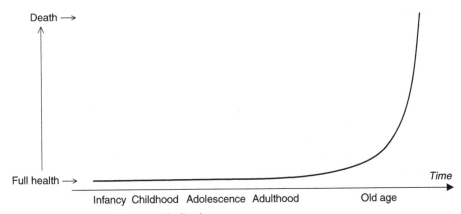

Fig. 6.1 Natural history of disease, idealized.

Tuberculosis provides an excellent example, illustrated in Figure 6.2, which shows the natural history in one hypothetical individual in a simple way. This person was exposed to the tubercle bacillus in early childhood, but the primary tuberculosis that followed hardly impaired his health. He harboured this illness through childhood but it recurred in adolescence (possibly because of other health problems at that time) with recovery. Then a second recurrence in early old age led to death. Figure 6.3 shows a typical path for the natural history of coronary heart disease (CHD). The causes exert their effect in early life and the development of atheroma usually begins in adolescence (or earlier). Disease may not be manifest until adulthood (often middle age). The first clinical occurrence may be angina or a heart attack, with partial recovery, until recurrence and death in later life.

While it is of vital importance, information on natural history is very hard to obtain. Reflect on the questions in Box 6.2 before reading on.

In practice, the natural history of diseases such as tuberculosis is interrupted as soon as possible either by treatment, or by immunization with Bacillus Calmette–Guérin (BCG). It would be ethically unacceptable anywhere in the world to observe the natural history of tuberculosis. Treatment is curative and cheap. As a medical diagnosis is essential to define the natural history of disease, the truth about it is seldom known for two major reasons. First, the act of diagnosis

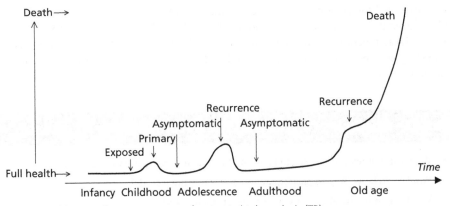

Fig. 6.2 Natural history disease: outcome of untreated tuberculosis (TB).

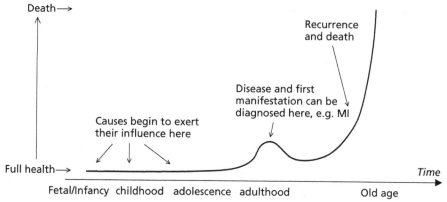

Fig. 6.3 Natural history of coronary heart disease (CHD).

and follow-up by a physician may initiate changes in the disease process, for example, through the placebo effect, or by changing the behaviour of the person observed. This principle is clear in the case of psychological disorders, say depression or anxiety, but probably applies to all diseases in a subtler form. For example, the observation of the natural history of CHD by repeat electro-cardiogram or Rose Angina Questionnaire in people is likely to raise awareness of the disease and induce some modifications of lifestyle. Second, the scientific objective of observing the natural history of disease clashes with the ethical medical imperative to act to alleviate, contain, or treat the disease. For medically qualified epidemiologists the ethical imperative is clear, but it is less so for non-medical ones, for there is no widely agreed and enforced ethical code for science (see section 10.11). (In cases of doubt, all epidemiologists should ensure that their work is cleared by an ethical committee.) Defining the natural history of most diseases in the modern world is, there-fore, problematic. Once a person is under medical care then outcome is likely to be influenced and is known as the prognosis. By contrast with natural history, prognosis is easy to study if patients can be followed up, with the problems being technical rather than ethical.

Studies of the natural history of disease are potentially ethically explosive. One infamous exam-ple was the United States Public Health Service's Tuskegee Syphilis Study (see Jones 1993), where 600 'negro' men, many with active syphilis, in the state of Alabama in the United States of America were followed up for a period of about 40 years. They were actively shielded from treatment by the investigators. The investigators believed that the scientific value of their observations on natural history exceeded the right of their subjects to therapy. There was no informed consent by the subjects. Even if there had been, the study would still be unethical, because it clashes with the medical ethical imperative to do good and not harm (this example is also discussed in Chapter 4 and in Chapter 10 because it is one of the defining chapters in the modern history of the ethics of medical science).

Box 6.2 Obstacles to studying the natural history of disease

- What difficulties can you see in studying the true natural history of disease?
- Would you be willing to participate in a natural history study?
- What might be the effect on you of being in such a study?

The ethical principles for epidemiological studies of natural history are that:

- these studies can only be done on informed individuals;
- studies are only permissible when there is no known effective therapy;
- if an effective therapy becomes available after the study starts then the study will need to be modified or abandoned.

The placebo group in some clinical trials is, potentially, an important source of information on the natural history (see Chapter 9). Placebos have an influence so, strictly speaking, even this is not the true natural history. The emerging principle for trials is that the control group should receive the best available therapy, and not placebo, so this source of data on the natural history of disease may dry up.

Follow-up, or cohort, studies are needed to define the natural history of disease (see Chapter 9 for a discussion of cohort studies). Repeated observation of the same individuals over long time periods is usually necessary in chronic diseases. Ideally, a disease-free population would be observed closely and repeatedly, until either the population is no longer at any risk of the disease or until death. For example, in an ideal study of the natural history of gestational diabetes, a representative sample of pregnant women would be followed, with observations to include tests of blood glycose levels. For those who did not develop diabetes in pregnancy, the observations could stop until the next pregnancy. For those who did develop diabetes, follow-up would continue after pregnancy, to assess whether it resolves and whether there are long-term adverse outcomes. In the latter case, the follow-up may be measured in decades, and in those with continuing diabetes and complications, until death. With this information we can decide whether gestational diabetes is a harmful phenomenon, and develop appropriate health services, on appropriate timescales. To take one simple question: does gestational diabetes herald type 2 diabetes in later life? If not, after pregnancy the woman need not be followed up, at least in relation to diabetes. If yes, such women may need to be followed up. In practice such cohort studies are rare, and long-term observations may prove costly or impossible. The natural history is usually pieced together from a mixture of observations, including those from single individuals (case reports) or from case series observed by clinicians, rather than in formal epidemiological studies. In Chapter 9, I show how each study design links to natural history.

The time between exposure to the agent and the development of disease is called the incubation period. It varies greatly in individuals but in populations the pattern can be defined both for broad categories of disease and for specific diagnoses. Diseases that have long incubation periods, usually measured in years and sometimes decades, generally have a long clinical course and, if so, by convention they are called chronic diseases (the label is embedded in medicine, even though it is problematic). An example of a chronic disease is chronic bronchitis. This disease is likely to have been caused by prolonged exposure to a mixture of agents including respiratory infections in childhood and adulthood, air pollution, and tobacco smoke. Chronic bronchitis is likely to run a clinical course measured in decades and the damage is usually irreversible. Other examples of chronic diseases include rheumatoid arthritis, CHD, diabetes, and most cancers.

Some chronic diseases, paradoxically, lead to sudden and unexpected death (e.g. a stroke or heart attack); the diagnosis is possibly made at a post-mortem. The label chronic disease is based on the natural history as defined in many individuals, not the clinical course in an individual. The opportunity to control and treat a chronic disease may be short, but the opportunity to prevent it will be prolonged.

Diseases with a short incubation period (days, weeks, and sometimes months) usually have a short course (say, less than a year), and by convention are known as acute diseases. These include most infections and many toxic disorders, for example, influenza, food poisoning, and carbon

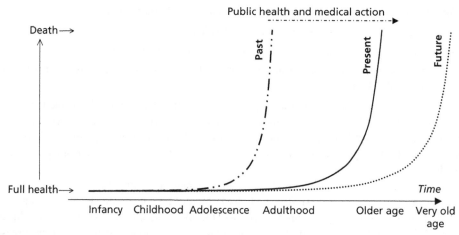

Fig. 6.4 Natural history of disease: giving purpose to public health and medicine.

monoxide poisoning. Paradoxically, the effects of acute disease may also be severe and prolonged, such as post-viral syndromes. Clearly, an acute disease can leave permanent (chronic) sequelae; for example, meningitis can lead to chronic deafness. The incubation period, together with minimal clinical information on the nature of the illness (e.g. a rash and fever), may be sufficient to identify the disease. This is particularly the case with infectious diseases. For example, vomiting within a few hours of eating a meal in a group of people is much more likely to be due to Staphylococcus aureus food poisoning than salmonella infection. This is an example of how epidemiology serves medicine and public health.

Knowledge of the natural history is vital for disease prevention policies, particularly for secondary prevention based on screening, and provides the underlying rationale for all medical practice. Indeed, the whole purpose of medicine is to influence the natural history of disease by reducing and delaying ill health. Figure 6.4 illustrates this. When this is achieved through deliberate actions by societies, the collective endeavour is public health.

The natural history concept applies to individuals but it has implications for thinking about disease in populations. First, changes in the natural history of disease in individuals do, of course, affect the population pattern. Improved general nutrition, for example, reduces the likelihood of an individual developing secondary tuberculosis. In turn this reduces the risk of person-to-person transmission, and hence the incidence of clinical tuberculosis and death. Second, the various paths to progression in individuals can be aggregated to produce a portrait of what alternatives may happen in a population. This is shown in Figure 6.5 and will be discussed in section 6.3.

6.2 **Population trends in disease**

The concept of the natural history of disease should not be (but is) confused with the changing pattern of disease in populations over time, for example, the decline in recent decades of gastric cancer or the rise of AIDS. It is commonplace to hear or read, for example, that the natural history of stroke has changed in the past hundred years. Such trends should not be referred to in this way. There is no widely agreed word or phrase to capture this concept, though the 'secular trend' in disease (secular in the sense of long term) is sometimes used. The secular trend is, however, a limited concept; it does not capture the point that the incidence of the disease may not change much, but the population pattern of disease occurrence may be radically altered. For example, the

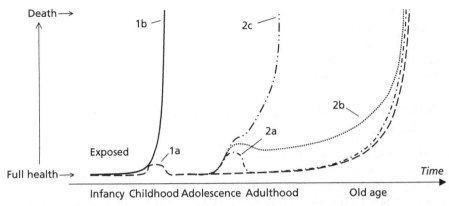

Fig. 6.5 Natural history of disease: pathways in tuberculosis. 1a: Primary infection with complete remission (death from other causes); 1b: fatal tuberculous meningitis; 2a: recurrence with successful treatment (death from other causes); 2b: TB with residual disability (and TB contributory or actual cause of death); 2c: recurrence with fatal outcome.

distribution of a disease across socio-economic groups may change, as it has for CHD which has become less common in wealthy, and more common in poor, populations. An appropriate phrase that captures this broader concept is the 'population pattern of disease' (PPOD), as it is more specific than a phrase that is often used—the epidemiology of disease. The main measure of PPOD is the disease incidence given over time, place, and person (see Chapter 7).

Clearly, changes in the natural history of disease and in the population pattern are linked. Before reading on, consider the exercise in Box 6.3.

Reducing the population's susceptibility would diminish the number of cases of overt, diagnosed disease, while enhanced susceptibility would have the opposite effect. The secular trend would change. If the changes in susceptibility are uneven across a population, there will be other changes in the PPOD too, for example, the change in inequalities in CHD referred to earlier in this section.

The duration of an episode of disease is likely to be linked to susceptibility, and hence the capacity to fight against the disease. A shorter course is also likely to have a better outcome, with less long-term morbidity or mortality. While the disease incidence will not be affected, the prevalence and case fatality is likely to be (Chapters 7 and 8). These changes will be reflected in the PPOD.

The length of the incubation period can affect disease patterns. If the incubation period lengthens in a chronic disease from 20 to 30 years, then the disease burden will decline, at least for some

---

Box 6.3 Interrelationship between natural history and population pattern of disease

Assuming there are no changes to exposure to the causal agent, what effect would changing the natural history have on the population pattern? Consider, for example, the effect of:

- reduced and enhanced susceptibility;
- a shorter or longer course of disease;
- a longer and shorter incubation period;
- a more severe or less severe disease.

time. The severity of the disease can also change, either as a result of changed virulence of the disease agent or changed susceptibility of the host. This will alter the balance between diagnosed and undiagnosed cases, changing the measured incidence and prevalence, and hence PPOD.

The idea that an exposure can lead to variants (and varying severity) of the same disease is the spectrum of disease (an idea that is sometimes confused with the natural history of disease).

6.3 Spectrum of disease: a clinical concept fundamental to epidemiology

The spectrum of disease captures the idea that diseases present with varying signs, symptoms, and severity. For example, if a hundred people are exposed simultaneously to an aerosol contaminated with the Legionnaires' disease bacillus, most (about 98%) will have no perceptible problems. The remainder will have disease which varies from a mild influenza-like illness to severe pneumonia. Of those who become ill, about 10–15 per cent will die unless effective treatment is given. The mortality rate will be higher in some settings and population groups, such as in nursing homes, or hospital outbreaks where the frail or elderly are. The period of time between exposure and first symptoms will vary from as little as two days in some people, to as much as 10 days in others. The symptoms and signs of illness will vary greatly; some people have an illness dominated by neurological problems, others by chest problems. Among survivors, some will recover fully, and others will be left with disability. This principle of variability of outcome applies to nearly all diseases, whether they be infections, toxic problems, or cancers.

Tuberculosis is a particularly good example and is illustrated in Table 6.1 and Figure 6.5, which combine the natural history and spectrum of disease concepts. Figure 6.5 develops this idea from a population perspective, where the collective observations on a number of individuals are summarized as possible pathways in the natural history. With some exceptions, children develop a mild illness (or a subclinical problem) from which they recover. This illness is not usually recognized as primary tuberculosis, but as a febrile illness of childhood. This progression is shown by line 1a in Figure 6.5. Rarely, this first exposure will lead to a serious infection, which may be systemic (i.e. affects the whole body). Tuberculous meningitis is one of the rare, potentially fatal outcomes of such infection (line 1b). More usually, the primary tuberculosis is followed by a lifetime of cohabitation by the agent and host with living organisms sealed off in the lymph glands of the patient (line 1a). In some cases, particularly when the natural defence mechanisms of the patient are weakened by other illnesses (e.g. AIDS, age, or other factors), the bacillus overcomes the defence mechanisms to cause secondary tuberculosis (line 2). The commonest form of this disease is respiratory, or lymphatic, but it may be a more general illness with fevers and weight loss. In most instances, the disease will respond to therapy (after which we are not observing the

Table 6.1 Spectrum of disease: tuberculosis

Primary tuberculosis	Secondary tuberculosis
No symptoms	Fever and weight loss
Minor self-limiting illness	Enlarged lymph glands
Grumbling illness with fevers	Persistent cough
Overwhelming illness such as tuberculous, meningitis	Skin rashes
	Septicaemia (miliary tuberculosis)

natural history but the prognosis) or heal spontaneously (line 2a). Some people will be left with permanent disability (line 2b), while others will die (line 2c).

The spectrum of disease is a concept with obvious and important implications for clinical medicine. Doctors who are not aware of the full spectrum of disease, particularly the less severe or rare forms, are likely to be misled. The variants within the spectrum of disease may differ in different population groups. For example, while pulmonary tuberculosis is the dominant mode of clinical presentation in European-origin residents in the United Kingdom, lymph node tuberculosis is the commonest form in UK residents of Indian subcontinent origin. Coronary heart disease is more likely to present as angina in women, and as a heart attack in men. In the elderly and in people with diabetes, in particular, CHD may present as a silent myocardial infarction, that is, a heart attack without chest pain.

Some diseases occur more than once. Presentation of the same disease may differ at different times. The first occurrence of malaria is likely to be far more severe than subsequent episodes. In chronic diseases, however, recurrences may be characteristic; for example, if a person develops pain in the jaw and tongue in one occurrence of angina, then that person is likely to have a similar pattern at recurrence, rather than, say, pain in the left arm.

The fact that diseases may be mild or even 'silent' are among the many explanations for undiagnosed disease in the community, even when people are served by an excellent health service, a phenomenon described by the metaphor of the iceberg of disease (see Last 1963) and developed as a pyramid by me.

6.4 **The unmeasured burden of disease: the metaphors of the iceberg and the pyramid**

Surprisingly, for most health problems and within all health-care systems, there are large numbers of undiscovered or misdiagnosed cases of disease. The exceptions to this generalization are the serious diseases that have obvious symptoms, which lead to a rapid and accurate diagnosis. Lung cancer is an excellent example of an exception, while prostate cancer is illustrative of the generalization. Lung cancer has characteristic symptoms, for example, cough, weight loss, and blood in the sputum, and, if untreated, it spreads and is invariably fatal. Prostate cancer may remain localized, with no signs or symptoms and in these circumstances poses little threat to health. Yet prostate cancer may also kill, and be diagnosed too late to cure. (See also Exemplar 6.1.) Serious and deadly disorders such as diabetes, atrial fibrillation, and hypertension are other good examples of this phenomenon. This principle applies alike to populations served by comprehensive, publicly funded health-care systems, and to those with private services only available to those who can pay. Obviously, the number of undiagnosed cases in relation to those diagnosed will be bigger where the health-care system is poor.

The metaphor for this phenomenon is the iceberg of disease and symptoms. The concept was brought to close attention with the publication in 1963 of a paper entitled *The Iceberg: 'completing the clinical picture' in general practice*, by John Last. Last pointed to the importance of the phenomenon for clinical practice, epidemiological methods, and screening. Surprisingly, he did not illustrate the paper with an iceberg.

Cases that have been correctly diagnosed are the tip of the iceberg, visible, and easily measured. In most diseases, as with the iceberg, the larger amount lurks unseen, unmeasured, and easily forgotten with potentially catastrophic consequences. Figure 6.6 illustrates this and also develops the iceberg concept as a pyramid of disease by using its clearer structure and shape. At the tip of the pyramid are the cases that are diseased, diagnosed, treated, and controlled. The next block is the diagnosed but uncontrolled cases. The failure to control the disease arises from either technical or organizational

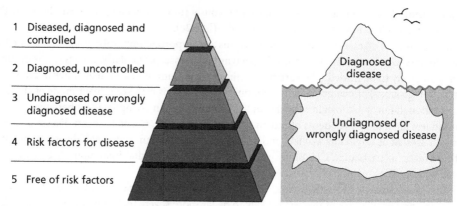

1 Diseased, diagnosed and controlled

2 Diagnosed, uncontrolled

3 Undiagnosed or wrongly diagnosed disease

4 Risk factors for disease

5 Free of risk factors

Diagnosed disease

Undiagnosed or wrongly diagnosed disease

Fig. 6.6 Iceberg and pyramid of health and disease.

factors or from the patient's preferences not to participate in therapy (so-called non-compliance or non-adherence). The third block comprises the patients with undiagnosed or misdiagnosed disease, which may be a reflection of the difficulties of making the diagnosis, or the failure to access health care. The fourth block is the population that harbours the causal factors for disease, but remains disease-free. The final block is the population free of both disease and causal factors. Blocks 1 and 2 correspond to the iceberg above sea level and blocks 3 and 4 to below sea level. The pyramid comprises both the diseased population and those potentially diseased (i.e. it is a whole population concept), while the iceberg relates only to the diseased population. The population with risk factors and free of risk factors could be considered as the sea from which the iceberg emerges.

There is a specific and minimal level of health care need at each level as shown in Figure 6.7. For block 1, the need is for vigilance and perhaps follow-up. For block 2, there is a need for review and effective and acceptable care. There may also be a need for more research to discover better therapeutic interventions. For block 3 there is, potentially, a need for screening to detect people with early disease. For block 4, there is a need for health education, health promotion, and health policy to control risk factors. For block 5, there is a need for health promotion to maintain this desirable state.

Epidemiology that forgets the iceberg phenomenon, and merely counts and studies cases actually seen by clinicians and diagnosed, is potentially misleading. Both for applied and causal

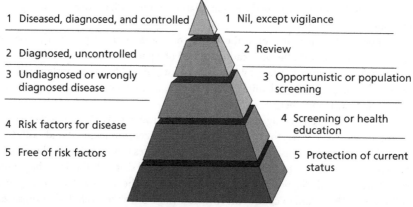

1 Diseased, diagnosed, and controlled

2 Diagnosed, uncontrolled

3 Undiagnosed or wrongly diagnosed disease

4 Risk factors for disease

5 Free of risk factors

1 Nil, except vigilance

2 Review

3 Opportunistic or population screening

4 Screening or health education

5 Protection of current status

Fig. 6.7 Pyramid (iceberg) of disease: potential health and health-care need.

research, epidemiology on data obtained from routine systems like hospital admissions is likely to be compromised. The missing cases thwart our efforts to assess the true burden of disease. This creates difficulties in judging priorities and assessing the need for health services. There are no easy rules or formulae to apply to judge the true burden of disease using data on those diagnosed. However, experience with type 2 diabetes mellitus indicates that, in the absence of opportunistic or systematic screening, about 50 per cent of the cases in the community are diagnosed at any point in time. The findings for hypertension are about the same. For less serious diseases (migraine, eczema, back pain, anaemia) or those which tend to get less attention (thyroid disorders, chronic bronchitis, peptic ulcer, and osteoarthritis) the proportion diagnosed would be lower. When health services, particularly primary care, are alert to this phenomenon and institute case-finding measures, then the proportion of undiagnosed cases declines, as has happened in affluent countries for type 2 diabetes mellitus. It is reasonable for researchers and health planners to assume that the true burden of disease is much higher than their data show, and unreasonable to reach conclusions without reference to the iceberg phenomenon (as is too often the case).

Unidentified cases may be different from identified ones, in terms of both the natural history and the spectrum of disease. For example, people with undiagnosed prostate cancer are less likely to have urinary symptoms or pain compared with those diagnosed. Where symptoms, disease progression, and outcome are related, the undiagnosed cases are likely to be less severe. For this reason a screening programme (see next section, 'Screening: early diagnosis of disease or disease precursors') may uncover not just cases of disease at an earlier stage of the natural history, but also less aggressive and severe cases. This may mislead the evaluation of screening programmes. In contrast, when symptoms and signs are not evident in the early stages of disease, as in high blood pressure or chronic glaucoma, undiagnosed cases may be just as severe as diagnosed ones.

Epidemiological studies of the burden, causes and consequences of disease should, ideally, be of representative cases. Studies based on selected cases from the tip of the iceberg may give an erroneous view. The study of the outcome of prostate cancer based on cases diagnosed in hospital would lead to the view that the disease is usually, if not always, progressive. Studies of unselected cases, however, show that prostatic cancer can be a static, or slowly progressive phenomenon. There is a view that causal research does not need representative cases. That is correct for proof-of-concept studies. The results will then need checking in other contexts. For example, the causes of prostate cancer in diagnosed hospitalized patients may be different from those in the undiagnosed people (probably with the slow growing variety of cancer).

Patients who are at the tip of the iceberg are more likely to have multiple health problems than others because these diseases bring them to medical attention, which in turn increases the diagnostic activity, leading to even more diagnoses. Their susceptibilities to various diseases, the causal pathway, and their outcomes may differ too. For example, people with cardiorespiratory problems and diabetes, and those living alone or in poverty, are more likely to be admitted to hospital than those without such a clustering of circumstances. False and misleading associations between diseases and life circumstances may be generated in studying only hospital cases. This is the basis of the bias known as Berkson's bias (Chapter 4).

6.5 Screening: early diagnosis of disease or disease precursors

6.5.1 Introduction: definition, purposes, and ethics

The principles and methods in this section are focused on screening populations in public health contexts. However, they mostly also apply to diagnostic tests in clinical care, to opportunistic screening in clinical care, and in the use of disease prediction models, algorithms, and questionnaires to evaluate risk. Here, the term *screening* should be understood to mean population screening, where the target population is invited to participate.

Screening is the use of tests to help diagnose diseases (or their precursor conditions) in an earlier phase of their natural history, or at the less severe end of the spectrum than usual. We hope that the diagnosis may be made long before (maybe years or decades) it would be normally. By contrast, clinical diagnostic tests aim to speed up and make more accurate the diagnostic process. In so doing, screening uncovers the iceberg of disease. On the pyramid model in Figure 6.7, screening is applied to block 3 and, less commonly, to block 4. The main aim is to reverse, halt, or slow the progression of disease more effectively than would normally happen. This is the only aim of screening that is unequivocally, ethically justifiable. Providing early knowledge about the diagnosis, whether to the patient or professional, is, on its own, insufficient reason for screening. The reason for this is that there are harms and costs of both screening and of knowing the diagnosis that may outweigh the health benefit of such knowledge.

There are, however, more controversial purposes of screening. Screening is also done to protect a society, even though the individual may not benefit, or might even be harmed. Screening potential immigrants at the point at which a visa is issued or at the port of entry (for both contagious and chronic diseases) is an example. Screening may be done to select out unhealthy people, for example, for a job. The police, fire brigade, armed forces, and airlines are employers that screen potential employees in detail. Screening is sometimes done to help to allocate health-care resources that are limited. The most extreme example is the practice of triage in wartime, when those unlikely to survive war wounds are left untreated so saving resources for those likely to survive. Screening may be done to identify disease at an early stage to help understand the natural history. In these circumstances, when the screening is not primarily for the benefit of individuals being screened, there are difficult ethical issues, particularly in genetic screening.

The ethical viewpoint, that the natural history of disease must be influenced favourably, sets limits on the scope of screening, and poses important challenges. This means that the natural history of the disease needs to be understood, there need to be effective interventions for treating or controlling the disease, and the screening test needs to detect the problem at a stage when the disease has not advanced beyond the stage of useful therapy. These aims of screening are summarized in Box 6.4.

Screening applies tests to people who have not actively sought clinical care or advice for the disease to be tested for. At best they have been invited and informed, and have consented to be screened, and at worst they may have been screened without their informed consent. This is the feature that distinguishes screening from normal clinical practice where the patient has initiated the contact. The ethical basis of screening is fundamentally different from testing in clinical settings, because who initiates the test and why is all-important.

Box 6.4 Aims of screening

♦ Better prognosis/outcome for individuals

♦ Protect society

♦ Rational, efficient allocation of resources

♦ Selection of healthy individuals

♦ Research (e.g. on natural history of disease)

6.5.2 **Choosing what to screen for: the lasting legacy of criteria of Wilson and Jungner**

Potentially, screening could be done for every disease for which there is a diagnostic test, or diagnostic signs and symptoms. Indeed, this idea often gains enthusiastic support, including from the media, but it is misguided. Screening is only rarely justified. Unfortunately, because of its superficial attractiveness, screening is implemented too early with little benefit and at great cost, not to mention harm.

To guide the rational development of screening programmes, there are several sets of criteria, usually variants of those of Wilson and Jungner (1968), as listed in Box 6.5. The criteria have had a lasting effect. The UK National Screening Committee website lists 22 criteria under four headings: 1. The condition; 2. The test; 3. Treatment; 4. The screening programme (examined June 2015).

The World Health Organization (WHO) Bulletin has revisited the original criteria in the era of the new genetics, including a synthesis of criteria proposed over 40 years (Andermann *et al.*, 2008). The original ideas of Wilson and Jungner still represent an excellent summary for our purposes. There are two issues in the revisions that struck me as especially noteworthy. First, screening, especially genetic screening, has implications for others, especially close family. The UK criteria say the test of genetic mutations should be acceptable to other family members. While this is worthy of debate it does draw to our attention that many screening tests may have implications for others, both in terms of their own health risks and also in other matters, for example, declaring such matters for health insurance. The second point, often forgotten, but even if not so, one that is difficult to apply; that is, that primary prevention efforts should have been implemented already. We know a great deal about how to prevent breast cancer (early age at childbirth, breast feeding, have several children, etc.) but none of them are acted on seriously, while many countries have implemented national breast cancer screening through X-ray examination of the breasts.

Box 6.5 The criteria of Wilson and Junger

1. The condition sought should be an important health problem

2. There should be an accepted treatment for patients with recognized disease

3. Facilities for diagnosis and treatment should be available

4. There should be a recognizable latent or early symptomatic stage

5. There should be a suitable test or examination

6. The test should be acceptable to the population

7. The natural history of the disease, including latent disease, should be adequately understood

8. There should be an agreed policy on whom to treat

9. The cost of case-finding (including diagnosis and treatment of patients diagnosed) should be economically balanced in relation to possible expenditure on medical care as a whole

10. Case-finding should be a continuing process, and not a 'once for all' project

Most lists of criteria are hard to remember, so I have condensed them to six questions:

1. Is there an effective intervention for those screened?
2. Does intervention earlier than usual improve outcome?
3. Is there a screening test that accurately recognizes disease earlier than usual?
4. Is the test available, affordable, and acceptable to the target population?
5. Is the disease one that commands priority?
6. Do the health and other benefits of screening exceed the financial and other costs in this society?

If the answer to these six questions is yes, then the case for screening is worth examining carefully. The final decision will, as ever, depend on availability of resources and the priority of this programme in relation to others. As population screening is in the public eye, the decision often involves the government, and not just health services.

Screening programmes need more careful evaluation than clinical care. The reasons for this include: screening is a professionally initiated activity whereas diagnosis is a response to a patient seeking care; the outcomes of screening are not easily measured for they accumulate over long time periods; the acceptability of a programme may change with time; the performance of the test may change over time, particularly if the frequency of disease changes; and screening is an expensive and difficult process, which is hard both to implement and to withdraw.

Opportunistic screening is the term used when people coming for health or other care for another reason are invited to take the opportunity to be tested. While they should be informed and give consent, this may well not happen explicitly. For example, people may go to see a doctor because of increasing deafness, but their weight and/or blood pressure is measured while they are there. This information may then be put into a cardiovascular disease risk prediction model to calculate the risk of a cardiovascular event over the next 10 years. Both steps are opportunistic screening.

Screening for hypertension illustrates the issues well. Hypertension is a common, major causal factor in stroke, CHD, heart failure, and in disorders of other organs, particularly the kidney. Mostly, the cause of high blood pressure in an individual cannot be found, and this type of disease is called essential hypertension, where essential really means 'of unknown cause'. In perhaps 5–10 per cent of cases there is an identifiable cause (e.g. severe kidney diseases leading to hypertension), and this form is known as secondary hypertension. Hypertension is not, strictly, a disease but a precursor of disease. Nonetheless, its importance and close association with diseases has led to it being considered, in practice, as a disease.

Hypertension usually occurs without symptoms and may first present as a stroke or heart attack. The challenge is to prevent this. As some of the changes induced by hypertension occur at an early stage of the natural history and may become irreversible, this is best done through screening. Before reading on, do the exercise in Box 6.6.

Box 6.6 Screening for hypertension

Even if your knowledge of high blood pressure is limited, assess this condition against the criteria in Box 6.5 (perhaps after a little extra reading). Now, apply the six questions on the previous page.

Wilson and Jungner's criteria are met and the answer to the six questions mentioned earlier is unequivocally yes. The problem is a priority. Effective, acceptable, and cheap treatments that improve long-term health outcomes are available. A screening test is widely available and acceptable, though it has some problems. The benefits of screening for hypertension far exceed the costs. The screening test is measurement of the blood pressure (BP), usually using a sphygmomanometer. This simple instrument consists of a cuff that is placed around the upper arm and inflated until blood flow is cut off. The pressure at which blood flow restarts is the systolic blood pressure, which is the maximum pressure as the heart beats. In healthy people, systolic pressure is about 110–120 mmHg (millimetres of mercury). The blood pressure when the heart is not beating is about 80 mmHg. Blood pressure is expressed as the systolic value over the diastolic, that is, usually about 120/80 mmHg. Sometimes two readings may be made, 5 to 30 minutes apart. The definitive diagnostic test is, effectively, repetition of the same test on several different occasions combined with a clinical history, examination, and other tests to check for other diseases, particularly those that cause specific forms of hypertension. A check is also made on whether the adverse consequences of high blood pressure have occurred (e.g. on the eyes, or kidneys).

Additional tests of high blood pressure are possible but are used infrequently, at least in screening, including 24-hour readings using equipment that permits measurement while the person is living normally. Blood pressure screening based on the sphygmomanometer is done in many settings: in routine clinical practice in primary care and hospital settings; in pre-employment physical examinations; in workplace health programmes, as part of a periodic check up; in well-woman/well-man clinics; in antenatal clinics; and even in pharmacies and supermarkets. As the equipment and expertise to do the test is so widespread, in many countries there is little need for a specially designed population-based screening programme. Nonetheless, people are missed, especially men who are most at risk. Therefore, this test is usually incorporated into health check population screening programmes, for example, the Vascular Checks Programme of NHS England.

The problem is that blood pressure measurement, like all screening tests is not 100 per cent accurate, which we will consider next.

6.5.3 Sensitivity, specificity, and predictive powers of screening tests

Screening will make blocks 1 and 2 in the pyramid of disease (Fig. 6.6) grow and block 3 shrink. The danger is that through incorrect false positive tests, people in blocks 4 and 5 are wrongly placed in blocks 1 and 2, and through incorrect false negative tests, people in blocks 1 and 2 are placed in blocks 4 and 5.

The ideal test would pick up all cases of hypertension in the population tested. This attribute of the test is known as high sensitivity (or, alternatively, as the true positive rate). To help remember this, remember that such a test would be sensitive to the presence of disease. Clearly, the ideal test would also correctly identify all people who do not have the disease. Think of this as the test being specific to those who have the disease. This attribute of the test is the specificity (or, alternatively, the true negative rate). The ideal test would, therefore, correctly identify both cases and non-cases.

In the ideal test, therefore, when patients undergo more detailed clinical examination, the screening test result is confirmed (i.e. a screening test predicts the final result). A positive test, in ideal circumstances, would predict with 100 per cent accuracy the presence of hypertension and, similarly, a negative test would predict its absence. These attributes of the test are known as the predictive powers.

There is, unfortunately, no such perfect test, whether for screening or for diagnosis. Similarly, all epidemiological measures are also imperfect. We can think of these measures as tests and evaluate

Table 6.2 The 2 × 2 table: assessing the performance of the screening test

Screening test	Disease (true/definitive test)		
	+ve	**−ve**	**Total**
+ve	a	b	a + b
−ve	c	d	c + d
Total	a + c	b + d	a + b + c + d

Sensitivity or true positive rate = a/(a + c). Predictive power of a +ve test = a/(a + b).
Specificity or true negative rate = d/(b + d). Predictive power of a -ve test = d/(c + d).

their accuracy in the same way as for screening tests. As 100 per cent accuracy is not attainable with any diagnostic procedures, we apply the best available means of diagnosis as the gold standard against which the screening test is compared.

These four measures—sensitivity, specificity, and predictive power of a positive and negative test—are the main way to assess the performance of a screening or diagnostic test. These and other measures of test performance can be calculated from the 2 × 2 table as shown in Table 6.2. The rows of Table 6.2 show the results of the screening test, the columns the disease status. The disease status is said to be the true status of the person based either on a definitive (gold standard) series of tests or on clinical observation, often made over long time periods (possibly checked post-mortem). As even the definitive test is never 100 per cent accurate, a screening test is being evaluated against another imperfect, albeit better, test.

Table 6.2 uses a standard notation and layout: the letter 'a' represents true positive results on the screening test, 'b' false positives, 'c' false negatives, and 'd' true negatives. The formulae for the four measures are in the table. The best way to understand these formulae and to learn how to interpret the data is through practice. Try the exercise in Box 6.7, before reading on.

The sensitivity (93.4%) and specificity (98.2%) of the test are very high, as shown in Table 6.3. (This level of accuracy is unusual in clinical practice.) In other words, in these circumstances the test will correctly identify most people who have the disease (a), and also correctly identify most people who are disease-free (d). Nonetheless, about one person in 20 who does have the disease will be misclassified as disease-free (c), and hence wrongly reassured. If the disease is serious and late diagnosis dangerous, this could be a problem. Far fewer people without disease will be misclassified as having the disease (b). This performance is reassuring from a population perspective, but it is not information of direct interest to individuals and their doctors who want to know

Box 6.7 Calculating sensitivity and specificity

Five hundred patients known on the basis of definitive diagnostic tests to have a particular disease were screened with a new test. The study was done to help evaluate this new test for its possible use as a screening tool. Five hundred controls without this disease were also screened. Of the 500 patients with disease, 467 had a positive test. Of the group without the disease, nine had a positive test. Create a 2 × 2 table based on Table 6.2 and reflect on the interpretation of the data especially by describing a, b, c, and d. Calculate the sensitivity and specificity of the test. Is this a good performance? What are the implications for those wrongly classified by the test?

Table 6.3 Calculation of sensitivity and specificity based on data in Box 6.7

Screening test	Diseased (true/definitive test)		
	+ve	−ve	
+ve	467 (a)	9 (b)	476 (a + b)
−ve	33 (c)	491 (d)	524 (c + d)
	500 (a + c)	500 (b + d)	1000 (a + b + c + d)

Sensitivity = a/(a + c) = 473/500 = 93.4%.

Specificity = d/(b + d) = 491/500 = 98.2%.

the implications of their individual results. They want to know what the definitive test is likely to show. In the special circumstance of an evaluation study, of course, they already know the true result but that would not be true of a screening programme. This is given by predictive powers (formulae in footnote of table 6.3). Reflect on Box 6.8 before reading on.

The predictive power of a positive test in the context here, where half of our population has the disease, is a/(a + b) = 467/476 = 98.1%; and of a negative test is d/(c + d) = 491/524 = 93.7%. In other words, only one or two per cent of those testing positive will have this result overturned by the definitive test. More of those with a negative test, however, will have this result overturned. This excellent performance is, however, a result of the artificial nature of the population, in which 50 per cent have the disease. That is, of course, unusual. The prevalence of the disease has a profound effect on the predictive power (but as considered later, not on sensitivity and specificity). Usually we consider a disease as common if one per cent or more of the population has it. You can think through the effects of change prevalence through the following reflection. Imagine that you take this test to a country where no one has the disease, that is, the prevalence of the disease is zero per cent. What will happen to the predictive powers of a positive and negative test? Now imagine the same for a population where 100 per cent have the disease.

If the prevalence of a disease is actually zero all screening test positive cases must, of necessity, be false positives (i.e. (b) in the notation in Table 6.3) and all screen negatives will be correct (i.e. (d) in the notation in Table 6.3). The predictive power of a positive test is zero since (a) is zero (and the predictive power of a negative test is 100%).

If the prevalence of a condition is 100 per cent then, logically, all screen positive cases will have the condition (and screen negatives will all be false), so the predictive power of a positive test is 100 per cent (and of a negative test zero). Predictive powers vary with disease/outcome prevalence, as shown in your exercise of the imagination above and in Figure 6.8. You can examine the effect of varying prevalence on predictive powers by doing the exercise in Box 6.9. In practice most diseases are uncommon, so the predictive power of a positive screening test tends to be low.

As the prevalence declines, as Table 6.4 and Table 6.5 show, the predictive power of a positive test declines, and the opposite is true for a negative test. When the prevalence is one per cent—a

Box 6.8 Predictive powers

If a man is positive on the screening test and asks what is his chance of eventually having the disease, that is, once all the definitive tests are done, what can we advise? Similarly, what do we advise if the test is negative on the screening test? From Table 6.3, calculate predictive powers.

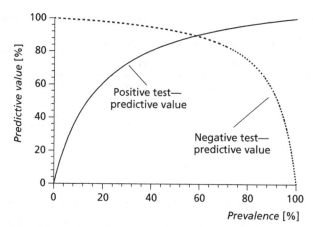

Fig. 6.8 Changes of predictive values with the prevalence of a disease (this example is calculated with a test sensitivity of 0.93 and a specificity of 0.85).

figure which actually represents a disease that is considered common in the community—the predictive power of this same test is 34.2 per cent; in other words, in 6.5 of 10 cases the screening test will be wrong, and those cases will possibly have been subjected to unnecessary anxiety and tests. It is vital that the performance of screening tests is evaluated in the context where they are to be used. Often tests are developed in research settings or hospitals, but applied in community settings. It should not be surprising that they do not work as well there.

Within any population there will be some subgroups with high, and others with low, prevalence of disease. For example, White Scottish people with Northern European origins have a high incidence of colorectal cancer, while people of Pakistani and Indian ethnicity in Scotland have low incidence. The colorectal cancer screening tests will not perform in the same way in these two populations. The performance is mainly in relation to predictive powers but we also need to beware of effects on sensitivity and specificity.

It is generally the case that the sensitivity and specificity of a test are independent of prevalence, but in practice they may not be. As the prevalence of the disease declines the accuracy of observers is diminished, reducing the sensitivity (Fowkes 1986). This is, of course, due to misclassification error. Furthermore, the principle that sensitivity and specificity are stable to changes in disease prevalence applies when there is a definitive test (gold standard) and not necessarily in other circumstances.

Box 6.9 **Varying prevalence: impact on predictive power**

Assume that the test in Table 6.3 is applied to (a) a population of 1000 patients attending general practice (primary care/family medicine), and that the prevalence of the disease is 10 per cent; and (b) in a community setting where the prevalence is one per cent. There will be 100 case of disease in (a) and 10 in (b). The sensitivity and specificity is as in Table 6.3. Prepare two 2 × 2 tables, complete the cells starting with (a + c), (b + d), and (a + b + c + d), and calculate the predictive powers. Now compare your answers with Tables 6.4 and 6.5.

Table 6.4 Predictive power (prevalence of disease = 10%)

Screening test	Disease (definitive test)		
	+ve	**−ve**	
+ve	93.4	16.2	109.6
−ve	6.6	883.8	890.4
	100	900	1000

Predictive power of positive test = a/(a + b) = 93.4/109.6 = 85.2%.

Predictive power of negative test = d/(d + c) = 883.8/890.4 = 99.3%.

There are many other measures for the performance of screening tests that readers will find in specialist literature. As with other summary measures, the precision of these screening measures should be demonstrated, for example, by providing confidence intervals.

Most screening and diagnostic tests do not give a positive or negative result but a measurement, which needs to be converted to a result using a cut-off, as discussed next.

6.5.4 Setting the cut-off point for a positive screening test: introducing the relation between sensitivity and specificity and the ROC curve

The sensitivity and specificity are profoundly affected by the 'cut-off', that is, the value of the measure at which a test is defined as positive. This is a very difficult decision. Try the exercise in Box 6.10 before reading on.

We could observe the disease outcomes associated with different cut-offs and see whether damage occurs. For blood pressure, we could take the cut-off value that is associated with a higher risk of disease. Because, by and large, low blood pressures are associated with lower rates of cardiovascular disease, this could mean a cut-off value less than 120/80 mmHg, the average in most industrialized populations. The problem with this low cut-off is that about half of the population would thereby be defined as hypertensive. For most people so defined, the additional risk of cardiovascular disease outcome would be very low.

Based on a low cut-off point, say 120/80 mmHg, the sensitivity of the test for adverse hypertensive disease outcomes would be very high, the specificity low, the predictive power of a positive test low, and the predictive power of a negative test high.

If we took the hypertensive cut-off value as 180/120 mmHg, few people would be defined as hypertensive and for those that were, the frequency of adverse disease outcome would be high.

Table 6.5 Predictive power (prevalence of disease = 1%)

Screening test	Disease (definitive test)		
	+ve	**−ve**	
+ve	9.3	17.8	27.2
−ve	0.7	972.2	972.8
	10	990	1000

Predictive power of a positive test = a/(a + b) = 9.3/27.2 = 34.2%.

Predictive power of a negative test = d/(c + d) = 972.2/972.8 = 99.9%.

Box 6.10 Setting a cut-off point: the example of high blood pressure

Continue with the example of screening for high blood pressure. How would you make this decision? What would be the consequences of choosing a low and high cut-off? Think of this both from the perspective of people screened and the effects on sensitivity and specificity. Also, think of screening here as a way to early detection of cardiovascular disease risk, with the aim of reducing the outcome.

Sensitivity for hypertensive disease outcomes would be low, specificity high, predictive power of a positive test high, and predictive power of a negative test low.

There is a price to be paid for each choice. The lower cut-off picks up nearly all future cases, but creates unnecessary anxiety and the risk of unnecessary treatment among those who were not destined to develop hypertensive disease outcomes (false positives). The higher cut-off, however, misses cases (false negatives).

Setting the cut-off point is a matter of difficult judgement, balancing the costs and benefits of false positives and false negatives. For blood pressure the clinically agreed cut-off point has been reducing over the years (from about 160/100 mmHg to 140/90 mmHg). This reflects the better therapies and better services available, and an increasing in tolerance to the adverse effects of high blood pressure. There is pressure to reduce this cut-off to 135 mmHg or even 130 mmHg systolic, especially in people at very high risk of adverse outcomes, for example, people with diabetes, and those who have already had a cardiovascular event. There are additional complexities because systolic blood pressure may be high while diastolic is not, and vice versa.

As the cut-off is reduced, sensitivity approaches 100 per cent and specificity approaches zero per cent. In Figure 6.9 (a) showing a stylized example of sensitivity and specificity in relation to cut-off points, we see that as one rises the other falls. We can use this kind of picture to make decisions. If we are content with picking up 50 per cent of cases (sensitivity), we can see that specificity will be 50 per cent. If we want to pick up 90 per cent of cases (sensitivity), we get 10 per cent specificity. There is a cross-over point. With this, we seem to have a point of balance. Imagine the relationship looked more like Figure 6.9 (b). Here, we can pick up 70 per cent of cases (sensitivity) with 30 per cent specificity. We might want to maximize sensitivity and specificity. The sum of sensitivity and specificity is 100. If we accept sensitivity of 10 per cent (specificity about 98%) then we have a sum of about 110.

We can also refine this kind of decision by plotting sensitivity against specificity, or more commonly 1 minus specificity, or 100-specificity when using percentages. This creates a graph with one line. For historical reasons, a graph of sensitivity in relation to 1 minus specificity is known as a receiver operating curve, or ROC for short. (This term comes from the world of radar.)

Now try the exercise in Box 6.11.

Now do the exercise in Box 6.12 before reading on and looking at the figures.

Figures 6.10 (a) and (b) are, obviously, showing the same data and they indicate the interrelationship between each pair of sensitivity and specificity for detecting left ventricular hypertrophy (LVH) at various cut-points of BP, with an X marking the intersection. The line drawn between the points is clearly artificial, but it makes the point. At any BP all cases of LVH would be picked up so sensitivity is 100 per cent, but specificity is zero so all people would be declared at high risk of LVH. At the other extreme, at a BP cut-off of ≥150 mmHg the sensitivity is only 40 per cent, but now specificity is high at 85 per cent.

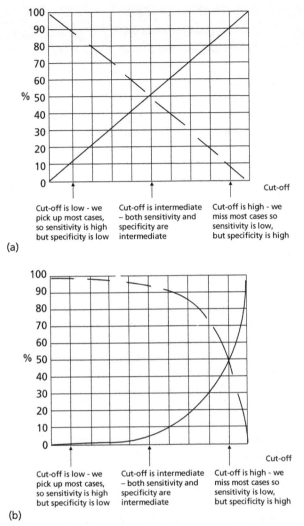

Fig. 6.9 Stylized relationship between sensitivity and specificity. (a) Simplified relationship between sensitivity (broken line) and specificity (solid line) and cut-off point. (b) Simplified but more realistic relationship between sensitivity (broken line) and specificity (solid line).

By convention these data are not graphed as in Figure 6.10 (a) but as in Figure 6.10 (b), which is simply a plot of sensitivity (true positive rate) and 1-Specificity (false positive rate). Figure 6.10 (b) adds another line, which is the one expected by chance if the test had no value at all; that is, it was the same as guessing the outcome. If so, the true positive rate would be the same as the false positive rate (i.e. there is a 50:50 chance of guessing the outcome correctly). This format (10b) is known as the receiver operating characteristic (ROC) curve. (The receiver, originally, was the person reading radar signals.) The area under the line of a completely ineffective test is 50 per cent of the square, that is, that below the diagonal line. The area under the line of a perfect test is 100 per cent. In Figure 10 (b), the area under the line is about 75 per cent. Therefore, the test is midway being perfect and useless. (The measure is the c-statistic, given as a probability, here about 75% or

Box 6.11 Calculating sensitivity, specificity, and 100-specificity— blood pressure and LVH

In a study of 500 people, examining blood pressure and disease, the outcome was an enlarged heart (left ventricular hypertrophy, or LVH for short). The outcome was, let us assume, based on a perfect measure. The results were as follows:

Blood pressure (mmHg)	True outcome		
	LVH	No LVH	Totals
< 120	5	95	100
≥ 120–129	10	90	100
≥ 130–139	15	85	100
≥ 140–149	30	70	100
≥ 150	40	60	100
Totals	100	400	500

What proportion of all the cases is correctly defined as LVH if we set the blood pressure cut-off at ≥120 mmHg, that is, what is the sensitivity? Do the calculations for each potential cut-off (i.e. ≥120, ≥130, etc.). To do this prepare 2 × 2 tables (like Table 6.2) for each cut-off point. Now, what proportion of no-LVH people is correctly assigned, that is, specificity, at each cut-off. Calculate 100-specificity also. Compare your results with Table 6.6 and the Appendix, which shows the 2 × 2 table underlying the results (Table A6.1).

0.75). Just from a visual examination and from a general understanding of the problem at hand (BP and LVH) we may choose a cut-off of about 140 mmHg accepting a 70 per cent sensitivity, 77 per cent specificity (23% 100-specificity, or false positive rate). The decision on cut-points is open to discussion. ROCs help this discussion. As the line is often a curve, it is common to write area under the curve (rather than line).

If we were also assessing electrocardiogram (ECG) as a screening test for LVH, we might wish to compare that with high blood pressure. This graph-based approach is particularly helpful for comparing several different screening tests for the same outcome. The layout of the ROC graph

Table 6.6 Sensitivity, specificity, and 100-specificity for left ventricular hypertrophy (LVH) at varying cut-off points for blood pressure (see Appendix 6.1 for 2 × 2 tables)

Cut-off (mmHg)	Sensitivity (N = 100)	Specificity (N = 400)	100-Specificity
Any blood pressure (mmHg)	All 100 cases picked up = 100%	None of 400 – no LVH group declared negative = 0%	100%
≥120	95 cases = 95% (5 in < 120 range missed)	95 –ve = 24%	76%
≥130	85 cases = 85%	185 –ve = 46%	54%
≥140	70 cases = 70%	270 –ve = 68%	32%
≥150	40 cases = 40%	340 –ve = 85%	15%

> **Box 6.12 Graphing the relationship between sensitivity and specificity, and sensitivity and 100-specificity**
>
> Now graph your results of (a) sensitivity and specificity, and (b) sensitivity and 100-specificity using the figures in Table 6.6. Place sensitivity on the y-axis of your graph and specificity (and for (b), 100—specificity) on the x-axis. Add the cut-off points for each pair of sensitivity/specificity and sensitivity/100—specificity. Compare your results with Figure 6.10 (a) and (b), and interpret this graph.

permits the easy calculation of the area under the curve (AUC), which gives a summary number. This number can be compared for several tests. A single graph may show the ROC curves associated with several potential tests. The curves do not tell us the 'right' cut-off, or the right test, but help us choose. There are numerous other useful measures of the performance of screening and diagnostic tests that are in more advanced textbooks.

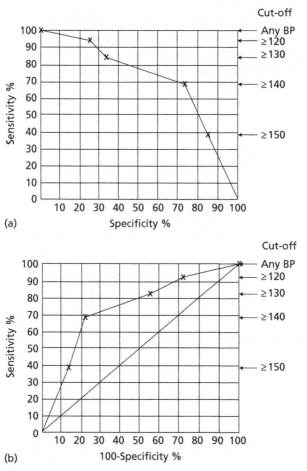

Fig. 6.10 (a) Relationship of sensitivity and specificity based on exercise in Box 6.10 and results in Table 6.6 (b) Relationship of sensitivity and 100-specificity based on exercise in Box 6.10 and Table 6.6.

6.5.5 **Distributions of the outcomes we are screening for—explaining the relations between sensitivity and specificity**

Why do sensitivity and specificity have a relationship where one rises while the other falls? There is a fundamental reason that is one of the axioms of screening and diagnostic tests.

The underlying reason for the reciprocal nature of sensitivity and specificity is that cases and non-cases belong to one, not separate, distributions of values of the factor being screened for. Figure 6.11 shows blood pressure on the x-axis and a three (trimodal) distribution of the adverse outcome—diseases caused by high blood pressure. The level of risk in the three populations is shown by shading. In Figure 6.11(a), there are three distributions that could be described as low, medium, and high risk of hypertensive, end-organ disease. If the objective were to sepa-rate Group A from C, then cut-off points are comparatively easy to set. A value of 150 mmHg systolic blood pressure would clearly separate the high (Group C) and low risk (Group A) groups. Misclassification would be uncommon in distributions like Figure 6.11 (a). At a cut-off of 150 mmHg one can see that a few people at high risk of disease (shaded as grey) are missed; mostly they belong to Group B. Extremely few people who belong to Group A will be wrongly judged as at high risk of hypertensive disease (by being placed in Group B or rarely in Group C). Even with this artificial distribution— the screener's ideal—there is some misclassification error. At a cut-off point of 150, sensitivity and specificity will, however, both be close to 100.

Figure 6.11(b) shows a more realistic, but still rarely seen, so-called bimodal (two peak), dis-tribution. The distribution implies there are two groups of people—one with high blood pressure and high risk of disease (Group E) and the other with low blood pressure and low risk of disease (Group D)—with overlap between them. Setting the cut-off point to separate the two groups here

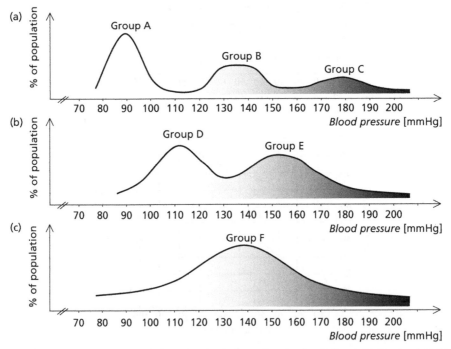

Fig. 6.11 Blood pressure: three distributions of values. Darker shading indicates higher level of risk of adverse outcome.

Box 6.13 Setting the cut-off

Looking at Figure 6.11 (c), where would you set the cut-off point? What would you like to know to help you in the task? Do you think the cut-off point will be the same for all populations?

is more problematic. Setting it at 150 mmHg will lead to many people at high risk of disease being missed, and setting it at 120 mmHg to many people who are actually at low risk being screened as positive. There is a natural and visually compelling, though not necessarily correct, cut-off value which divides groups D and E at about 130 mmHg.

Figure 6.11(c), however, is the picture portraying the distribution of the risk for many common disorders including stroke and CHD (risk factor being high blood pressure as here), diabetes (risk factor being blood sugar), and glaucoma (risk factor being intraocular pressure). There is no natural separation between people at high risk of disease and at low risk. The cut-off point is set solely on a judgement balancing the importance of avoiding false positives (achieving high specificity) versus avoiding missing true positives (achieving high sensitivity). Try the exercise in Box 6.13 before reading on.

Four types of information would help to define the cut-off point. First, we need a clear understanding of the natural history of the disease (untreated) at each level of the risk factor. Second, we need to know the adverse and beneficial consequences of treatment. Third, we need to know the sensitivity, specificity, and predictive powers of the screening test in the population to be screened. Fourth, we need to know interacting risk factors. For example, a blood pressure of 150/100 mmHg is likely to pose a greater risk of heart disease for a smoker, a person with diabetes, someone with high cholesterol, and someone who is genetically susceptible to CHD. A person's risk of adverse outcomes, shown as grey shading on the distribution curve (Fig. 6.11), is determined by a combination of environmental and genetic factors and not just the blood pressure level. Therefore, the correct cut-off may be different for different subpopulations. There are many problems in screening, as described next.

6.5.6 Some problems in screening: the example of blood pressure, with potential solutions

There are errors in measurement of blood pressure, and true variations in blood pressure relating to the environment and the biology of the person. Errors also occur in the recording and interpretation of the results. The relation between a screening test result and the disease outcome may differ between individuals and populations. These kinds of problems, illustrated in relation to hypertension here, can be generalized to most screening tests.

Some of the problems with screening for hypertensive disease based on sphygmomanometry are these:

- Hypertensive disease is a consequence of long-term raised pressure of blood inside a complex vascular system. In screening we measure the pressure at one or a few time points, using an indirect measure of the true intra-arterial pressure, usually at one place in the vasculature, that is, the arm. This may not reflect the situation in the whole body.

- Individuals and groups are differentially susceptible to the consequences of a particular level of blood pressure. We generally ignore this.

- Blood pressure is variable, changing from minute to minute in response to stimuli including smoking, external temperature, exercise, emotional stress, and posture. Blood pressure also shows a 24-hour (circadian) rhythm, and in healthy people is much lower at night than during working hours.

◆ In most populations, blood pressure rises with age. A measure at one time (or even two or three times) is no more than a snapshot of highly variable blood pressure across decades.

◆ The measurement of blood pressure by manual sphygmomanometry requires some skill, including the ability to choose and apply the right cuff in the right way, release the pressure in the cuff, and coordinate what is heard (Korotkoff sounds) while watching a falling column of mercury (or a digital display) and taking the readings at the appropriate moment. Observer errors are common, ranging from crude ones such as those caused by deafness to the subtler ones such as preference for particular numbers, usually those ending in 5 or 0, so causing rounding errors. Automated methods also have problems. Automation removes the problem of observer error, but machines can also go wrong.

◆ Poorly maintained equipment is a common cause of measurement errors. Sphygmomanometers are robust instruments but they go wrong, and need regular calibration and occasional repair.

These sorts of problems, which arise in many screening programmes using a variety of tests (from questionnaires to blood tests), can be partially solved by following these principles:

◆ Study and quantify the relationship between the screening test (here occasional measures of blood pressure by sphygmomanometer) and the underlying measure of interest (here intra-arterial blood pressure over long periods). In this way, you can confirm whether, in principle, the screening measure is a good indicator of the underlying phenomenon to be measured.

◆ Study and quantify the relationship between the screening test result and disease outcome in the population as a whole and in population subgroups.

◆ Standardize the measurement. For blood pressure, as a minimum, the person must be sitting, at rest for five minutes, and the cuff used needs to be of specified and appropriate size for the body build of the person screened. Ideally, the repeat blood pressures would be taken at the same time of day, in a controlled physical environment, and the subject should not have smoked for at least 20 minutes. In research, more stringent criteria are usually necessary.

◆ Training needs to be provided to those doing the screening, and skills need to be regularly updated and checked.

◆ Equipment needs rigorous quality checks.

Even with everything in place, we need to show that screening achieves its goals in practice.

6.5.7 **Evaluating a screening programme: biases and options**

How good, in practice, is a population-based blood pressure screening programme? This question requires careful evaluation, which is a complex subject beyond the scope of this book. Table 6.7, however, gives a sketch of the main ways that screening programmes are evaluated, the study designs usually used, and some of the potential problems. This table provides a foundation for further reading.

There are three important biases (Table 6.8) that are vitally important in interpreting data from non-trial-based evaluations. The solutions given are only partial ones.

Screening programmes are often implemented before there is unequivocal evidence of benefit (this is also true of diagnostic tests). The reason why this happens is not wholly clear, but screening often seems good on common-sense grounds. Clinical practice, with screening on an ad hoc basis (so-called opportunistic screening), may long precede the implementation of a formal

Table 6.7 Evaluation of screening programmes: options, designs, and problems

Option	Design	Problem
Examination of trends in morbidity/mortality	Before/after screening programme comparisons	Natural fluctuations in disease occur over time making interpretation difficult
Geographical comparisons in trends in mortality and morbidity	Regional/international comparisons of places with and without screening	Variation in diagnostic and treatment practices between places makes interpretation difficult
Audit/surveillance of cases to assess the stage of disease when diagnosis is made	Case series analysis over time (see Chapter 9)	Screened cases are probably self-selected volunteers, have higher social class, present at an earlier stage of disease (lead time bias—see Table 6.8), and may have less severe disease
Comparison of incidence, case fatality, and mortality in screened vs. unscreened populations within the same population at a particular time or time period	Population case series, case-control, and cohort studies (see Chapter 9)	Differences between screened and unscreened groups are many; apparent benefits may be due to this
		Unscreened cases are those missed by screening, in those who refused uptake, in those lost to follow-up, and cases picked up between screenings. They may be different—probably with more aggressive diseases—to those diagnosed at screening (Table 6.8)
Experimental implementation of screening	Trials (see Chapter 9)	The ethical, practical, and financial constraints of organizing effective, large trials are great (but need to be overcome). Trials are essential

screening programme. This may make rigorous evaluation based on a randomized controlled trial (Chapter 9) impossible. Figure 6.12 illustrates why rigorous evaluation is essential. A vast amount of costly work is entailed in screening. There are side effects both in terms of health and finance. The effectiveness and cost-effectiveness of screening programmes changes as the population pattern of disease changes and as health care evolves, so evaluations need to be updated.

Table 6.8 Three biases in non-trial evaluations and their partial solutions

Bias	Solution
Self-selection, i.e. those accepting screening are different from those declining it	Match comparison populations for all the important characteristics
'Lead time' bias, i.e. screened cases are picked up at an earlier stage	(a) Adjust survival data for estimated lead time (b) Stage disease and compare morbidity/mortality within stages
Speed of disease progression, i.e. 'length bias': cases picked up by a screening may be less severe, and slowly progressive compared with others	Awareness of this possibility

6.6 **Applications of the concepts of natural history, spectrum, population pattern, iceberg/pyramid of disease, and screening**

Health policies can be formulated and evaluated in terms of their expected influence on the natural history, spectrum, and population pattern of diseases. Simply put, the purpose of all health policy would be to shift the natural history of disease to the right and alter the spectrum, so disease is less severe (Figs 6.4 and 6.5). This will alter the population pattern, with reduced disease compressed into the later stages of life. Public health and medical action spearhead the attack against ill health and disease (Fig. 6.4). The natural history of disease concept focuses attention to the long timescales in disease causation and prevention, and hence the potential for screening.

Figure 6.3 illustrates the challenge in relation to coronary heart disease. The main adverse outcomes are angina and heart attack in middle and old age. However, as the causes exert their influence from conception onwards, a policy for heart disease control should work across the life course and would therefore need to be seen as a 50–75-year plan. One surprising, and yet predictable, consequence of the decline in heart disease mortality is a rising prevalence of angina and heart failure. The spectrum of this disease has changed; as fewer people die from heart attack mainly because of better treatment, more develop the less serious consequences. Instead of heart attack being a disease of late middle age, often ending in death, it is becoming one of old age. Both circumstances enhance the prospects for effective screening. Enormous research, policy and service efforts have, unfortunately, shown that screening does not make much difference. The reason is, probably, that screening does not lead to adequate behaviour change. More effective behaviour change interventions are needed for screening to work well.

Knowing the natural history of disease can radically alter the organization of health care. With this knowledge care can be proactive, in relation to disease control, screening, rehabilitation, and long-term surveillance. It may also provide the scientific rationale for health-care agencies to seek partnership with other agencies such as education, housing, and social services. For example, knowing the role of early life events in the genesis of heart disease and diabetes fundamentally alters our approach to these problems. Suddenly, these diseases are not seen as a matter for adult health care alone. The rationale for cross-disciplinary working within health care (primary health care, paediatrics, obstetrics, nutrition, and adult medicine) is clear. The need to influence the policies that foster good education and the health of mothers and their infants unites people in health care, housing, employment, agriculture, and nutrition.

The period between exposure, pathogenic effect, and disease may be decades (indeed, sometimes the disease never occurs because of death from other competing causes), making the discovery of causes difficult. Scientists studying people with disease may need to obtain information about the life circumstances of the patient in childhood and even in utero (the fetal or developmental origins hypothesis), as for CHD (Fig. 6.3). Information may be needed for the period even before the conception of the patient or even before the patient's parents' conception! This strains most scientific methods. Epidemiological methods that require people to recall information on causal factors are severely limited by lack of quality data. How can we ask, reliably, a 60-year-old patient with a heart attack about her life circumstances in infancy (e.g. birthweight) and in the teenage years, say on her diet? This challenge is leading to the development and testing of new methods, such as the life-grid approach where questioning is linked to memorable life events, for example, smoking habits at the time of marriage, or at the birth of the first child. It also spurs the development of birth cohort studies, so such data can be collected along the life course.

Prospective epidemiological methods entail delay, measured in the same order of time as the natural history of the disease. A cohort study (Chapter 9) to study the full range of known and

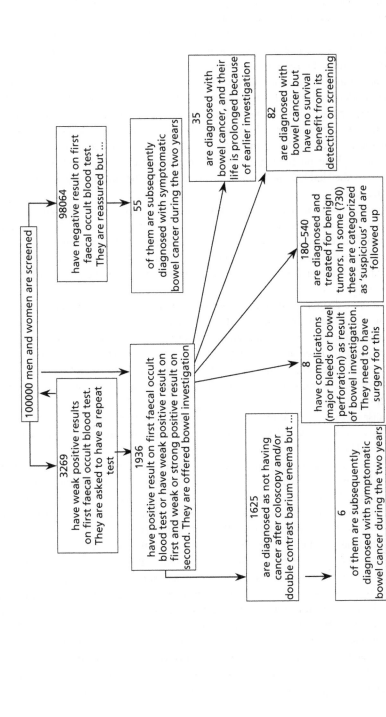

Fig. 6.12 Screening: example of colorectal screening based on faecal occult blood.

postulated risk factors for coronary heart disease would need to last for about 70 years, and even then would not provide information about the causes and course of the disease in very old age. Furthermore, the ethical basis of research that observes people without intervening is increasingly questioned. For these reasons the natural history of most human diseases is patchily understood, and that of coronary heart disease will probably never be fully grasped.

Prevention of disease is dependent on understanding the natural history of disease. The timing of prevention interventions is critically important, for in some diseases the pathogenic effects are irreversible. Natural history of disease is also essential to diagnosis, therapeutics, and prognosis. For example, in managing the care of a child presenting for the first time with an epileptic fit, the physician needs to understand what the likely course of events is and whether this child is likely to have epilepsy long term or whether this episode is likely to be a single one. This knowledge will affect both therapy (are preventive drugs necessary?) and general care (can the patient be discharged from specialist care or does the patient need long-term review?). The parents and child will put great emphasis on the long-term outcome, which cannot be easily or accurately predicted for the individual but is usually based on the aggregated natural history in past patients (i.e. epidemiological data).

The level of need for health services is often underestimated. New services designed to meet demands commonly find that new demands emerge to again outstrip supply. This may perplex and frustrate health planners, who conclude that the demand for health care is infinite, when the simple explanation is that some of the previously unidentified cases (the iceberg below the sea) are coming to light as a result of the extra service, or cases are being identified at an earlier point in their natural history.

The iceberg of disease phenomenon underpins the idea that health policy should be based on a realistic estimate of the size of the unidentified population of cases and those at risk. This principle is easy to state, but hard to implement. First, estimating the true size of the disease iceberg is not easy, and requires representative population-based surveys, which have their own limitations and costs. Some diseases, especially rare ones such as multiple sclerosis, or those with a very short natural history such as transient ischaemic attacks, are not suitable for study using survey methods, and rely on disease registers which can only list diagnosed cases. Second, not all those with identifiable disease in the context of an epidemiological survey will, in practice, ever be identifiable by a routine service. Services designed on the true number of cases could be wasteful. An example of this would be the number of people who have diabetes.

The WHO definition of diabetes includes a glucose tolerance test in standardized conditions. Such a test can be done in research conditions, but is not easy in routine practice (hence it is being replaced by other tests). The results for an individual may change over relatively short periods of time, so a single test is insufficient. Some people with diabetes would not wish to avail themselves of the services even once the diagnosis was made in this way. Basing services for diabetes on epidemiological surveys of the true size of the iceberg of this disease could, therefore, lead to over-provision. Population-based surveys are, therefore, complementary to information on service utilization.

By combining health utilization statistics, epidemiological survey data, and their own experience, clinical staff can assess the level of service needed. Clinicians need to take an active approach to identifying cases in the submerged part of the iceberg and work both with epidemiologists in assessing the true population burden of the disease, and with primary care staff to understand the specific clinical requirements of these cases. Health promotion's primary role is to attack the submerged parts of the iceberg of disease. This is done by organizing society and the environment to protect the whole population, by a combination of education and early detection of disease through screening targeted at blocks 3, 4, and 5 as conceptualized in the pyramid of disease (Fig. 6.7).

6.7 **Epidemiological theory: symbiosis with clinical medicine and social sciences**

In pointing to epidemiological theories underpinning this chapter, it would be futile to seek to disentangle them from other clinical sciences. Epidemiology has been pre-eminent in promoting the theory developed by many medical and biological sciences that many diseases are initiated by events acting years, or decades, before any clinical manifestation. This has created a subspecialty of life-course epidemiology. Epidemiology has emphasized, and contributed greatly to, building the picture of both the natural history of disease, and the spectrum of disease. The spectrum concept has illustrated that diseases may manifest themselves in many ways, including asymptomatic yet sometimes still damaging forms. Shifts in diseases' natural history and the spectrum partly underlie changes in population patterns of disease and help to explain the iceberg concept of disease. In trying to understand why some people with symptoms and signs of disease seek care, and hence are diagnosed, while others do not, epidemiology crosses to the social sciences, linking into theories of illness-seeking behaviour. These theoretical constructs have immense practical significance, both in terms of prevention, early detection, and management of disease, and in terms of managing health services, for example, explaining why demand rises as health-service capacity increases. Screening is an application of epidemiology, but it rests on other theoretical concepts, particularly the natural history of disease. Epidemiology has shown, irrefutably, that disease patterns are consistently shifting in populations. Epidemiology will never, therefore finish its work.

6.8 **Conclusion**

Understanding the interrelated concepts of the natural history, incubation period, spectrum, population pattern, and iceberg of disease and their relation to screening is crucial to epidemiology. Exemplar 6.1 takes prostate cancer as an example of the concepts of this chapter, illustrating them in the context of one of the most important contemporary cancers, for which screening is controversial. Natural history is usually pieced together from an understanding of causes and their effects, and outcomes of disease, and hence lies at the heart of epidemiology. Rational health policy, health care, and health promotion require a knowledge of the natural history. The ethical and technical difficulties of studying natural history are a deterrent, however, and the necessary work is rarely done. The model of the natural history of disease provides a unifying common purpose for all the medical sciences, and all branches of the healing and caring health profession: to influence the natural history of disease by reducing or delaying exposure to the causal agents; to promote resistance to these agents; to detect the pathogenic effects early on while disease onset can be prevented or delayed (often through screening); and to manage disease onset to minimize complications and long-term effects, including delaying death. This is a mission that engages everyone in the health professions.

Exemplar 6.1: **Prostate cancer: population patterns, spectrum, iceberg, natural history, and screening**

Background biology

The prostate gland is found in men and is below the bladder and in front of the rectum. (There is a female equivalent gland known as Shene's gland—the female prostate—which is not pertinent to this account.) It is important in male reproduction as it produces fluid that is an important part of semen. The urethra runs from the bladder through the prostate to the penis, ejecting both urine and semen.

Natural history

The natural history of prostate cancer is very difficult to study because it is usually a very slow growing tumour. Autopsy and other kinds of study show that at death many men have a prostate cancer that has been present for a long time—perhaps several decades—and has not done any harm. Yet, prostate cancer can be aggressive and deadly. The circumstances which explain these differences are unclear. It is likely, however, that prostate cancer develops over very long periods—several decades. Watching and waiting—a requirement for natural history research—is not an option, given the potential dangers.

Spectrum

Given the natural history it is unsurprising that the spectrum of symptoms, signs, and outcomes is extremely wide—from no problems of any kind during life, to rapidly spreading cancer and serious illness.

Iceberg

Prostate cancer (and its benign cousin, enlargement of the prostate) is like a large iceberg. The tip is dramatic and important, but most of the burden is hidden from view.

Population pattern of disease

Prostate cancer is becoming more common. There are three reasons for this:

1. it occurs mostly in older people and there are more people surviving to the age when this cancer becomes common
2. the causes of the cancer, though unclear, may well be more common than before (e.g. certain kinds of diet)
3. earlier diagnosis, especially through screening.

In comparison with White European-origin populations, prostate cancer occurs more commonly in African American and African and Caribbean-origin populations living in the United States of America, and Europe, respectively. By contrast, it is less common in South Asians and Chinese-origin populations. These ethnic variations are unexplained but potentially important to both screening and understanding causation. The risk is raised in those with a family history of prostate cancer.

Screening

Given its long natural history, prostate cancer should be an ideal candidate for screening, early detection, and early treatment. There have been two massive problems that have hindered successful screening; that is, that screening picks up prostate cancers that were not destined to cause any problems, and, that available tests are not sufficiently sensitive and specific.

The main screening test available, other than reported symptoms, are rectal examination to feel the prostate gland and the prostate specific antigen (PSA) test. In some countries, and with some health insurance schemes, a rectal examination is done. A rectal examination is also a generic test for other problems. So, here we will only concern ourselves with the PSA. PSA has been a controversial test, though it has been used on hundreds of millions of men. The way to help resolve the controversy over whether there should be a routine, national screening programme using this test is to undertake randomized controlled trials (see Chapter 9). Currently the use of the test is considered a matter of individual level decision-making at the doctor–patient level.

The rest of this exemplar panel will consider a recently reported trial.

Study

Schröder, F.H, Hugosson, J., Roobol, M.J., *et al.* (2014) Screening and prostate cancer mortality: results of the European Randomized Study of Screening for Prostate Cancer (ERSPC) at 13 years of follow-up. *Lancet*, Volume 384, Issue 9959, pp. 2027–35.

This trial started in 1993, enrolling 50–74 year olds, and screening them at four-yearly intervals using PSA. The cut-off was set at 3.0 ng/ml, so above this level a biopsy of the prostate was done. The primary outcome was prostate cancer mortality, though all-cause mortality data were collected.

A total of 72 891 people were in the screened group and 89 352 in the control group. The focus was on men 55–69 years old. This study showed reductions in prostate cancer mortality at 11 years of follow-up, but over-diagnosis and side effects of treatment were continuing problems precluding clear decisions on population-based routine screening. At 13 years of follow-up, the prostate cancer mortality was 0.43/1000 person-years in the intervention group and 0.54/1000 person-years in the control group. The relative risk was 0.79. All-cause mortality did not differ. To avert one prostate cancer death, 781 men were invited to take the test. The mortality reduction did not occur in Finland. Over-diagnosis was estimated at 40 per cent of cases, who were, therefore, treated unnecessarily.

The benefit in this trial was not seen in another US-based trial (Prostate, Lung, Colon, and Prostate Cancer Screening Trial). The authors conclude that the evidence is not sufficient to implement population-based routine screening.

Concluding remarks

PSA was first measured in the blood in 1980 and shown to enable early diagnosis of prostate cancer in the 1990s. PSA has been adopted in many places in clinical practice. As with many technologies, the evidence of benefit in relation to harms and costs is not commensurate with current practice.

Prostate cancer exemplifies the complexities of moving from the promise of early detection as reflected in the natural history of disease, and prioritized by population trends, to successful screening. Even with this enormous effort only a fraction of deaths were averted. There is promise but the screening strategies need much more refinement.

Summary

The natural history of disease is the uninterrupted progression of disease from its initiation by exposure to the causal agents to either spontaneous resolution, containment by the body's repair mechanisms, or to a clinically detectable problem. Natural history includes the long-term course of that problem, but without treatment. The natural history is seldom known, for the act of diagnosis and treatment influences it. Genuine studies of natural history impose profound ethical difficulties. As the causes of some diseases act decades before the disease is diagnosed, often the only way of studying the natural history of disease is to do follow-up (cohort) studies. The impact of knowledge about the natural history of disease is often profound. For example, understanding that coronary heart disease, a killer in middle and old age, is influenced by factors acting in the uterine and early childhood environment significantly alters the strategy of prevention. The primary purpose of public health and medicine is to influence favourably the natural history of disease.

The natural history of disease is related to (and influences), but is not synonymous with, the changing pattern of disease in populations, or the different levels of severity with which a disease may present (spectrum of disease). One aspect of the natural history is the incubation period, which is the time between exposure to the cause and disease onset. For chronic diseases, this is long and for acute diseases, it is short. In some infectious diseases the incubation period is highly informative for diagnosis.

For many health problems, the number of cases identified is exceeded by those not discovered. An illustrative metaphor for this is the iceberg. Correctly diagnosed cases are represented by the tip of the iceberg visible above sea level, and undiagnosed ones by the larger presence below sea level. An alternative metaphor, the pyramid of disease, develops this into a population concept. The iceberg phenomenon thwarts epidemiological efforts to assess the true burden of disease and creates difficulties in accurately judging the need and demand for services. Since unidentified cases may be different from identified ones, it is often impossible to identify truly unselected and representative cases for epidemiological studies.

Screening is the application of tests to diagnose disease (or precursors) in an earlier phase of the natural history of disease, often in well people or in a less severe part of the disease spectrum than is achieved in routine medical practice. Screening uncovers the iceberg of disease. Screening tests are not usually diagnostic but they may be, and if so, this is usually by repetition of the test (e.g. in screening for high blood pressure). The key to successful screening is a simple test that can be applied to large populations with minimum harm and has a high degree of accuracy in separating those who need more detailed investigation from those who do not. The ideal test would have high sensitivity (i.e. it picks up cases) and specificity (i.e. it correctly identifies non-cases). A person positive on the screening test would have a high probability of being confirmed as a case. A person negative on the screening test would have high probability of being confirmed as problem-free. The potential of screening is vast but there are important limitations such as the inability to influence the natural history of many diseases, either because of lack of effective interventions or lack of services to deliver them. There is a need to balance the benefits of earlier diagnosis against penalties such as engendering anxiety, the danger of side effects, and costs of further tests and treatments. The concepts in this chapter are are highly interrelated.

Sample questions

Question 1 Define what is meant by natural history of disease and explain why this is difficult to study in epidemiology.

Answer The natural history of disease comprises the processes and outcomes that arise following exposure to the disease and which lead to either resolution, disability, or death. The concept implies that there has been no interference with this process.

Natural history is difficult to study because of ethical, policy, and legal requirements to treat people whenever possible, or at the least to alleviate their problems when there is no treatment. So human studies of the natural history of disease are extremely difficult.

Question 2 Define screening and briefly outline its principal benefits.

Answer Screening is the use of tests to help diagnose diseases (or their precursor conditions) in an earlier phase of their natural history or at the less severe end of the spectrum than is achieved in routine clinical practice. In so doing, screening attempts to uncover the iceberg of disease. The main aim is to reverse, halt, or slow the progression of disease more effectively than would normally happen.

Screening is also done to protect society, even though the individual may not benefit, or might even be harmed. Screening may be performed to select out unhealthy people (e.g. for a job). Screening is also sometimes done to help allocate health-care resources that are limited.

Screening may be done simply for research, for example, to identify disease at an early stage to help understand the natural history.

Potential benefits of screening

◆ Better prognosis/outcome for individuals

◆ Protect society from contagious disease

◆ Rational allocation of resources

◆ Selection of healthy individuals

◆ Research (natural history of disease)

Question 3 A hospital laboratory is asked to test 200 specimens of urine, of which 100 are known to contain glucose; the remaining 100 being free of glucose. The laboratory reports 130 with glucose, 90 of which were known to contain glucose.

  i. Create a 2 × 2 table for this data

 ii. Calculate sensitivity and specificity for the laboratory's test results

iii. What can be said about the test's performance? What are the consequences of using this test for a screening programme to detect glycosuria, that is, glucose in the urine, which may be seen in diabetes mellitus in (a) hospital settings and (b) community settings, where prevalence of glycosuria will be lower? (Table 6.9)

Answer ii. Sensitivity = a/a + c = 90/100 = 90.0%; specificity = d/b + d = 60/100 = 60.0%.

Answer iii. The performance of this test is poor. The laboratory's glycosuria test shows a sensitivity of 90.0 per cent and specificity of only 60.0 per cent. These results suggest that about 1 in 10 true cases will be misidentified as not having glycosuria, which is worrying as patients are falsely reassured. On the other hand, the relatively low specificity suggests the laboratory will mislabel as positive a large number (4 out of 10 cases) of true negatives, and therefore overestimate the number of cases. This creates much unnecessary anxiety to people.

Table 6.9 Table in response to Q3, part (i)

Laboratory results	Actual glucose status		Total
	Present	**Absent**	
Present	90 (a)	40 (b)	130 (a + b)
Absent	10 (c)	60 (d)	70 (c + d)
Total	100 (a + c)	100 (b + d)	200 (a + b + c + d)

The prevalence of disease influences the yield or number of cases detected by a screening programme.

- In a high-prevalence population such as in a hospital, the percentage of tests found to be positive (assessed using the positive predictive value) is likely to be high.
- In a low-prevalence population, the positive predictive value will be lower, and a much higher proportion of those with positive screening results will be found not to have the disease upon further diagnostic investigation. The test will be less effective in the community.

Question 4 Why is the concept of the iceberg of disease important for epidemiological research describing the burden and distribution of disease and in health-care planning?

Answer The iceberg of disease is important because:

- Epidemiological research describing the burden of disease will underestimate the problem, sometimes by a great amount. For common disorders such as recurrent headache, the true burden may be 10 times or more that which is recorded or noted in records. For serious disorders such as diabetes mellitus, the true burden may be double that known. Studies of the distribution of disease by time, place, or person (the epidemiological triad) may reach wrong conclusions. For example, investigators may conclude that disease incidence is rising over time, but in reality the incidence is stable, but the iceberg of disease is being uncovered by more doctors using new technologies being more able to diagnose disease, especially in community settings.
- If a service is planned for the known amount of disease, there will be insufficient resource. If additional resources are made available (e.g. an additional doctor), more of the iceberg of disease will be uncovered. The service to the community is likely to be improved, but again there may be pressure for additional resources as the number of known patients rises.

References

Andermann, A., Blancquaert, I., Beauchamp, S., *et al.* (2008) Revisiting Wilson and Jungner in the genomic age: a review of screening criteria over the past 40 years. *Bulletin of the World Health Organisation*, **86**, 241–320.

Fowkes, F. (1986) Diagnostic vigilance. *Lancet*, **i**, 493–4.

Holland, W. and Stewart, S. (1990) *Screening in Health Care*. London, UK: Nuffield Provincial Hospitals Trust.

Jones, J. (1993) *Bad Blood. The Tuskegee Syphilis experiment*, 2nd edn. New York, NY: Free Press.

Last, J. (1963) The iceberg 'completing the clinical picture' in general practice. *Lancet*, **ii**, 28–31.

Mausner, J.S.K.S. (1985) *Epidemiology—An Introductory Text*, 2nd ed. Philadelphia, PA: W.B. Saunders.

Schröder, F.H., Hugosson, J., Roobol, M.J., *et al.* (2014) Screening and prostate cancer mortality: results of the European Randomised Study of Screening for Prostate Cancer (ERSPC) at 13 years of follow-up. *Lancet*, **384**, 2027–35.

Wilson, J.M.G. and Jungner, G. (1968) *Principles and Practice of Screening for Disease*. Geneva, Switzerland: World Health Organization.

Appendix 6.1

The 2 × 2 tables underpinning Table 6.6 (Table A6.1).

Table A6.1 2 × 2 tables for ROC curve data in Table 6.6

	Disease			
	Test	**+**	**−**	**All**
Cut-off > 120	+	95*	305**	400
	−	5	95	100
		100	400	500

Sensitivity = 95% Specificity 24% 1-Specificity = 76%

	Test	**+**	**−**	**All**
Cut-off > 130	+	85	215	300
	−	15	185	200
		100	400	500

Sensitivity = 85% Specificity 46% 1-Specificity = 54%

	Test	**+**	**−**	**All**
Cut-off > 140	+	70	130	200
	−	30	270	300
		100	400	500

Sensitivity = 70% Specificity 68% 1-Specificity = 32%

	Test	**+**	**−**	**All**
Cut-off > 150	+	40	60	100
	−	60	340	400
		100	400	500

Sensitivity = 40% Specificity 85% 1-Specificity = 15%

*95 is the sum of the LVH cases in Box 6.11 except in those with BP < 120, i.e. 10, 15, 30, and 40.

**This is the sum of + non-LVH cases in these groups, i.e. 90, 85, 70, and 60.

Chapter 7

The concept of risk and fundamental measures of disease frequency: Incidence and prevalence

Objectives

On completion of the chapter you should understand:

- that risk is the chance (probability) in a defined population and time period of developing a disease or risk factor;
- that epidemiology measures the quantity of disease in populations (absolute or actual measures) and how this quantity compares between populations (relative measures);
- that a risk factor is a characteristic that is associated with a disease and, possibly causally (also called the exposure variable);
- the meaning and applications of the words rate, ratio, and proportion in everyday and epidemiological language;
- that the fundamental measures of disease frequency in epidemiology are the incidence rate and prevalence proportion;
- the differences and similarities between the incidence rate estimated using a person–time denominator and using a population denominator;
- the interrelationship between incidence and prevalence;
- that there are great challenges in accurately measuring the events (numerator) and populations at risk (denominator) needed to calculate incidence and prevalence;
- the advantages of using subgroup-specific, as opposed to overall, rates.

7.1 Introduction: risks, risk factors, and causes

In everyday language, risk is the possibility of suffering harm or danger. A person at risk from an environmental or behavioural factor is someone endangered. This everyday concept of risk factors is clearly a causal one, that is, a risk increases a person's chances of harm, or danger, or indeed, of contracting a disease.

Risk in epidemiology usually refers to the chance (i.e. probability), of dying or developing a disease, or its precursors, so the word is used similarly to everyday language. In epidemiology, our prime interest is in the association between the risk of the outcome and those environmental, individual, and social characteristics which influence the risk. The influencing characteristics are called risk factors. Reflect on the question in Box 7.1 before reading on.

In epidemiology the term *risk factor*, perhaps in contrast to everyday language, does not necessarily imply that the characteristic has a causal effect (association is not causation). In Chapter 5 we considered the difficulties in demonstrating an association is causal. This principle is known,

Box 7.1 Risk factors and causes

Reflect on the phrases 'risk factor' and 'cause of disease'. What is the difference between them?

albeit often ignored, by epidemiologists. It is not known by the general public and the mass media. The problem in the communication of science is that this principle is too often forgotten.

The term *risk marker* is sometimes used in preference to risk factor, simply to emphasize that no causal relationship is presumed. This term has no logical advantages and it wrongly implies that a risk factor (rather than marker) is causal.

Some risk factors may be agreed to have more than a statistical association with disease. When a causal relationship is agreed, the term *causal factor*, or simply *cause*, is used. For example, we say smoking is a cause of coronary heart disease (CHD). For most CHD risk factors (e.g. hyperhomocystinaemia, low levels of high-density lipoprotein cholesterol (HDL), high C-reactive protein, job strain) we may imply, but rarely claim, a causal role and use the phrase risk factor. Much of epidemiology concerns the search for causal risk factors, as covered in Chapters 3–5.

In contemporary epidemiology there is imprecision in the interpretation and use of these vital terms. The confusion leads to attribution of cause where it is merely association, and alternatively the failure to speak of an association as causal when it is. Such confusion has led to much criticism of epidemiology. In the sixth edition of *A Dictionary of Epidemiology*, there is a change in the long-standing definition of risk factor, as we have reflected on just now. Risk factor is said to be causally related to a change in risk of an outcome. This change is not in line with usage and I do not recommend it. If a factor is a cause, call it a causal factor. (The dictionary also introduces the term *risk indicator* to include both risk factors and risk markers, but this is an unnecessary addition.) Chapters 3, 4, and 5 explain the difficulties involved in achieving causal understanding, and the reader will appreciate that a cautious approach is usually to be applauded rather than criticized.

As already discussed, associations are rarely causal, but their analysis is the starting point of causal understanding in epidemiology. This chapter and the next two consider the basic epidemiological tools needed to obtain, quantify, and summarize information for this task.

7.2 Quantifying disease frequency, risk factors, and their relationships: issues of terminology

The *numerator* is the upper number of a fraction and the *denominator* is the lower number, that is, as in $^a/_b$ where a is the numerator and b the denominator. From this simple arithmetic we construct virtually the entirety of quantitative epidemiology. Epidemiology has developed a terminology based on, but not corresponding exactly to, everyday and mathematical words for similar ideas. This is a potential cause of difficulty, for which there is no easy remedy. Indeed, there has been a great deal of debate over the last 20–40 years that readers may wish to access (see, for example, Elandt-Johnson 1975). I refer to it briefly here.

Before reading on, try the exercise in Box 7.2.

Dictionaries show there are many meanings and even those relating to mathematics overlap. Understandably, *A Dictionary of Epidemiology* leaves room for interpretation. To put it simply, a ratio is any number in relation to another number, so all fractions are ratios. A rate comprises the numerator in relation to the denominator in a specified time and is, therefore, a type of ratio.

Box 7.2 Terminology

Define the following terms, using a general dictionary and one on statistics, mathematics, and epidemiology if necessary.

- Ratio
- Rate
- Proportion

Proportion is a part in relation to the whole and is hence, also, a ratio. So, how do we apply these terms in epidemiology? There is no simple, fixed, or universally agreed approach, not least because usage has been changing and that people coming into epidemiology from different disciplines and eras will use the terms differently. So, take care, and interpret words thoughtfully by gaining an understanding of what was actually done. In the following account, I have summarized both currently recommended and actual usage of words.

The word *ratio* is commonly used in epidemiology, but is usually reserved for summarizing the division of one ratio by another ratio. This is explained in Chapter 8 in the discussion of the proportional mortality and morbidity ratios, standardized mortality ratio, and odds ratio.

In epidemiology, the word *rate* is often used for a ratio where the numerator and denominator have different qualities, for example, deaths/population. This kind of fraction, of numerator divided by denominator, is commonly called the rate in demography, epidemiology, public health, and medicine. The dictionary meaning of the word *rate*, which corresponds best to this use, is a quantity measured with respect to another quantity. This is the way the word is used in many journals (including some specializing in epidemiology), books, the media, and verbal discourse. It is also in line with its use in allied disciplines, for example, sociology, economics, and demography. Currently there is strong emphasis in epidemiology that rates must have a time dimension. Some flexibility and awareness of the issues are required, as many writers do not adhere to this recommendation. I refer to this later in the chapter.

A *proportion* in epidemiology is usually a ratio where the numerator is a part of the denominator, so both have the same qualities. For example, deaths due to one cause/deaths due to all causes. This corresponds to the dictionary definition of one part in relation to the whole, though the word has many other meanings that overlap with rate and ratio.

Epidemiological studies collect, measure, summarize, present, and interpret data on the frequency of death, illness, disease, and risk factors. (Epidemiology also measures health states and functions, e.g. wellbeing, height, weight, haemoglobin, etc. These kinds of measures are important, but not to the focus of this chapter.)

The epidemiological question usually is, in what quantity does the disease occur in a population (absolute measures) and how does this compare with other populations (relative measures)? Table 7.1 lists the main measures that answer these questions and that are to be discussed here and in Chapter 8. The epidemiological strategy for working out causes of disease works best by using the comparative (relative) approach, while that for assessing a population's health needs works best by examining that population's actual health pattern (absolute approach).

While there are many measures, two underpin virtually all epidemiology: known in shorthand as *incidence* and *prevalence*. These are discussed in detail in this chapter. Table 7.2, which is a variant on Table 1.4, gives brief definitions of incidence and prevalence and indicates the type of studies (discussed in Chapter 9) from which such data are derived.

Table 7.1 Some epidemiological measures in relation to whether they provide absolute (actual) or relative (comparative) frequency

Numbers of cases	Absolute
Proportional mortality	Absolute
Proportional mortality ratio	Relative
Overall (actual or crude) prevalence proportions and incidence rates	Absolute
Specific prevalence proportions and incidence rates	Absolute
Standardized rates	Absolute/relative mix
Standardized ratios	Relative
Relative risk	Relative
Odds ratio	Relative
Attributable risks	Absolute
Numbers needed to treat and prevent	Absolute
Life years lost	Absolute
Disability-adjusted life year (DALY)	Absolute
Quality-adjusted life year (QALY)	Absolute

The patterns of diseases (and of their risk factors) are constantly changing, mainly because the environment within which populations live is changing. Frequency data must, therefore, be described in the context of the population, the place, and the time of the study. Many published reports and papers omit this information. They also need to give the number and characteristics of disease cases, and of the population from which they come. Numbers of cases, or people with the risk factors, usually comprise the numerator, while the population from which they come is usually the denominator.

Table 7.2 Introduction to incidence rates and prevalence proportions (sometimes, in practice, also called rates)

Measure	Key features	Type of study	Formulae*
Incidence	Count of new cases over a period of time in a population of known size defined by characteristics (age, sex, etc.), and place and time boundaries	Disease register Cohort Trial	New cases ÷ population at risk (cumulative incidence) or New cases ÷ time spent by the study population at risk (incidence rate)
Prevalence (point prevalence)	Count of cases (new and old) at a point in time in a population of known size defined by characteristics (age, sex, etc.) and place	Cross-sectional Disease register in combination with population counts	All cases ÷ population at risk

*The resulting fraction is multiplied as discussed later

From basic data on disease, death, risk factors, and population counts, many summary measures of health status and risk, some of which are listed in Table 7.1, can be calculated as shown here and in Chapter 8. Different ways of presenting the same data have a major impact on the perception of the results and, in particular, relative and absolute measures of frequency portray dramatically different priorities. Epidemiological data should be presented, wherever possible, to indicate both relative and actual frequency, as discussed in Chapter 8.

The following principles in the analysis of differences and changes in disease frequency apply to all epidemiological measures but are explained and emphasized for incidence rates. However, the likelihood of artefacts explaining differences and changes in disease frequency is greater with prevalence measures than with incidence, simply because the former are more complex, being influenced not only by disease occurrence but also by death, migration, and recovery.

7.3 **The concepts of person–time incidence rate (incidence rate) and cumulative incidence rate (or proportion)**

The meaning of *incidence* in everyday English is broad, which explains why this word is so commonly used to mean different things, even in epidemiology. Readers cannot assume the writer has used the term in a technical way, so examine the data carefully—often incidence and incidence rate are used generally to mean disease frequency, including prevalence. The meanings of the word *incidence* in epidemiology that correspond to its general definition are: the act of happening, and the extent or frequency of occurrence.

In epidemiology, incidence rate is the frequency of *new* occurrences of an event in a population at risk of the event, in a period of time (Table 7.2). The word *new* is the key defining feature. The meaningful interpretation of disease incidence requires the number of new cases (the numerator), the population at risk (denominator), the time period, and the place of study. For simplicity, the discussion here assumes the event is a disease but it could be some other outcome. Some writers simply say incidence instead of incidence rate. I have done this sometimes. Strictly, however, the incidence (without the word rate) of a disease is a count of new cases unrelated to a denominator, and therefore it is not a rate.

The incidence rate is a fundamental measure in epidemiology and yet the concept underlying it and the terminology have evolved in recent decades. Presently there are two main variants: the person–time incidence rate and cumulative incidence (Table 7.3 summarizes some of their qualities). One reason for confusion is the use of several terms that convey much the same underlying concept. Some recommend cumulative incidence proportion rather than cumulative rate, but in practice the traditional use has continued, so I use it here. Person–time incidence is known simply as incidence rate. Person–time incidence rate ranges from zero to infinity, as many deaths might occur over a short period of time.

Cumulative incidence is usually referred to as incidence rate, but is also known as incidence proportion, cumulative incidence, and cumulative proportion. Cumulative incidence rate is also often used synonymously with risk (i.e. probability). The cumulative incidence rate varies from 0 to 1 (or 0–100%). Readers will need to become accustomed with, and alert to, these two related concepts and their synonyms. (The complexity of these issues is reflected in the relevant entries in the sixth edition of *A Dictionary of Epidemiology*.) For simplicity, I will use one phrase—incidence rate—to capture two conceptual approaches, one based on a population denominator, the other on a person–time denominator. When readers are examining incidence data, they should check which concept is in use.

The need for these two approaches is best understood by an example. Remember, the denominator is the population at risk. Assume the occurrence of a disease is 20 per cent per year and we

Table 7.3 Qualities of the incidence rate obtained using the person and person–time denominator (numerator is identical)

Person denominator (cumulative incidence rate or proportion, or very often simply incidence rate)	Person–time denominator (or usually incidence rate)
Ranges from 0 to 1*	Ranges from zero to infinity
Measures absolute risk (probability) of new disease*, e.g. 500 new cases/10 000 people per year = 5%	Not clearly interpreted as a measure of absolute risk, e.g. 50 cases per 1000 person-years
Can be used to construct relative risks	Can be used to construct relative risks (or strictly, relative rates)
Can be calculated with population estimates, e.g. from a census	Person–time incidence rates usually cannot be calculated in population estimates, e.g. from a census
Can only be used in cohort studies where study participants are enrolled at about the same time	Can be used either when enrolment is at about the same time or when enrolment is spread over time

*When the denominator is the population at the beginning of the study.

follow-up 100 people. Let us also assume that the disease occurs evenly over time. After 6 months, on average, 10 people will develop the disease. If there are no deaths from this disease, and the disease does recur and there is no immunity, then the denominator (i.e. the people at risk) remains 100. We would expect, on average, another 10 cases in the next 6 months.

There might, however, be deaths or immunity in cases. After one year, we might expect that even in these circumstances, 20 new cases will occur. Do you agree? How many new cases occur by the first six months, on average? Then, how many new cases will occur in the second six months?

On average in these circumstances of death and immunity, we would expect a little fewer than 10 cases at the six-month point. For diseases that occur only once or lead to death these cases are no longer at risk after their occurrence. This would certainly be true for many infectious diseases that are followed by lifelong immunity. This would also apply to those chronic diseases that only occur once and persist. When the outcome of interest is death, then these cases are no longer at risk.

The denominator is, we now see, 100 only at the beginning of the study. In theory, for first-event only studies for example, death, as each case occurs, should be subtracted from the denominator. So, in our example, the denominator would be slightly more than 95 at the three-month stage, about 90.25 (not 90) at six months, about 85.7 (not 85) at nine months and about 81.5 (not 80) at 12 months. The detail of this is not important here but the concept—that the denominator may diminish, is vital.

In a large population, and a common disease, the denominator would be diminishing almost continuously. To take this fully into account we would need to measure incidence rate in very small increments of time. There are theoretical measures of the occurrence of disease over a period of time approaching zero. Figure 7.1 illustrates this point. The formula is given in *A Dictionary of Epidemiology* under the entry, 'Force of Morbidity'.

Closely linked concepts relating to the incidence rate at a point in time are described by these phrases—forces of morbidity and mortality, hazard rate, instantaneous incidence density, instantaneous incidence rate, disease intensity, and person–time incidence rate. In practice, epidemiologists mainly work with the last of these. The person–time approach provides

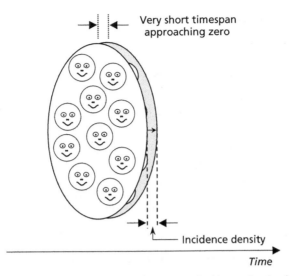

Fig. 7.1 Incidence rate in a period of time approaching zero—incidence density, forces of mortality/morbidity, hazard rate, disease intensity: a pictorial representation.

an easy way of handling the aforementioned diminishing denominator problem, as we will now discuss.

The person–time denominator is simply the amount of time that the study population as a whole has spent at risk (disease-free, or alive, in the case of mortality studies).

The formula for this is:

$$\text{Person-time incidence rate} = \frac{\text{New occurrences of outcome over a period of time}}{\text{Time spent by the study population at risk over this period of time (person-years of observations)}} \quad (7.1)$$

$$\text{Or more simply (after Rothman)} = \frac{\text{Disease occurrences}}{\text{Sum of time periods}} \quad (7.2)$$

Figure 7.2 illustrates this formula; we start with a population of 10 people in the denominator (smiling faces) and none in the numerator at the top. In the first year, there are no cases so the incidence rate is $^0/_{10}$ years of observation. In the second year, one case occurs. We do not know exactly when this case occurred. What can we do in these circumstances, which are not uncommon? We assume that cases are occurring evenly over time. Some will occur early in the period, some later. On average, therefore, each case contributes 0.5 years of observation. In this illustrative example, there is only one case but we will assume it reflects the average. If we know the exact amount, say, the case occurred at three months, we would add 0.25 of a year but here we do not. Therefore, in this second year, the 10 people have contributed 9.5 years of observation, 19.5 in total. So, the incidence rate is $^1/_{19.5} = 0.0512$ per year of observation = 51.2 cases per 1000 years of observation. Here, the fraction is multiplied by a thousand but the choice is arbitrary. This procedure continues until the end of the study, here three cases and 35.5 years of observation = $3 \div 35.5 = 0.0845$ per year of observation, or 84.5 cases per 1000 years of observation. This formula provides investigators with great flexibility, particularly in cohort studies where investigators

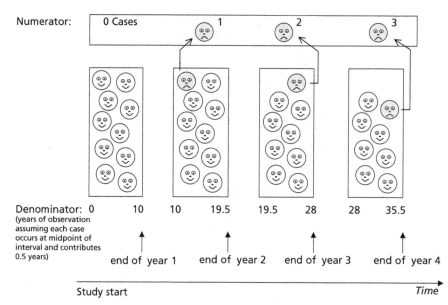

Fig. 7.2 Incidence rate—three cases per 35.5 person-years—estimated using the person–time denominator: a pictorial representation.

know, for each person, the date of entry into the study, and the date of onset of disease or death, or exit from the study. Its flexibility also allows study subjects to enter the study at different times, and it makes handling losses to follow-up and death easy (for these simply contribute less time to the denominator).

This approach does have some disadvantages. First, it does not give an easily interpreted direct measure of risk, that is, probability; the incidence rate will be expressed, for example, as 84.5 cases/1000 years. This is not a problem for relative measures, but it is for actual or absolute ones as it is hard to grasp or convey to the public or health professionals. Secondly, there are assumptions underlying this estimate that the incidence rates in those entering and leaving the study at different times, and those lost to follow-up, are the same as in others in the study population. Neither of these assumptions are self-evidently true. Most diseases, however, present different risk at different ages and in different calendar periods.

Thirdly, the formula assumes that the disease occurs evenly over time, as the time periods contributed by those in the study for a short time are given the same weight as those contributed by people in the study for a long time. This gives the person contributing 50 years to a study five times the weight of a person contributing 10 years, and 50 times the weight of those contributing one year. A study with a large number of people with small time contributions may, if the assumption does not hold, come to a conclusion different from that of a study comprising mostly people with large time contributions.

The number of people in the person–time denominator can be judged only from a knowledge of the average time period of observation, which is only a reasonable estimate if there is no skew in the distribution (so investigators need to give population size information and the distribution of time contributions).

In historical, and much current, epidemiological practice, the problem of the diminishing denominator of those at risk has been sidestepped. Where the denominator is not altering, or is not altering much, or cannot be adjusted for lack of data on timing of deaths and disease, the person denominator and cumulative incidence is usually used. The standard, and time-honoured, formula for incidence rate is:

$$\frac{\text{New occurrences of outcome over a period of time}}{\text{Population at risk over that period of time}} \qquad (7.3)$$

The resulting fraction, as with person–time incidence rate, is usually multiplied by an appropriate number; for example, by 100 to give a rate per hundred which is a percentage, or by 1000 to give a rate per thousand. International statistics for diseases by the World Health Organization (WHO) are usually expressed per 100 000.

When the baseline population is the denominator, this measure is commonly referred to as *cumulative incidence rate* or *cumulative incidence proportion* (the latter is not popular, though accurate). It is a direct measure of the probability of a new event occurring in a population, and hence the risk of that event.

In this formula, the person-based denominator is fixed at one point in time, usually at the beginning or middle of the time period; for example, if the study is one year long, the denominator might be the baseline population. If the disease is recurrent, and the investigator is interested in all, and not just new occurrences, then using a baseline denominator is correct, for the whole population remains at risk of the event of interest. Deaths and exits from the study for other reasons should, however, be subtracted from the denominator if possible. When the person denominator is so adjusted, the cumulative incidence and person–time rates converge. However, as most outcomes are rare it is not usually done.

Particularly in studies of the causes of disease, investigators often choose to study only first occurrences. If so, when the disease is common, adjusting the denominator is usually advised. If the incidence of the disease or death was low, say only 0.5 per cent per year, then on practical (but not theoretical) grounds the investigator might argue that adjusting the denominator is unnecessary, for it would only decrease from 100 to about 99.75 at the six months stage, and have no important effect on the calculation.

In many studies the denominator is not adjusted either because the information is not available to do this, the investigators have not thought to do so, the outcome is too rare for it to matter, or because investigators are interested in all events.

Do the exercise in Box 7.3 before reading on. To prepare you may wish to read the relevant sections on case series (section 9.3) and on cohort studies in Chapter 9 (section 9.6) first. (This is not, however, essential.)

Box 7.3 Two approaches for measuring incidence rate in two kinds of study

(a) Imagine a cohort study with follow-up over five years to answer the question: what is the incidence of coronary heart disease in 45–74-year-old people? Consider the advantages and disadvantages of the two approaches for measuring incidence rate.

(b) Imagine a study of the incidence of coronary heart disease (or mortality) based on a register of diseases (or deaths) compiled for five years. Again, consider the advantages and disadvantages of the two approaches for measuring incidence.

In the cohort study—(a) in Box 7.3—the decision on which formula to use will, in theory, depend on the design of the study. If the cohort is assembled at one short period of time—say all people born on one day, or army personnel retiring in a particular month of the year—then there is an open choice. In the case of CHD in 45–74 year olds, we could enrol all people of this age from a general practice or other population registers providing age. The participants would then be followed up over time to observe the outcome. The denominator could be the study population at the beginning or the midpoint of the interval of time in question. This will be apt, particularly when absolute or actual rates are the prime output of the analysis, that is, risk data are needed. This approach will work if the follow-up period is short, say, a year or two.

If the study sample in the cohort is recruited over a prolonged period of time, say over three years, then a population denominator is not appropriate and a person–time approach is much better. When relative measures are the prime output the elegant choice, in both instances, is the person–time denominator. Generally, and increasingly, person–time denominators are preferred in cohort studies.

Mostly, incidence rates are calculated by setting up registers of deaths or disease—as in (b) in Box 7.3—and using census or other estimates of the size of the population from which the cases arose for the denominator. Information on migration, and other means by which a person is effectively lost from the system capturing data for the register, is not usually available on all the individuals making up the denominator. The assumption is made that the population is fairly stable and usually the midpoint of the time period is used. If the disease were uncommon, as is usually the case, adjusting the denominator to remove the new cases would make little difference to the result. If the disease is common, the denominator could be adjusted by assuming that the cases occur evenly through the year, so reducing the denominator by 50 per cent of the number of cases. In this kind of study, with no information on each individual in the denominator, there is often no added value to a person–time-based denominator. Table 7.4 summarizes the advantages and disadvantages of the two types of denominator. (In the first analyses of the Framingham cohort study—see Exemplar 1.1 in Chapter 1—the authors used the population denominator; they refer to some of the difficulties with this.)

These concepts and algebraic formulae require reflection, but putting the concepts into practice in measuring the incidence of disease accurately is a still greater challenge. The following discussion of measuring events (numerators) and population (denominators) is applicable to all measures of the frequency of the outcome in epidemiology.

7.4 Numerator: defining, diagnosing, and coding disease accurately and the challenge of using others' data

The greatest challenge in epidemiology is accurate data collection. The difficulties start with the numerator, that is, for incidence of the number of new cases. Epidemiological studies are usually based on diagnoses made by someone else, not the investigator. There have been some notable exceptions, mainly work by solo clinical investigators such as the general practitioner William Pickles who described the pattern of occurrence and natural history of several diseases in his own patients (Pickles 1939). With multidisciplinary, team-based health care, the specialization of medical practice, and the need for large studies, epidemiologists rarely make their own diagnoses. How can epidemiologists ensure that the diagnoses are accurate? After all, epidemiologists must take responsibility for the validity of the data, including the diagnosis. Their confidence should be based on research to establish the accuracy of the data. It is not acceptable, but it often happens, that epidemiologists do not know the accuracy of the data but assume it is accurate (it is not).

Table 7.4 Main advantages and disadvantages of person and person–time denominators in the context of (a) cohort and (b) register-based studies of incidence rates

	Advantages	**Disadvantages**
(a) Cohort study Population denominator	Measures risk directly Choices of time periods to present incidence data on, e.g. over 1 year, over 5 years, etc. Year of onset of outcome is usually enough	Requires everyone in the study to be enrolled at about the same time Not easy to account for losses to follow-up Baseline population becomes an inaccurate estimate of the population at risk for common diseases
Person–time denominator	Very flexible in coping with people entering and leaving study at different times Study population can be enrolled over long periods of time	No easily interpreted direct measure of risk Assumes disease occurrence is evenly spread across time Ideally, requires information on date of disease onset and date of entry and exit from study
(b) Register-based study Population denominator	Can use population size data from census and other sources if necessary Can use population at midpoint of interval of study follow-up as estimate Otherwise as for cohort studies	Accurate census or population register-based estimates of denominator are required Routine population data may give inexact denominator size Otherwise as for cohort studies
Person–time denominator	Not usually applicable, but when it is, then as for cohort studies Adjustments to denominator can be made by estimating exits, disease occurrence, and deaths	Information on individuals to calculate person-years is not usually available

Clearly, epidemiologists cannot be sure, but their confidence will be increased by a valid case definition, information on symptoms, signs, and tests relevant to the case definition, and health-care staff who have been trained well in diagnosis.

An information system is needed to hold the clinical data. Since neither the basic clinical information, nor the diagnosis, is likely to be recorded in unambiguous and consistent words, a means of judging the evidence to make or confirm a diagnosis is needed. A patient may have several diseases in the course of one illness.

Imagine, for example, a person who has a feverish illness diagnosed on laboratory tests as influenza, who develops cough and shortness of breath shown to be the result of pneumonia, followed by a deep venous thrombosis (a blood clot in the veins). The doctors suspect that pulmonary embolus (a blood clot in the lungs) has occurred but before it can be confirmed by tests, the patient collapses and dies unexpectedly. Assume that there is no post-mortem because the relatives refuse permission. These diagnoses will need to be extracted from a complex set of medical records, traditionally handwritten, though increasingly typed and held electronically. Which diagnoses will go on the death certificate (and ultimately our research database) and in what order? Do the exercise in Box 7.4 now. This exercise is particularly relevant to readers who are not doctors and have not completed death certificates.

Box 7.4 Entering diagnosis on a death certificate

Complete the specimen death certificate in Box 7.5 for the person just described. Take care to order the causes as instructed. Later you can compare your judgement with mine.

Compare your completed certificate with mine, which follows next.

1a Pulmonary embolus

 b Pneumonia

 c Influenza

11 Deep venous thrombosis

If you disagreed with me, then your experience is true to life.

Imagine that you are an epidemiologist who acquires 600 000 such death certificates on all causes of death and that you wish to study the incidence of mortality from pulmonary embolus. The task of extracting a list of cases of death due to pulmonary embolus is not a trivial one. One problem will be differences in writing style and words, with some doctors using pulmonary thrombosis, some lung embolus, some omitting it altogether from the death certificate.

One solution, which makes both the choosing of diagnoses and the handling of data easier, is a list of codes for disease. There are several such sets of codes but the most important one is the International Classification of Diseases (ICD) of the WHO. This is now in its tenth edition (WHO 2016).

The order of the causes of death on the death certificate is important, for there is a long tradition that only the underlying cause of death is coded, entered into computer, analysed, and published. This tradition has been overturned recently in the United Kingdom and the United States of America, and all the causes are now coded and available for analysis but it is still commonplace to focus on the underlying cause. Before reading on, do the exercise in Box 7.6.

My chosen codes are I26, J18, J10.0, and I80.1. If yours are different, then this variance reflects reality. In studies of disease incidence there is the complication, which does not apply to death, that a decision needs to be made on whether the case is a new case or an old one, and whether the person is at risk. The investigator with 600 000 death certificates (or hospital records) has to turn these into useful epidemiological information, including the accurate count of relevant cases.

Epidemiologists commonly use such existing data sets, particularly if the coding and computer entry has already been done. This is efficient as the costs of collecting new data are high. It is a

Box 7.5 Specimen death certificate

CAUSE OF DEATH

The condition thought to be the 'Underlying Cause of Death' should appear in the lowest completed line of Part 1.

I (a) Disease or condition directly leading to death
   (b) Other disease or condition, if any, leading to 1 (a)
   (c) Other disease or condition, if any, leading to 1 (b)

II Other significant conditions CONTRIBUTING TO THE DEATH but not related to the disease or condition causing it

Box 7.6 Coding of diagnosis

- ◆ Based on your completed death certificate, code the causes of death (see Table 7.5 for some codes).
- ◆ Reconsider your choice of order of causes of death after reading the coding rule from the ICD (see footnotes of Table 7.5).

Table 7.5 Selected codes from ICD-10, with brief notes on coding rules*

Chapter IX	Diseases of circulatory system	I00–I99	
	Hypertension	I10–I5	
	Ischaemic heart disease	I20–25	
	Cerebrovascular	I60–69	
	Phlebitis and thrombophlebitis	I80	I80.0 of superficial vessels of lower extremities
			I80.1 of femoral vein of other lower extremities (deep vein thrombosis)
	Other venous embolism and thrombosis	I82	
	Varicose veins of lower extremities	I83	
	Pulmonary embolism	I26	
Chapter X	**Disease of respiratory system**	**J00–J99**	
	Influenza due to influenza virus	J10	(J10.0 with pneumonia)
	Influenza, virus not identified	J11	(J11.0 with pneumonia)
	Viral pneumonia, not elsewhere classified	J12	
	Bacterial pneumonia, not elsewhere classified	J15	
	Pneumonia, organism unspecified	J18	
	Respiratory failure, not elsewhere classified	J96	

Chapter XVII Symptoms, signs, etc. not elsewhere classified

Respiratory arrest (cardiorespiratory failure)	R00–R99
	R09.2

*Note: The causes of death to be recorded are all those that resulted in or contributed to death, and the circumstances of accident or violence which produced injury.

The underlying cause of death is (a) the disease or injury which initiated the train of events leading directly to death or (b) the circumstances of the accident or violence which produced the fatal injury.

Source: data from World Health Organization, *International Statistical Classification of Diseases and Related Health Problems, 10th Revision (ICD-10) (WHO Version for 2016)*, 'http://apps.who.int/classifications/icd10/browse/2016/en', accessed 01 Feb. 2016. Copyright © 2016 WHO.

common mistake, however, to analyse such data sets as if they consisted of valid, complete data. Epidemiologists have a duty to understand the weaknesses and limitations of such data sets, for they are responsible for data accuracy and interpretation of everything they publish. If mistakes are made the authors, not those supplying data, are responsible.

Two examples, lower limb amputation and Legionnaires' disease, provide contrasting perspectives on the problem of achieving accuracy in the numerator.

The words 'lower limb amputation' convey the essence of the case definition, and it is a small step to define it further in terms of anatomy, that is, what part of the limb is amputated. There is no great need for the diagnosis to be confirmed by a doctor or by checking medical records. The amputee will almost certainly have been treated by the health service and probably have been hospitalized. The obvious place to look for data is the hospital admissions or discharges information system, or the operating theatre records or the limb-fitting centre. It seems straightforward.

Figure 7.3 shows the result of a study. Of the 291 cases identified, only 17 were recorded in all three information systems. If the authors had relied on operation records alone, which seems a reasonable strategy, 192/291 (66%) of cases would have been identified. Even for such a straightforward diagnosis, the difficulty in defining the numerator accurately is extreme. This kind of observation is commonly made, and it continues to surprise us. The lesson is generalizable and reminds us of the iceberg of disease (Chapter 6); the system usually underestimates the burden of disease.

There is a worldwide movement for health care to be planned rationally based on data from routine sources. This is a good idea but is often unworkable for lack of accurate data. The resources for a 'needs'-based service for amputees, planned using 'routine' information from the hospital discharge data, would have been depleted rapidly. It is best to incorporate information on past resource requirement in planning health services. When information is available from several independent sources, the capture–recapture technique, originally designed for measuring the size

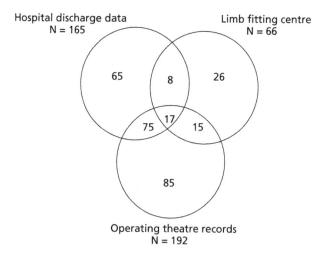

Fig. 7.3 Use of routine information to measure the number of people with limb amputation: ascertainment based on three data sources. Data from Leeds Health Authority (England), July 1992 to December 1993. Total number of cases of LEA = 291.

Source: data from Bodansky HJ, Airey CM, Chell SM, Unwin N and Williams DRR. The incidence of lower limb amputation in Leeds, UK: setting a baseline for St Vincent. International Diabetes Federation Meeting. *Diabetologia*, Volume A1850, Copyright © 1997.

of animal populations, can sometimes be used. Discussion of this technique is beyond the scope of this book.

In contrast with lower limb amputation, Legionnaires' disease is complex. This pneumonia cannot be differentiated from other forms of pneumonia clinically, and has a wide spectrum of presentation (see Chapter 6); some patients have minimal illness, and others a wide variety of signs and symptoms. Most patients are likely to be cared for in the community (as a flu-like illness or pneumonia) rather than be admitted to hospital. The challenge is for the physician to consider this diagnosis and order the necessary laboratory tests. The tests are often difficult to interpret, especially as culture of the organism is only successful in a minority of cases. There was, until the publication of ICD 10 giving the code A48.1, no specific ICD code for this pneumonia—so information about cases could not be extracted by searching in routine information systems, including those for hospital inpatients. This meant that for epidemiological studies a specific register of cases had to be maintained. Since the diagnosis requires both clinical and laboratory information, a register cannot be maintained from laboratory records alone. As it is a rare disease, incidence studies require the participation of a large number of physicians in supplying information to a registry. Add to this the need to protect the confidentiality of clinical information and it is not surprising that there is a huge 'iceberg' effect for this (and similar) diseases. Fewer than 10 per cent of all cases are counted in most registers. The reader should ponder on the difficulties of measuring the incidence rate of this and similar diseases.

To calculate the incidence rate of disease, the procedures for registration of cases will need to include rules to judge whether a case is new or old, and decide whether to include recurrences. For example, in a study of the incidence of bronchiolitis, the common cold or acute myocardial infarction, the investigator needs to decide whether only the first occurrence is included as a new case or whether each occurrence is to be included. As there is no general rule, each study will need to make this decision in the light of its aims. These decisions are not always easy except for the incidence of mortality, diseases which are irreversible (e.g. amputation of a limb), diseases which usually occur only once (e.g. measles), or diseases agreed by definition or convention to be lifelong diseases (e.g. diabetes).

Where the prime purpose of the study is to measure the frequency of disease to assess its importance or assess need for services, all cases must be included. Where the aim is to make comparisons between populations to develop or test causal hypotheses, there is a choice but we usually study new cases. In measuring the incidence of stroke, for example, all new and recurrent cases will probably be included if we are doing the study to measure the need for services or evaluating interventions. In a study of whether cholesterol is a causal risk factor for stroke, possibly based on studying groups of subjects with low and high cholesterol, there is a choice. Interpretation of the findings of such a study is usually easier if first occurrences only are included. The simplified rule is this: for burden of disease and health needs— study all cases; for causes of disease study new cases.

There is a truism that epidemiology is the science of denominators but that is simplistic and perhaps just wrong. The accurate collection of numerator data is an enormous, underestimated problem in epidemiology.

7.5 Denominator: defining the population at risk and the problem of inaccurate data

The quality of the data in the denominator (the lower number in a fraction) is crucial. Our first need, for incidence rates, is to know the number of people at risk of disease. As a simple rule, if people are at risk of being in the numerator, the population from which they came should be the

Box 7.7 Defining the denominator

◆ What might be your denominator for a study defining the incidence rate of

  (a) infant mortality;

  (b) the sudden infant death syndrome (cot death); and

  (c) myocardial infarction (heart attack)?

◆ What information would you need to make a rational choice?

denominator. Clearly, women are not at risk from testicular cancer, or men from cancer of the cervix. In these cases, the denominator would be sex-specific. It is common practice in epidemiology to consider men and women separately for most analysis, for their disease patterns are often different. If their patterns are demonstrably not different, data can be combined. Often, the choice of denominator is common sense but sometimes it is not. Try the exercise in Box 7.7 now.

The key is to understand the definition of the health problem under study. The infant mortality rate is by definition the number of deaths within the first year of life. The word *infant*, actually meaning a very young child, has been given a more precise meaning here. The logical denominator would be the population of 0–1 year olds, or the person-years of observation of a cohort of newborns (which is less than the population size because of deaths, migrations, and losses to follow-up). By definition, however, the denominator for infant mortality rate is the number of live births. The reason is a practical one, for this information is easy to obtain, accurate, and up-to-date. Effectively, this defines a cohort for which outcomes are obtained from mortality data. In contrast, to know the size of the population of 0–1 year olds would require an annual census or only occasional data analysis (the population census is mostly done every 10 years). To measure person-years of observation would need follow-up of members of our cohort individually. Since infant mortality rates are less than one per cent in industrialized countries, to follow-up individuals to collect 100 deaths would need a study of more than 10 000 infants. This is not worth doing given the costs. The formula for infant mortality rate in a particular year can now be seen as a pragmatic, low cost, and sensible compromise, and is:

$$\frac{\text{Number of deaths in infants under one year in year X}}{\text{Number of liveborn in year X}} \qquad (7.4)$$

To choose a denominator for sudden infant death syndrome (SIDS) we need to know the definition of the disease, for example:

> Sudden death of an infant under one year of age, which remains unexplained after a thorough case investigation, including performance of a complete autopsy, examination of the death scene, and review of the clinical history.

> US National Institute of Child Health (Willinger *et al.* 1991)

The denominator is infants less than one year old. The denominator choice here is driven by the definition of the disease, for identical deaths after the first year would not be called SIDS or 'cot' deaths. Older children are not at risk of SIDS by definition. Again, it is reasonable to use live births.

For the incidence rate of myocardial infarction, the denominator would be those at risk. It would be reasonable to exclude children and adolescents, for myocardial infarction is extremely rare in these groups. There is no scientific rationale for excluding the elderly, one sex (sometimes women are excluded), or particular ethnic groups. If the numerator comprises only selected cases based on age, sex, or ethnic group then the denominator will need to reflect this. In research focusing on the causes of disease those who have already had a heart attack before, and are therefore no longer at risk of having a *first* attack, might reasonably be excluded. The cause of a recurrent myocardial infarction may be different from a first one, and hence deserve separate study. If the information is to be used for priority setting or health needs assessment, the study should measure the incidence of first, recurrent, and total infarcts.

Where are we going to get the denominator data from? Although myocardial infarction is a common problem, if we were to study it in men and women aged 18 upwards there may only be a few cases per thousand of the population per year. To get enough cases for study needs either very long follow-up of study populations, or the study of large populations using disease registry data. The latter is the usual action in this case and then the denominator data need to come from a census or a population register. Now, the epidemiologist has to establish the accuracy of the denominator data. Census and other population registers are inaccurate and may be out of date. Typically, censuses are done every 10 years and even though they may be compulsory, they may be incomplete. There may be gaps for example, inner city inhabitants. Young people, men, and ethnic and racial minority groups and migrants tend to be underrepresented in such population counts. Though updated estimates are derived using births, deaths, and migration statistics, there may be errors. The epidemiologist needs to be acquainted with, and alert for, denominator errors. As with numerator data, the epidemiologist may be dependent on others' data but remains fully responsible for published errors.

The principles in terms of establishing the numerator and the denominator, discussed in the context of disease incidence studies, are similar but are even more complex in relation to prevalence.

7.6 Prevalence and prevalence proportion (but still often called rate)

Prevalence is the extent to which something exists. In epidemiology (Table 7.2) prevalence is the number of people with the factor of interest in the study population. The key features of prevalence are given in Table 7.2. For simplicity, let us assume the factor of interest is a disease, but it could be something else, such as a behavioural trait or an abnormal value in a blood test. The prevalence is usually expressed in relation to a population at risk, but sometimes another type of denominator may be chosen. For example, the prevalence of congenital abnormalities is usually expressed in relation to the number of live births. The term prevalence rate, the traditional phrase when rate was used generically, is in continuing usage but, as discussed earlier, a rate should have a time dimension.

Readers are advised to be aware they may read of prevalence rate, prevalence proportion, and/or simply prevalence, all meaning the same. The term *prevalence proportion* is correct but it has not become popular. The sixth edition of *A Dictionary of Epidemiology* has sidestepped the issue by simply calling the ratio prevalence without further qualification (but this is not correct either).

There are three types of prevalence proportions: point, period, and lifetime.

The *point* prevalence proportion comprises all the cases of the factor in a place at a point in time. The denominator is chosen to represent those at risk. The population at risk is often specifically recruited into the study so this number may be known. In studies where the investigators have not recruited the population, the denominator is usually derived from population estimates.

It is unlikely that such estimates will exist for a point in time (e.g. they are usually mid-year estimates, from the census). Inaccuracy in estimating prevalence is, therefore, likely in such studies.
In a study of the prevalence of, say, menstrual irregularity, the denominator would be women
who are menstruating, and a focus on a group of women 15–45 years of age might be a reasonable
choice rather than on all women. For prevalence proportion, unlike the incidence rate, we ought
not to exclude from the denominator those people who already have the factor. As the denominator includes the numerator, the result is a proportion and ranges from 0 to 1 (or, 0–100%). The
formula is simple:

$$\text{Point prevalence proportion} = \frac{\text{All cases of the factor of interest at time X}}{\text{Population at risk at time X}} \tag{7.5}$$

In practice, population at risk will be estimated and may well be the population at the start of
the study or the mid-year estimate. The resulting fraction is multiplied to get a whole number,
usually by 100 or 1000.

Period prevalence is a way of recognizing and overcoming the limitations of prevalence studies
done at a point in time. All cases whether old, new, or recurrent, arising over a defined period,
say a year, are counted. The denominator is the average population at risk over the period (or
midpoint estimate). Period prevalence, which combines incidence and point prevalence, is particularly useful in gauging the burden of episodic, recurrent diseases such as depression, anxiety,
or migraine. Both point prevalence and incidence, alone, tend to underestimate the size of such
problems, so a combination is desirable. The formula is:

$$\text{Period prevalence proportion} = \frac{\begin{array}{c}\text{All cases (old and new) of the factor}\\ \text{of interest during a time period}\end{array}}{\begin{array}{c}\text{Average population at risk during}\\ \text{the time period}\end{array}} \tag{7.6}$$

While the denominator is the average population, in practice the investigators may use other
easily available denominators.

Lifetime prevalence is the ultimate extension of the idea of period prevalence, and is the proportion of the population who have ever had the factor of interest. This can be derived systematically
from a birth cohort study (where people are followed up from birth). We can derive the proportion of the population who have ever had asthma by the age of 5, 10, 15, 30, and 45 years or more
until all are dead. Lifetime prevalence has value for drawing attention to how common some
disorders are. For example, over a lifetime mental health problems are extremely common. The
formula is:

$$\text{Lifetime prevalence} = \frac{\text{All cases who ever had the factor of interest during lifetime}}{\text{Population at risk (at the beginning of the time period)}} \tag{7.7}$$

In this measure, the only denominator that logically makes sense is the number in the birth
cohort. However, for some outcomes that mainly, or even only occur at certain ages, it is not practical. For example, dementia is very rare under the age of 40 years so it is reasonable to study a cohort
of age 40 and above. For most infections, skin disorders, etc., a life course cohort approach is needed.

The algebraic formulae for prevalence proportions are simple but, as with incidence rates, the
measurements underlying them are problematic. Most of the principles discussed in relation to

---

Box 7.8 Defining the numerator and denominator for the prevalence proportion of type 2 diabetes mellitus

In general terms, consider the steps you will need to take to count the numerator and denominator to measure the population prevalence proportion of type 2 diabetes.

---

incidence rates apply to prevalence proportions; for example, the need for a valid case definition and information to judge whether a case qualifies, a system for collection of information on the numerator, and defining and measuring an appropriate denominator. Imagine we are interested in measuring the prevalence proportion of type 2 diabetes. Now try the exercise in Box 7.8 before reading on.

The first and crucial step is to decide on the definition of type 2 diabetes. For this step, you will turn to current clinical guidelines wherever possible. The usual choices are:

◆ The WHO definition of a plasma glucose of, or more than, 11.1 mmol/L two hours after a standard oral glucose tolerance test. To meet this definition your study population will need to undergo this test which involves fasting overnight, having a blood test, then drinking the standard 75 g glucose drink and having blood taken 120 minutes later. This will require a special study, for such information does not exist in routine information systems. Since such a test is potentially dangerous or inadvisable in those with diabetes, not everyone will be able to do it. Despite its difficulties, this is still the test of choice in research settings and some clinical settings.

◆ The definition of the American Diabetes Association, now adopted by WHO, of a fasting plasma blood glucose level of more than 7 mmol/L. Again this information does not exist in routine records so a special study will be needed. This test is simpler than the glucose tolerance test but will lead to a different list of people being diagnosed and a different prevalence proportion than the aforementioned definition.

◆ In 2011 the WHO agreed that another test, of glycosylated haemoglobin (i.e. HbA1c), would be diagnostic if the value exceeded 6.5 per cent (48 mmol/l).

◆ Definitions based on a mixture of symptoms, signs, and of a variety of diagnostic strategies, including tests used in normal clinical practice. This approach is relatively easy, for the cases can be identified from medical records or registers, but is likely to underestimate the prevalence. Sometimes access to medical records and doctors will not be possible, leaving the investigators to rely on doctors' diagnosis reported by the study participants at interview or by questionnaire. This will underestimate the prevalence even more, for some participants will fail to report such a diagnosis. There are also other ways of diagnosing diabetes but the four mentioned here are sufficient to emphasize the point that there is no single correct measure of the numerator. These four definitions give substantially different results. Combining all three is likely to lead to an inflated estimate.

The second step is to select an appropriate population at risk. Identifying unbiased sample populations, and enlisting their cooperation in prevalence (cross-sectional) studies is a formidable task which will be discussed more fully in Chapter 9. Prevalence studies are usually of survivors. With the rare exception of prevalence studies including autopsy data, deaths are not included. This causes survivor bias. The reason for underestimating the burden and severity of the disease in a community-based study is that due to their disease, many people have either died or are in institutions (hospitals, nursing homes). Very often, the denominator is the number of people recruited into a study (as would be the case for the first three definitions of type 2 diabetes mellitus above, that is, the number who had the test). Sometimes, prevalence data can come from a register, for example, the Scottish Diabetes Register is based on in-service diagnosis (definition 4 in the previous list). By using the denominator of the Scottish population estimated at the census, the prevalence proportion (and as necessary incidence rate) can be calculated.

The duration of the prevalence study depends on what it measures: point, period, or lifetime prevalence. Point prevalence studies should take place on a particular day or narrow time interval; for example, a survey of the proportion of people in a hospital who are bedbound, or have an ulcer, or a hospital-acquired infection. In practice, observations on hundreds, sometimes thousands, of people cannot be made in this way and measurements take place over months or even years. Figures 7.4 and 7.5 are simple illustrations of the effects this can have.

Figure 7.4 is a study of a common permanent condition in 20 people, divided into four groups to make fieldwork easier, and spread over the year. The lines show the onset of the disease. The shading in the figure, which shows the fieldwork periods, is simply to help the counting. Do the exercise in Box 7.9 before reading on.

The point prevalence proportion with a denominator of 20 is 10 per cent in January (two cases exist, numbers 1 and 15), 20 per cent in July (four cases, numbers 1, 3, 15, 18), and 25 per cent in December (numbers 1, 3, 12, 15, 18). The (cumulative) incidence rate for the year is 16.6 per cent (three new cases/18 at risk; two already had the disease). Of course, the incident cases (especially case 12) may not be recognized in the field, so assume there is a registration system to pick them up.

The period prevalence is the sum of initial prevalent cases (2) plus incident cases (3) divided by the denominator (20), so 25 per cent. Here the denominator is again 20, the entire population under study. We cannot calculate lifetime prevalence on these data; we need to know what will happen to our study population until they die.

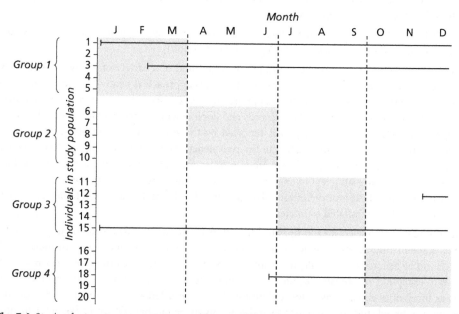

Fig. 7.4 Study of a common permanent problem. Each horizontal line denotes a case and shading the fieldwork order.

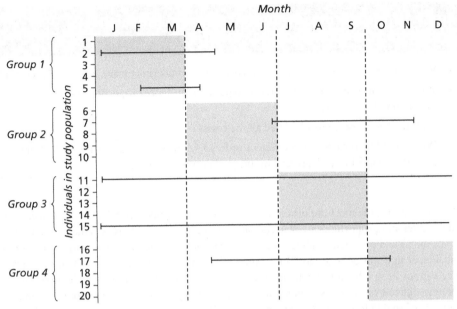

Fig. 7.5 Study of an impermanent problem, for example, taking up an exercise programme.

Of these cases only one (no. 12) will be missed by the fieldwork team; the fieldwork is before the date of onset. If the fieldwork order was changed, for example, group 4 first (January–March), group 3 second (April–June), group 2 third (January–September), and group 1 last (October–December), case no. 18 would also be missed (in addition to case 12). In the study, as actually conducted, one case is missed and the prevalence is underestimated. It is obvious that when studying factors that vary gently over time, especially seasonally, investigators should design their work to avoid this problem.

Figure 7.5 represents a study of a changeable condition, say, taking up an exercise programme. Do the exercise in Box 7.10 before reading on.

The point prevalence proportion is 15 per cent in January (3/20, numbers 2, 11, 15), 20 per cent in July (numbers 7, 11, 15, 17), and 10 per cent in December (numbers 11 and 15). The cumulative incidence rate of exercise uptake is 3/17, which is 17.6 per cent (numbers 5, 7, 17)—note that the three people already taking exercise are excluded from the denominator here as they are not at risk of taking up exercise. The period prevalence is 30 per cent. On this occasion, our fieldwork team misses no cases. If the fieldwork order had been group 4, 3, 2, 1, then cases 2, 5, and 17 would have been missed. Now try the exercise in Box 7.11 before reading on.

Box 7.9 Measuring prevalence proportion and incidence rates in a permanent condition

In Figure 7.4 what is the point prevalence proportion in January, July, and December? What is the cumulative annual incidence rate? What is the period prevalence proportion? What is the lifetime prevalence proportion? Have the fieldwork team identified all cases? What would be the effect of doing the study in a different order, say if group 4 went first, group 3 followed, etc.

Box 7.10 Measuring incidence rates and prevalence proportions in a changeable condition

- What is the point prevalence proportion of exercise uptake in January, July, and December?
- What is the cumulative incidence rate and period prevalence proportion of exercise uptake by the end of December?
- Have the fieldwork teams identified all the cases?
- What would be the effect of a different order of fieldwork, say group 4 went first, that is, January, group 3 in April, group 2 in July, and group 1 in October?

In this example, the most important information is the counts of incident and prevalent cases and the rates and proportions are of secondary interest. In other words, it is the incidence (new cases counts) and prevalence (all cases counts) that matter. A denominator may or may not be available, or may not be required. This example illustrates why the words incidence and prevalence cannot be a substitute for incidence rate and prevalence proportion. The first and surprisingly difficult task, as is so often true in epidemiology, is to define and count angina. The diagnosis of angina is a clinical one with no definitive signs or symptoms and no specific diagnostic test. The sensitivity and specificity of the main approaches to diagnosis in the community, that is, clinical history or electrocardiogram (ECG), are low. As a result, substantial proportions of people with CHD and chest discomfort are not given the correct diagnosis and others who do not have angina are incorrectly given it. The former situation may occur because tests such as an exercise ECG were negative, the latter because another health problem (e.g. gastritis or oesophagitis were mimicking the symptoms of angina). The health authority could be advised to use data based on numbers of people seen by the service in previous years. As there is an iceberg of angina in the community, some people, often with the severest disease and destined for sudden death or heart attack, will be missed.

The second difficult task is to differentiate those people with angina who would benefit from surgery from those who would do as well on medical therapy or just general health advice. The usual way to do this is by coronary angiogram, an invasive procedure whereby the narrowing of the coronary arteries is displayed using X-ray techniques. The dangers of this procedure are sufficient to preclude its use in epidemiological surveys of apparently healthy populations. For this

Box 7.11 Incidence and incidence rates and prevalences and prevalence proportions in the context of planning a service

A health authority (or an equivalent body such as an insurance agency, or a managed care organization) serving 500 000 people wishes to cost and plan a service for the medical and surgical management of angina in the population, with particular emphasis on the numbers of cases requiring surgery. Angina is a typical symptom of coronary heart disease characterized by chest pain on exertion.

You are invited to assist. Consider the general principles that you would apply to the task.

Consider the relative merits of measuring incidence and incidence rates, as well as point prevalence, period prevalence, and lifetime prevalences and proportions.

reason, a preliminary test—the exercise ECG—is often performed, and those rating as positive on this receive the angiogram.

The investigator needs to define angina for the purpose of this task set by a health authority, and design a study to estimate the number of all cases and the fraction of cases that will require surgery. Since angina is rarely a problem in the young, it could be reasonable to limit the investigation to adults, perhaps aged 35 years or more. The incidence rate is not helpful for planning here because it hugely underestimates the burden of the problem. The point prevalence estimate is the number of people with angina in the community, but is not sufficient. Period prevalence (say over a year) is probably the most useful measure, for it informs the planner of the number of people in the community that will require some service in that year. Lifetime prevalence is of no immediate value here. The period prevalence could be measured by a combination of clinical examinations and tests, and a register of cases. If denominator data are available, rates and proportions can be calculated to provide a neat data summary for the population. Once the population of angina patients has been identified, further tests, including exercise ECGs and angiography, will help to identify the need for surgery or medical management. These numbers can be expressed as a proportion of the total angina cases; for example, 40 per cent need surgery and 60 per cent non-surgical management.

Incidence and prevalence are clearly related, which is discussed next.

7.7 **Relationship of incidence and prevalence**

There is a close relationship between incidence and prevalence. The relationship is shown in simple form in Figure 7.6, as the 'bath' model. The tap inflow is the incidence, the bath water the prevalence (pool of cases). The prevalence pool is changed by the rate of inflow (incidence), death, recovery, or emigration (the outflow). Figure 7.7 develops this simple model in relation to a population. The population reservoir is enhanced by births and immigration, and diminished by deaths and emigration. This population reservoir is the water supply to the bath. Some incident cases die before reaching the prevalence pool, such as sudden infant death syndrome cases. The recovered cases rejoin the main population reservoir unless they are by definition chronic, lifelong problems.

There is a mathematical relationship between incidence and prevalence in fixed populations. Imagine a fixed population of 100 newborn infants, all of whom survive for the duration of the study, say five years. The number of new cases over five years (five-year cumulative incidence) of

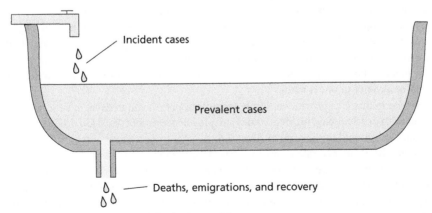

Fig. 7.6 Incidence, prevalence, and the 'bath' model.

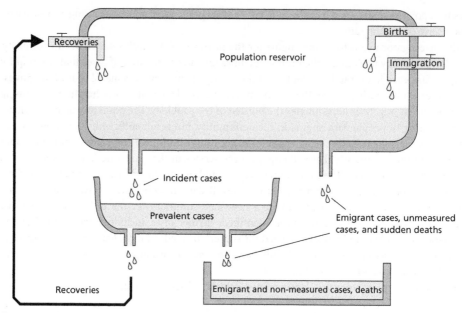

Fig. 7.7 Incidence, prevalence, and the 'bath' model in a population reservoir context.

a chronic, but non-fatal disease, and the total number of cases (prevalence) at the end of the study (five-year period prevalence) are identical. Therefore, if two new cases occur per year we will have 10 at the end of the study. The cumulative incidence rate, and the period prevalence proportion will be 10 per cent. The point prevalence proportion at the end of five years will also be 10 per cent.

If the duration of the disease is less than five years, then the prevalence at the end of five years will be smaller than the five-year cumulative incidence.

In fixed populations, when the incidence rate is low, the prevalence proportion is approximately equal to the incidence rate multiplied by the average duration of disease. It follows that incidence rate is approximately equal to the point prevalence proportion ÷ duration; and duration is approximately equal to the point prevalence proportion ÷ incidence rate. Exact formulae are also available (see Appendix 7.1). In practice, in the calculation of incidence rates and prevalence proportions our populations are complex and changing. For example, they are mostly dynamic with constantly shifting sizes and characteristics and changing incidence too.

In a dynamic population, the prevalence of a disease cannot be predicted from knowledge of the incidence (or vice versa) because of migration into and out of the population, deaths, changing disease rates, changes in prognosis, and error in measuring the incidence (or prevalence) accurately. In practice, both the prevalence and incidence are measured rather than mathematically estimated, or a choice of one is made.

The exercise in Box 7.12 provides a simple example to permit you to develop your understanding of, and skills in calculating incidence rates and prevalence proportions. Do this exercise before reading on. You will find the answers in Table 7.6.

The cumulative incidence rate of myopia, based on the denominator at the beginning of the study, is 100/10 000 per year = 1 per cent. The alternative is to take the population at risk at the midpoint of the time interval, at six months. By then 50 people will be myopic and hence no longer at risk. The incidence rate then is 100/9950 = 1.005 per cent. The incidence rate estimated by the person–time denominator of myopia is identical but expressed differently, that is,

Box 7.12 Incidence rates and prevalence proportions of myopia—short-sightedness

Imagine a population of 10 000 new school children, aged 5 years. Your interest is in the incidence rates and prevalence proportions of short-sightedness (myopia). Assume myopia is permanent. You follow the children for one year. All of the study population survive, all medical and eye test records are available, and all are available for interview and examination. Assume that the occurrence of myopia is spread evenly throughout the year, and that at recruitment none had myopia. Over the year, you find that 100 recruits had newly developed myopia.

- What is the one-year cumulative incidence rate of myopia? Calculate this with the baseline denominator of the children at risk. Also, re-do this calculation with the estimated at-risk population at the midpoint of the time interval of the study, that is, exclude those who have developed myopia and are not at risk any longer.

- What is the one-year incidence rate per 10 000 years of observation based on the person–time denominator? Remember, this denominator is not the same as the population at the start of the study. You can estimate it using the assumption that cases occurred evenly over time.

- What is the point prevalence proportion of having had myopia at the beginning, middle, and end of the year?

- What is the period prevalence proportion over the year?

- If the cumulative incidence rate remains the same over time (1% per year), and assuming a fixed denominator of 10 000, what is approximately the period prevalence proportion of myopia by the end of five years? (In practice it will be lower as the denominator will diminish as children develop myopia, so the number of cases will decline each year.)

- What is the estimate of the point prevalence of myopia at the midpoint of the five-year period?

- What is the estimated average duration of myopia by the end of the five years?

- What is the estimated point prevalence proportion using the approach of the above formulae?

- What is the estimated cumulative incidence rate based on the approach of the above formulae (section 7.7, paragraph 3)?

per person-years of observation. The total person-years of observation is 9950 (9900 given by those not myopic, and 50 by those 100 people who are myopic for they give, on average, 0.5 years of time to the study—if we had the exact time we could use that instead). The result is 100/9950 person-years, that is, 100.5 per 10 000 person-years.

The point prevalence at the beginning is zero, and at six months, on average, half of all cases will have occurred, so it is 50/10 000 (0.5%), and by the end of the year it is 100/10 000 (1%). The period prevalence at one year is also 100/10 000 (1%). We made a simple, unlikely assumption of no myopia cases at baseline. In reality, some children will already have this at school entry so these cases would need to be added on to prevalence figures.

The actual duration of myopia among cases is, on average, half of the time of follow-up. The prevalence is low and the population is fixed, so our simple formula will give a good estimate. The average duration of myopia is approximately point prevalence proportion at the midpoint

Table 7.6 Answers to questions in Box 7.12 on incidence rates and prevalence proportions of myopia

Cumulative incidence rate of myopia	$= \dfrac{100 \text{ new cases}}{10\,000}$	$= 0.01$	$= 1\%$
Cumulative incidence rate using midpoint estimate of population at risk	$= \dfrac{100}{9950}$	$= 0.01005$	$= 1.005\%$
Incidence rate using person–time	$= \dfrac{100 \text{ new cases}}{(10\,000 \text{ years} - 50 \text{ years}) = 9950}$	$= 0.01005$ cases per 10 000 years of observation	$= 10.5$ cases per 10 000 person-years

Prevalence Proportions

– beginning	$= \dfrac{0}{10\,000}$	$= 0$	
– middle	$= \dfrac{50}{10\,000}$	$= 0.5\%$	
– end of year	$= \dfrac{100}{10\,000}$	$= 1\%$	
Period prevalence over the year	$= \dfrac{0 + 100}{10\,000}$	$= 1\%$	
Period prevalence over 5 years	$= \dfrac{0 + (100 \times 5)}{10\,000}$	$= 5\%$	
Point prevalence at midpoint (2.5 years)	$= \dfrac{\text{Cases at midpoint interval}}{10\,000}$	$= \dfrac{250}{10\,000}$	$= 2.5\%$
Average duration of myopia (years)	$= \dfrac{\text{Point prevalence at midpoint}}{\text{Annual incidence rate}}$	$= \dfrac{2.5\%}{1.5\%}$	$= 2.5$ years
Point prevalence over 5 years based on formula	$= \dfrac{\text{Annual incidence rate} \times \text{duration}}{10\,000}$	$= \dfrac{100 \times 2.5}{10\,000} = \dfrac{250}{10\,000}$	$= 2.5\%$
Incidence rate based on formula	$= \dfrac{\text{Point prevalence proportion}}{\text{Duration}}$	$= \dfrac{250/10\,000}{2.5}$	$= 100/10\,000 = 1\%$

of the interval ÷ incidence = 2.5 per cent ÷ 1 per cent = 2.5 years. The predicted approximate point prevalence at 5 years = annual incidence × average duration × years of observation = 100 per 10 thousand × 2.5 years = 250 per 10 000 or 2.5 per cent. The incidence rate based on the formula is, approximately point prevalence proportion ÷ duration = 250/2.5 = 100 or 1 per cent.

The prevalence and prevalence proportion as calculated here slightly overestimates the reality because there will be a decreasing number of cases in each successive year, as those who develop myopia would be removed from the denominator.

A better estimate of the period prevalence proportion at 5 years is 490.1/10 000 (or 4.9%), as follows:

- 1st year incident cases = 100, leaving 9900 at risk
- 2nd year incident cases = 1 per cent of 9900 = 99, leaving 9801
- 3rd year incident cases = 1 per cent of 9801 = 98.01, leaving 9702.99
- 4th year incident cases = 1 per cent of 9702.99 = 97.03, leaving 9605.96
- 5th year incident cases = 1 per cent of 9605.99 = 96.06, leaving 9509.9 cases

The total number of cases is 490.1 compared with 500 in Table 7.7. The period prevalence proportion then was 490.1/10 000 = 4.9 per cent rather than 5 per cent.

The reader may wish to calculate the 5-year cumulative incidence based on the baseline and midpoint denominators, and the person-years of observation, and try the formula in Appendix 7.1.

7.8 **Choice of incidence or prevalence measures**

For studies of the causes of disease, mostly the incidence rate is preferred because it is a simpler, purer measure that is not affected by variation in treatment and case-fatality, so differences between populations are easier to interpret. For studies of the burden of diseases of short duration (e.g. measles, influenza, diarrhoea, transient ischaemic attacks, ankle sprains, acute low backache), incidence is also preferred because point prevalence would seriously underestimate the problem. The point prevalence figure would miss the recovered or dead cases.

The prevalence proportion is generally preferred as the measure of burden for long-lasting diseases, even when these are rare (e.g. multiple sclerosis, renal failure). For health behaviours and other disease risk factors, prevalence proportion is almost invariably the preferred measure.

Prevalence measures are sometimes perceived in epidemiology as inferior to incidence ones. They are not. Both measures have inherent weaknesses and strengths, and different value in various circumstances. Both measures are prone to the numerator and denominator errors discussed in sections 7.4 and 7.5. However, there are circumstances, as I have just described, where one measure is preferred to the other.

7.9 **Presenting rates: overall (actual or commonly crude) and specific**

Rates can be presented for the whole population under study or for subgroups of that population. For example, the estimated population of Scotland in 1999 was 5.195 million, and there were 60 277 deaths, giving an overall mortality rate of 60 277/5 195 000 = 0.0116 = 11.6 per 1000. Such an overall rate is commonly referred to as the crude rate. This phrase distinguishes the rate from an adjusted (or standardized) rate as explained in Chapter 8. Adjusted rates deal with confounding factors, especially age and sex. As the word *crude* has negative connotations, perhaps even perceived as useless, a better term is *actual*. The actual (crude) rate definitely has value, especially in health-care planning. The actual rate can be subdivided by any characteristic of the population of epidemiological interest (e.g. age, sex) and calculated for different places and times. Such subdivided rates are called specific rates (e.g. age- or sex-specific rates) and this is called *stratified analysis*.

Commonly used variables for subdivision of rates include age group, sex, ethnic group, race, social class, educational status, and marital status. Such variables are often referred to as epidemiological variables (discussed in Chapter 1). Obviously, to calculate specific rates we need to be able to subdivide the population denominator counts by these variables. We need to know, for example, the number of people in each ethnic group in the underlying population before we can calculate ethnic group specific rates. Such information may not be available, especially in small geographical areas and at times other than the census year.

Specific rates permit rational and easy comparison of disease patterns in different places and times for they can be directly compared with each other, and questions asked about why differences might occur. The answers are usually complex and elusive. Simple observations of difference in disease rates may lead to inspiration, as in the example of Semmelweis's hypothesis of a transmissible cadaverous particle, arising from his reflection on mortality in two clinics (discussed in Chapter 5). More often, the observations are merely noted or give rise to untested hypotheses. For example, long-standing observations of greater lifespan (and lower mortality rates) in women compared with men are largely unexplained in specific biological or social terms, as are differences in chronic diseases at different ages. Explaining differences in disease rates is exceptionally difficult epidemiological science.

Imagine that we observe that an English seaside resort town such as Bournemouth has a higher actual (or crude) overall mortality rate from stroke than, say, a city such as Bristol. The likely explanation is one of low scientific interest; the seaside resort has more elderly people, for it is a place people move to after retirement. The overall higher rate, though true, is usually adjusted to take account of these differences in age structure of the population of the two cities using methods discussed in Chapter 8. We would not usually investigate the role of age in causing differences in stroke between these cities because it is a basic explanation of little epidemiological interest nowadays. That is not to deny the continuing interest in the question of how ageing alters biology and disease.

Although there are still intriguing and unexplained differences in disease by sex and age, these variables are usually treated as confounding variables. It is good practice, however, to check for effect modification before treating these variables as confounders. Examination of age- and sex-specific data (counts of cases and rates) are part of sound epidemiological practice. This allows the investigator to get a good understanding of the data set, as well as making observations on the pattern of diseases. The problem is that the tables showing such data are typically large. An example of such a table is 8.17. These kinds of tables are only rarely published in journal articles, but are often found in reports or websites. There are good reasons for their inclusion in online supplementary tables supporting journal articles.

7.10 **Conclusion**

Epidemiology is a practical and pragmatic science that is focused on measuring and explaining the pattern of disease in populations. This requires three distinct types of data in context of time and place: on diseases; on the factors that potentially cause disease; and the size and characteristics of the populations under study. Obtaining these data with a high degree of accuracy is a serious obstacle to epidemiology, even in the most economically advanced populations. Many of these challenges are considered in Exemplar 7.1.

The art of epidemiology lies in making judgements on the appropriate interpretation of, inevitably, incomplete and inaccurate data. Epidemiological and other theories of health and disease, and frameworks for data analysis and interpretation, are vital to guide such judgements.

Theoretical considerations around measurement and presentation of risk, and mathematical and statistical ideas on measurement of disease occurrence, underpin the practice of data collection. These are the factors that have driven change and advancement in an aspect of epidemiology that is based on mathematics. The increasing use of the person–time denominator, rather than the traditional population size denominator is one example of such change.

Rate of disease, where a measure of the quantity of disease over a time period (the numerator) is considered in relation to a measure of the quantity of population (the denominator), lie at the core of the epidemiological method. We also need measures of the risk factors for diseases, which are usually described by prevalence proportions. These measures are the hammers, screwdrivers, and spanners of the epidemiological toolbox. Two types of counts and proportions are dominant in epidemiology: incidence and prevalence. The two are clearly distinguished by being concerned with either new events (incidence) or events old and new (prevalence). Epidemiologists should examine these building blocks of their data extremely carefully, questioning the veracity of the numerator and denominator. Although others may provide such data, epidemiologists remain fully responsible for the results. Numerous false starts and misleading turns would be avoided by careful scrutiny of the quality of the data underlying the proportions and rates. Only when these fundamentals are sound should more complex data analysis proceed. These two measures are manipulated in epidemiology to produce a multiplicity of perspectives on population patterns of health and disease—and that is the subject of the next chapter (Chapter 8).

Exemplar 7.1: Collecting and analysing incidence data in the Scottish Health and Ethnicity Linkage Study: insights from public health epidemiology (Fischbacher *et al.* 2007)

The Scottish Health and Ethnicity Linkage Study (SHELS) has produced many statistics, including on incidence and prevalence, for Scotland. As the chief investigator, I can share insights into the decisions underpinning its methods. I will demonstrate how the measures varied by outcome, how outcomes were defined, and how measures changed over time. This example also emphasizes that the investigators, and not those supplying the data, are responsible for their accuracy. This may be the first ever study to link an entire national census to virtually the entirety of the hospitalization and mortality records.

The problem to be solved that led to the study

As in many countries, Scotland has anti-discrimination legislation that imposes duties on public bodies to (a) provide equitable services, and (b) demonstrate that they have done so. The latter requires quantitative data. Scotland is renowned for its health data systems but around the year 2000, these only provided information on two of the characteristics protected by legislation, that is, sex (but not gender) and age. For race, ethnicity, religion (and other characteristics such as disability, sexual orientation, etc.) there were no relevant data, mainly because the health services had not collected sufficiently complete data to permit analysis. The collection of sufficiently complete and accurate data is a massive epidemiological challenge globally.

The key solution: data linkage

Of a number of approaches tested in pilot studies (2002–2005) the most promising was data linkage. Ethnicity was collected in the 2001 Census of Scotland. Health-care utilization and mortality data had already been linked by NHS Scotland and held in a database called SMR01 (Scottish Morbidity Record 01). Could we link these data sets? There were many hurdles in the way.

Surmounting the hurdles

Conceptualizing a secure method for linkage

In Scotland there is no unique citizenship number. There is a number on the census record and another one on most health service records (Community Health Index—or CHI—number).

Therefore, an exact linkage was not possible. We proposed a computer-driven probability match using name, address, postcode (zip code), sex, and date of birth as these were in both census and health records. The census number was also extracted, as was the CHI number. These numbers were encrypted. Once the match was done, the personal data were removed leaving the encrypted census and CHI numbers. These could be used to re-link to both census and health records, without further need for personal data.

Insight: conceptualizing the method in detail is essential and may be a lengthy process.

Ethics and privacy: gaining permission

The census is held every 10 years and is legally compulsory. The head of household is required to gather the information to complete it. It is strictly confidential with a 100-year guarantee by law. Yet, the Registrar General who heads up the responsible organization has a legal duty to produce statistics using the census to inform the public. The health data held by Scotland are also strictly confidential.

On the basis that the only practical, timely way to respond to the Race Relations Amendment Act 2000 was data linkage we obtained permission from the following, given here in approximate order of negotiations: Registrar General of Scotland; Council for Racial Equality, Scotland; Chief Medical Officer, Scotland; National Resource Centre for Ethnic Minority Health; Research Ethics Committee, Scotland; Privacy Advisory Committee, Scotland; and Community Health Index Advisory Group, Scotland.

For some other specific outcomes, we also had to obtain permission from the Caldicott Guardian (of clinical records), the Mental Welfare Commission, and individual general practices (family medicine centres).

Insight: gaining permissions may be a major component of any data collection exercise, whether using new original research or existing data.

The pilot study: myocardial infarction (heart attack)

The numerator We started with a public health priority where important ethnic differences were expected. We obtained an extract of all hospitalizations and deaths from acute myocardial infarction (MI). We used ICD ninth and tenth editions. The codes were 410 to 414 in the ninth edition and I20 to I25 in the tenth edition.

The extract held all the coded causes of death on the death certificate, and outpatients and inpatient discharges with up to six coded diagnoses.

Our definition for the numerator was this: the first event of either hospitalization or death from MI following the 2001 census in April 2001 to December 2003. We used any of the six diagnoses on the hospitalization record but only the underlying cause of death.

How did we separate first events from recurrent events? We examined the SMR01 database for 10 years before April 2001. If a person had no prior record of MI we made an assumption that this was a first event. This seems like a reasonable assumption although it is possible that a person had an event earlier than 1991. We accepted potential error of this kind.

What about the quality of the diagnostic data? All doctors in Scotland have access to national guidance on diagnosing and recording MI. Laboratory tests are an important part of the diagnostic process, thus reducing diagnostic bias. We examined quality of data reports indicating 90 per cent of diagnoses for CHD were accurate. We thought this was reasonable and that it would be higher for MI, which is a serious manifestation of CHD. We did not know whether diagnostic accuracy was similar across ethnic groups but assumed it was.

Therefore, our data captured all events of MI or MI death recorded in Scottish hospitals and on death certificates in Scotland. What could be missing from the numerator? There may have been cases that were hospitalized or died without a correct diagnosis being made. There may have been cases managed in the community, though that would not be acceptable practice in Scotland. People may have been out of the country when they developed MI. They may have been admitted to a private hospital that did not submit their data centrally, though that is most unlikely in Scotland for this outcome, especially as private hospitals are required to submit data centrally.

We can see the limitations of the numerator data but also its strengths. For example, many cases of MI lead to near instant death in the community, but by combining deaths in and out of hospital and hospitalizations without deaths we get a truer picture of the burden across ethnic groups. It is plausible that hospitalization rates may not be equivalent across ethnic groups.

Insight: clarifying the numerator and the limitations of the data are important and difficult matters. This is especially so when using others' data.

The denominator This pilot study was conducted to compare MI in South Asian and White Scottish populations. White Scottish is straightforward because this is one of the ethnic group labels offered on the census form. South Asian is an academic term not on the census. We knew that, desirable as it was, we did not have enough events to examine each South Asian group separately, so we combined the census categories of Pakistani, Indian, Bangladeshi, and other South Asian groups to create the category South Asian.

We analysed for men and women separately because disease rates are much higher in men. This was a big decision because it reduces the number of overall outcomes for analysis by splitting them across sex specific groups.

We excluded people under the age of 25 years when MI is very rare. This was done because small numbers (and zeros in some age groups) make age standardization unreliable.

So what do we know about the accuracy of the denominators? The census office knew that 4.9 million of Scotland's estimated 5.2 million people completed census returns. The census office's studies indicate men, the young, and ethnic minority groups are the least likely to participate in the census, so we worried that our South Asian denominator, especially in men, might be underestimated, thus spuriously increasing disease rates.

Of these 4.9 million people in the census, 4.62 million (95%) were linked, that is, we obtained a match with an NHS CHI number. Was linkage equivalent across ethnic groups? We had anticipated that linkage would be more difficult in South Asians, for example, the names were less likely to match in the census and health records because of different spellings. We set a quality standard, based on our collective judgement that linkage needed to be at least 85 per cent. For the South Asian group together this was achieved, but the linkage at 85.4 per cent was lower than in the White Scottish (95.1%). This was another issue to consider in data interpretation.

Insight: decisions need to be taken in the light of the amount and quality of the data. Some of these decisions have benefits and weaknesses, for example, analysing men and women separately.

The calculations

We calculated the cumulative incidence rate using baseline denominators. This means we did not adjust the denominator—the number of outcomes seemed too small to matter. We analysed by 10-year age groups, and then calculated the all-age crude (actual) rate before standardizing for age using the direct method, as explained in Chapter 8.

Insight: there are many routes in the analysis and investigators need to choose to maximize the benefits in the light of the goals.

Interpretation of results We found that South Asian men and women had a higher incidence rate of hospitalization and mortality than White Scottish people. This seemed unlikely to be a result of the potential errors in numerators and denominator, even though we were not able to check this quantitatively.

This pilot study demonstrated the potential value of the methods, and subsequently the study was expanded and the methods refined.

Insight: perfection cannot be achieved in epidemiology. These results achieved the study goal (i.e. demonstrating the methods worked and were worth pursuing).

Next steps in SHELS and refinements to calculating incidence rates

In addition to obtaining longer-term outcomes (numerators) and a wide range of health outcomes, SHELS also made the following changes to numerators and denominators in later analyses.

Numerators: for some recurrent outcomes (e.g. asthma), we included all cases, without doing a lookback, that is, the cases were both recurrent and first hospitalization (and deaths).

Denominators

In the pilot study, the follow-up time period was only about 30 months. This meant the number of outcomes was small. In later phases for different outcomes, we had 7, 9, and even 13 years of follow-up data. These longer timescales, however, meant we could not be confident about the denominator being stable over time. The population sizes would be declining because of deaths and migrations. The only indicator of migration we had was that NHS Scotland's records had been requested by the NHS elsewhere in the United Kingdom. We wanted to adjust our denominator to account for these departures. The cumulative incidence rate method, though still feasible, was not convenient for this so we changed to a person–time incidence rate. The time contributed to the denominator was reduced by taking into account the date of death and the date of medical records being requested by other part of the UK NHS. For conditions where only the first event was under study, we also used date of onset to censor further observations on that person.

We also checked whether the rates made sense by examining rates across the time period (by examining three-year periods and running averages).

We were still unable to adjust the denominator for deaths abroad, hospitalizations outside NHS Scotland, and emigration outside the United Kingdom. We acknowledged these limitations when interpreting data.

The complexity involved in working with these longer periods was compensated by the larger number of outcomes. For example, in later analyses of MI we presented data for Indians, Pakistanis, and other South Asians separately rather than as an aggregation of South Asians. There were big differences in rates for these populations.

Insight: methods may continually evolve and improve, so investigators should periodically scrutinize the analysis plan.

Conclusion

The calculation of disease frequency measures is not a mechanical or routine exercise. Rather, it requires careful thought on the sources, quality, validity, and stability of numerator and denominator data. The limitations need to be pinpointed. The method of calculation depends on the data and the purposes of the study. The stratification of data (here by sex and ethnic group) should relate to the goals of the study and the possible uses of the results. SHELS also calculated other summary measures including prevalence, but the principles applied were similar. In Chapter 8, we will return to SHELS when we discuss standardization and relative measures.

Concluding remarks

The formulae underlying much of the epidemiology are simple, but obtaining the necessary data, resolving data problems, and interpreting the results is complex.

Source: data from Fischbacher, C.M., Bhopal, R., Povey, C., *et al.* Record linked retrospective cohort study of 4.6 million people exploring ethnic variations in disease: myocardial infarction in South Asians. *BMC Public Health*, Volume 7, pp. 142, Copyright © 2007 Fischbacher *et al.*

Summary

Risk is the possibility of harm. In epidemiology, risk refers to the likelihood, or in statistical language, the probability of an individual in a defined population developing a disease or other adverse health problem. In epidemiology, the association at the population level between risk of disease and variation in both individual and social characteristics (risk factors) is often the starting point for causal analysis. Epidemiological studies measure, present, and interpret disease frequency, usually by comparing the patterns in one population relative to another. The prime measures of disease frequency that provide the basis for such comparisons are incidence rates and prevalence proportions.

The incidence rate is the number of new cases in relation to a population, time, and place. Two forms of incidence rates are in common use, usually distinguished by terms such as cumulative incidence and person–time incidence rate (or simply incidence rate). In cumulative incidence the denominator is the population; in person–time incidence the denominator is the sum of the time periods for which the individuals in the population have been observed.

Prevalence proportion measures a disease or a risk factor in a population either at a particular time (point prevalence) or over a time period (period prevalence, lifetime prevalence). There is a mathematical relation between the two measures, such that in a fixed population prevalence is approximately equal to the incidence multiplied by the duration of the disease. As epidemiology concerns dynamic populations, this relationship is seldom useable.

Rates and proportions are most accurately presented by age and sex groups ('specific' rates and proportions), but for ease of interpretation they may be grouped as overall, actual (crude) rates. The collection of both disease and population data to achieve accurate figures of incidence rates and prevalence proportions is problematic, and remains a major challenge. Epidemiologists need to rigorously examine the quality and completeness of data underpinning rates and proportions, especially in the analysis of data collected by others.

Sample questions

Many of the questions in Chapters 8 and 9 are relevant to this chapter.

Question 1 Why are (point) prevalence proportions useful in epidemiology? List at least five factors which may either increase or decrease the prevalence

Answer Prevalence proportions indicate the burden of health problems and of their causes or risk factors. They point to priorities and help target priority groups for health and medical services. Prevalence proportions may also serve as baseline indices for subsequent evaluations of health services in the groups served.

The prevalence is increased by:

- immigration of cases
- emigration of healthy people
- immigration of susceptible people or those with potential of becoming cases, for example, the aged
- prolongation of life of cases without cure (increase in duration of disease)
- increase in new cases.

The prevalence is decreased by:

- immigration of healthy people
- emigration of cases
- improved cure of cases
- increased death rate of cases
- decrease in occurrence of new cases
- shorter duration of disease.

Question 2 Nine hundred residents in a retirement home (350 with low salt intake and 550 with high salt intake) who do not have hypertension participate in a study to assess the incidence of hypertension. Assume that the populations remain stable over one year of follow-up. Blood pressure is measured in everyone at the beginning of the year and again at the end. At the end of follow-up, 20 residents with low salt intake (low risk) and 70 with high salt intake (high risk) have hypertension. Assume the diagnostic methods are correct.

1. Place these data in an appropriate 2 × 2 table.
2. Calculate the incidence rate for high blood pressure using the person–time denominator (base your denominator on the estimated population at risk, that is, taking into account the best estimate of the time contribution of those with the outcome).
3. Briefly state and discuss why the person–time denominator may be preferred over the population denominator. In this instance, does it matter which denominator you use? Explain why.

Answer 1

Table 7.7 Results of the hypertension study presented in a 2 × 2 table

Risk factor	Hypertension		
	Yes	No	Total
High salt intake	70	480	550
Low salt intake	20	330	350
Total	90	810	900

Answer 2 Incidence of hypertension in high salt intake group:

$$\frac{70}{(70 \times 0.5) + (480 \times 1)} = \frac{70}{515} = 135.9 \text{ per 1000 person-years}$$

Incidence of hypertension in low salt intake group:

$$\frac{20}{(20 \times 0.5) + (330 \times 1)} = \frac{20}{340} = 58.8 \text{ per 1000 person-years}$$

Answer 3 Often people are followed for different lengths of time. Some drop out or come into the study at different times. In such cases, the calculation of the denominator is not easy using people. The accumulated periods of time for each person in the study is an elegant option. The person-years approach has been an effective method of utilizing information about each subject, even if the period of follow-up is short. It uses all the data on participants in a follow-up study.

The incidence rates are not the same using the two different denominators. When using the population at risk denominator, the following results are obtained: incidence rate in high salt intake group (70/550) = 127.3 per 1000; in the low salt intake group the incidence is (20/350) = 57.1 per 1000.

Question 3 Why is the count of the numerator in the rate of disease difficult to measure accurately?

Answer The numerator is difficult to measure because of the problems in accurately defining diseases; in accurately making the clinical and laboratory measurement to see whether the definition applies; in applying these measurements in population settings; in collecting, analysing, and interpreting the usually incomplete and imperfect data; and in keeping track of changes over time.

Acknowledgements

Figure 7.6 shows a diagram given to me by Ms Denise Howel, whose assistance I am most grateful for.

References

Bodansky, H.J., Airey, CM., Chell, S.M., Unwin, N., and Williams, D.R.R. (1997) The incidence of lower limb amputation in Leeds, UK: setting a baseline for St Vincent. International Diabetes Federation Meeting. *Diabetologia*, A1850.

Elandt-Johnson, R. (1975) Definition of rates: Some remarks on their use and misuse. *American Journal of Epidemiology*, **102**, 267–71.

Fischbacher, C.M., Bhopal, R., Povey, C., *et al.* (2007) Record linked retrospective cohort study of 4.6 million people exploring ethnic variations in disease: myocardial infarction in South Asians. *BMC Public Health*, 7, 142.

Pickles, W.N. (1939) *Epidemiology in Country Practice*. Bristol, UK: Wright.

Porta, M. (2014) *A Dictionary of Epidemiology*, 6th edn. New York, NY: Oxford University Press.

Willinger, M., James. L.S., and Catz, C. (1991) Defining the sudden infant death syndrome (SIDS): deliberations of an expert panel convened by the National Institute of Child Health and Human Development. *Pediatric Pathololgy*, **11**, 677–84.

World Health Organization. (1992) *ICD-10: International Statistical Classification of Diseases and Related Health Problems*. World Health Organization, Geneva, Switzerland.

World Health Organization. (2016) *International Statistical Classification of Diseases and Related Health Problems*, 10th revision (ICD-10) (WHO Version for 2016). Available at: http://apps.who.int/classifications/icd10/browse/2016/en', accessed 01 Feb 2016.

Appendix 7.1

The exact formula for the relationship between incidence rate and prevalence proportion only applies when the conditions are stable in a fixed population. The formula is a little more complex than the one in the main text as follows:

$$\frac{\text{Prevalence proportion (as \%)}}{100\% - \text{prevalence proportion (as \%)}} = \text{Incidence rate} \times \text{disease duration}$$

The left-hand side of the equation is the odds. So, the prevalence proportion odds are equal to the incidence rate times disease duration. When the prevalence proportion of disease if uncommon—let us say two per cent—then the odds are very close to two per cent, that is,

$$\frac{2\%}{(100\% - 2\%)} = \frac{2\%}{98\%} = 0.0204 = 2.04\%$$

So, our approximation works when the prevalence is low, which is true for most diseases but not true for most risk factors.

Chapter 8

Summarizing, presenting, and interpreting epidemiological data: Building on incidence and prevalence

Objectives

On completion of the chapter you should understand:

- the general process of constructing summary measures of health status;
- that the aim of data analysis is to summarize information and sharpen understanding of actual and relative frequency of disease;
- the idea behind, definition, strengths and limitations, and means of calculation of:
  - proportional mortality and proportional mortality ratio
  - directly and indirectly standardized rates (and the standardized mortality ratio)
  - relative risk
  - odds ratio
  - attributable risk, population-attributable risk
  - years of life lost
  - numbers needed to treat and prevent
  - the quality-adjusted life year, and the disability-adjusted life year;
- that the principal relative measure is the relative risk (or rate) while the odds ratio can approximate it in particular circumstances;
- that attributable risk and population-attributable risk are measures that help us to assess the proportion of the burden of disease that is related to a particular risk factor;
- that the term avoidable mortality (morbidity) refers to the potential to avoid death (morbidity) from the specified causes if the best possible health-care actions were taken;
- that the number of years of avoidable life lost measures the impact of avoidable mortality and helps us to assess the effectiveness of health care;
- how epidemiological data contribute to assessing the health needs and health status of populations;
- that continuous data (e.g. height), also contribute to both description of health status and to understanding of causal relationships;
- that different ways of presenting the same data have a major impact on interpretation, so epidemiological studies should provide both relative and actual, or absolute, risk.

8.1 **Introduction**

Epidemiological data can be manipulated easily and in many ways, with the purpose of summarizing information and/or extracting additional insights. Usually, but not always, the objective is to permit or sharpen up comparisons, whether over time, or between places and population groups. This chapter introduces the main ways in which data are manipulated, with a warning that the end results are often artificial measures that change (and sometimes distort) the perception and interpretation of risk, a matter of utmost concern to a science where communication between researchers, health professionals, and the public is critically important. There are many other ways of summarizing data, and new ways are constantly invented. However, the principles underlying them tend to be similar.

8.2 **Proportional morbidity or mortality ratio**

Sometimes the only reliable data we have are on a series of cases. Comparisons are difficult without population denominators (to construct rates), but these may not be available or they may be inaccurate. For example, there are usually no accurate, stable population denominators for comparing disease and mortality outcomes by workplace or hospital, because most workplaces and hospitals do not draw their workers and patients, respectively, from a specific and defined population. Studies of ethnicity and health in the United Kingdom (and similarly in many countries) are thwarted by the fact that ethnic code has been collected only at three censuses (1991, 2001, and 2011) and that records providing information on disease do not record ethnicity accurately. For example, the death certificate in England has country of birth but no ethnic code and in hospital admission records, the ethnic code is often missing. In Scotland in 2012, ethnicity was included in the death registration process, but not in the rest of the United Kingdom. Furthermore, some record systems and studies that do provide an ethnic code use a different classification from that in the census. In these kinds of circumstances, a denominator-free method is needed.

The proportional morbidity or mortality ratio (PMR) is commonly used to study disease patterns by cause where population denominators are not available, as illustrated here using mortality, although exactly the same approach is followed for other outcomes.

The total number of deaths (not the population) is used as the denominator, and the deaths from each specific cause as the numerator. The proportional mortality (PM) is the resulting fraction, a proportion, usually expressed as a percentage. The formula is:

$$PM = \frac{\text{Number of deaths due to cause X}}{\text{Total number of deaths}} \qquad (8.1)$$

Multiplying this fraction by 100 is the convention and this provides the PM as a percentage. The PM can be calculated by sex, age group, or any other appropriate subdivision of the population. These figures can be compared between populations, places, or time periods by calculating the PMR, which is simply the ratio of PMs in the two comparison populations, that is,

$$PMR = \frac{\text{PM in population A}}{\text{PM in population B}} \qquad (8.2)$$

In this formula population A is usually the study population of interest, population B the standard, reference, or comparison population. The latter supplies the information on the expected proportion. Conventionally the study population—the one of special interest—is placed in the numerator, the reference population in the denominator, though sometimes this convention is not followed.

The PMR examines differences in the proportion of deaths attributable to disease X in one population compared with a second population. (Obviously, all-cause PM or PMR is always 100%.) The PMR (formula 8.2) can then be reconsidered as:

$$PMR = \frac{\text{Observed proportion of deaths from a specific cause}}{\text{Expected proportion of deaths from a specific cause}} \quad (8.3)$$
$$\frac{\text{(study population)}}{\text{(from the standard population)}}$$

Either the proportion in the overall standard population can be applied to obtain the expected proportion in all ages (the actual or crude PMR), or the age-specific proportions can be applied. If the latter is adopted, the expected proportion is calculated for each specific age group, with the group-specific figures being summed (in effect standardizing for age, as explained in section 8.3). The denominator may also be cause-specific. For example, we could look at deaths from coronary heart disease (CHD) as a proportion of deaths from stroke, or cancer, or accidents, rather than all causes.

PM and PMR are quite simple as you will find when you do the calculations in the exercise in Box 8.1.

In this simplified example, the PMR was 30 per cent higher in the second time period in the city under study. One explanation, of many, is that the underlying population is getting older and pneumonia is more likely to occur in old people. Another is that the phenomenon is general and not specific to this hospital. The results for the second hospital do not show the same pattern going against the second of these explanations.

The stage has been set for a deeper investigation. We will now look at a real study where PMR helped to resolve a difficult question and represents a creative use of the measure.

Box 8.1 Calculating PM and PMR

Doctors in a hospital observed that the number of patients being admitted for pneumonia and related serious infections of the lung was very high and rising. They had no reliable denominator data on the population the hospital served. They examined the hospital computerized records in two five-year time periods—2000–2004, and 2005–2009. They also compared their results with another similar city 20 miles away. The results were as follows:

Calculate PMs, and PMRs for the two comparisons, that is, over time and between the two hospitals. Were the doctors right? What explanations can you think of for what you observed? The answers are in Table 8.2 and the text above.

		City under study	City of comparison
2000–2004	Pneumonia	1000	1400
	All admissions	13 000	16 000
2005–2009	Pneumonia	1200	1500
	All admissions	12 000	17 000

Table 8.1 Proportional morbidity ratio (PMR) for ischaemic heart disease in male immigrants born in the Indian subcontinent and the African New Commonwealth

	Observed deaths	PMR
Standard population		100
Indian subcontinent-born		
With Indian names, presumed Indian ethnic origin	605	119
Without Indian names, presumed White British ethnic origin	535	121
African New Commonwealth-born		
With African names, presumed African ethnic origin	28	56
With Indian names, presumed Indian ethnic origin	23	120
With British names, presumed White British ethnic origin	39	84

Source: data from Marmot, M.G. *et al. Immigrant mortality in England and Wales 1970–78: causes of death by country of birth. (OPCS studies on medical and population subjects No. 47)*. London, UK: HMSO. Copyright © 1984 Crown Copyright.

Marmot and colleagues (1984) were interested in whether people of Indian, Pakistani, Bangladeshi, and Sri Lankan ethnic origin (South Asians) living in England and Wales have a higher rate of mortality from CHD than the population as a whole. They studied mortality rates around the years of the 1971 census when ethnicity was not collected. The preliminary answer on the basis of mortality rates by country of birth was—possibly so. The problem was that some people born on the Indian subcontinent were of European ethnic origin. Further, some South Asians were born in England and Wales. This creates a misclassification error (see Chapter 4), so the resulting calculations would be imprecise. Neither the 1971 census nor the death certificate recorded ethnic group, only country of birth. The solution Marmot *et al.* adopted was to calculate the age-adjusted PMR (see Table 8.1). They tested the hypothesis that the PMR in those with South Asian names (an indicator of ethnic group, not just birthplace), was different from that in those born in the Indian subcontinent without such names (probably White British peoples), and from African New Commonwealth-born, and from the whole population of England and Wales. The PM of the whole population of England and Wales provided the standard. A PMR of 100 per cent would, therefore, reflect no difference between the ethnic groups and the standard population. Before reading on, do the exercise in Box 8.2.

The PM reflects not only on the number of deaths from the cause under study but also the number of deaths from other causes. In comparing PM between populations, therefore, differences might arise from either differences in the disease under study, or differences in other

Box 8.2 Assumption behind, and interpretation of, the PMR

Examine Table 8.1. How do the PMRs in the Indian subcontinent group based on name compare with both the standard population and the African New Commonwealth-born?

♦ What is the fundamental assumption that underpins valid comparisons between populations using PMRs?

♦ Were Marmot *et al.* correct in inferring that ischaemic heart disease was comparatively more common in the South Asian, Indian subcontinent-origin populations?

Table 8.2 Answers to the exercise in Box 8.1 on PMRs

	City under study		Comparison city	
	2000–2004	2005–2009	2000–2004	2005–2009
A PMs	1000/13 000 = 7.7%	1200/12 000 = 10%	1400/16000 = 8.8%	1550/17000 = 8.8%
B PMR within hospital	10%/7.7% = 1.30		8.8%/8.8% = 1.00	
C PMR across hospital	7.7%/8.8% = 0.88	10%/8.8% = 1.4		

diseases. In South Asians, for example, cancers are less common than in the population as a whole, so the high PMR could be due to either a higher level of CHD or a lower one of cancer. While the data in Table 8.2, showing a high PMR for Indian named people whether born on the Indian subcontinent or the African New Commonwealth, favour the view that ischaemic heart disease is comparatively common in an Indian-born population, the result is not conclusive (at least, not on its own). People without Indian names born on the Indian subcontinent, presumed White British, also had a high PMR, which is interesting.

The PMR can be considered as a preliminary, or corroborative, analysis tool. This is because its fundamental assumption, that the distribution of deaths from causes other than the one under study is the same in the two populations, is often unlikely. When it does hold, the standardized mortality ratio (SMR—see section 8.3) and the PMR are related, according to the formula given in Roman *et al.* (1984) and in Appendix 8.2.

Clearly, proportional mortality is a simple and potentially useful way of portraying the burden of a specific disease within a population, and the PMR provides a way to compare populations. PMRs can be used to examine the association between an exposure and a cause of death. In our example of Marmot *et al.*'s study (Table 8.1), the exposure is South Asian ethnicity and cause of death CHD. The PMR then is one measure of the strength of the association, but for reasons already discussed in relation to the exercise in Box 8.2, a potentially flawed one.

8.3 Adjusted rates: direct standardization and the calculation of the SMR (indirect standardization)

In this section, I will use the word *rate* in a general and traditional sense. The principles here apply equally to proportions (and person-years) and so are relevant to prevalence and incidence data. Let us assume we are using cumulative incidence rates.

When numerator and population denominator data are available on a large scale, age- and sex-specific rates can be calculated and compared between times, places, and subpopulations (Chapter 7). These rates provide a view of the disease patterns in a population. Wherever possible, these rates should be presented. For simplicity, it might be enough to only show data for a few age and sex groups. It is arguably true that age- and sex-specific rates are the all-important fundamental building blocks of epidemiology and hold primacy in our discipline. This kind of analysis is often impossible because the number of outcomes is too small to produce precise, statistically stable rates.

When sex-specific rates are imprecise, the resulting data set may pose difficulties in interpretation. Age- and sex-specific tables are usually large and difficult to assimilate (e.g. Table 8.19).

Nonetheless, for reasons given in Chapter 7, epidemiologists need to examine such data carefully before summarizing them. The obvious answer is to calculate a summary figure such as the overall, actual (crude) rate. The result is then truly reflecting the burden of the disease under study in that population. This may well be the number that the health service and health professionals need, for example, to work out how much service will be needed next year.

For comparative research, however, overall, actual (crude) rates may be misleading. The usual problem is that the age and sex structure of the compared populations differs, in other words—age and sex are confounding variables (see section 4.2.4). We may conclude that the compared populations have very different disease rates when there is a simple explanation, for example, if one population is older than the other. The simplest way to consider this is to adjust (or standardize) the rates for age, sex, or both, as discussed next. This is usual and good epidemiological practice. There are a few exceptions to this principle. Where the comparison populations are virtually identical in age and sex structure, age and sex adjustment will not alter the results. When age and sex differences in populations are potentially interesting or important explanatory factors for population disease patterns, rates should not be adjusted and age-specific and sex-specific data should be shown.

Adjusted rates have become the norm, but are not true population-based rates, and do not relate to the health status of a real population; therefore, resulting estimates of health-care needs are wrong. For example, the age-adjusted rate for stroke in places that attract the recently retired may be lower than in major commercial cities such as London, but this is quite misleading. London's need for stroke services per unit of population is actually less than a place like a retirement resort.

Summarizing a set of age-specific rates into one age-adjusted figure loses information, which is particularly important when differences are not consistent across age group or sex. For example, Table 8.3 shows that the overall SMR, one method considered in section 8.3.2, for lung cancer in women living near industry (zones ABC) was higher than in the control area (S). (Study details are in Exemplar 4.1.) The summary figure (SMR all-ages) disguises the fact that mortality rates in the under-65-year-olds were much higher, while rates in over-75-year-olds were actually lower, in zones ABC than in zone S. Potentially important information is lost in the all-ages (standardized) SMR.

Where there are major differences in age and sex structure between populations, when adjustment is most needed, the method leads to the most distortion between the actual and adjusted

Table 8.3 Standardized mortality ratios (SMRs) for lung cancer in women at all ages and by age group in an area near industry (zones ABC) compared with an area in Sunderland (S) (populations from 1991 census)

Age group	Area ABC (N = 40 332 women)		Area S (N = 22 321 women)	
	SMR	N (cases)	SMR	N (cases)
All ages	217	288	173	152
0–64	287	136	170	55
65–74	190	98	165	56
75 +	161	54	192	41

Standardized to England and Wales population with 5-year age groupings. N is the observed number of population or deaths; SMR, standardized mortality ratios.

Adapted from Pless-Mulloli T, Phillimore PR, Moffatt S, Bhopal R, Foy C, Dunn C, and Tate J. Lung cancer, proximity to industry, and poverty in Northeast England. *Environmental Health Perspectives*, Volume 106, Issue 4, 189-196, 1998.

rates. These limitations also apply to the same population being compared at different time periods; for example, CHD in the United States of America in 1994 compared with 1940. Until recently USA CHD mortality data were adjusted using the 1940 age structure, but for the 1996 analysis the population structure of the year 2000 was used. The calculation for 1996 based on the 1940 structure gave a rate of 86.7/100 000, compared with 187.1/100 000 using the 2000 structure (the explanation for this extraordinary result is given next). Having signalled the pitfalls, it is necessary to note that standardization is vital in making comparative epidemiology work. The pitfalls apply to all methods of adjusting for age, sex, and other confounding factors—and these include multiple regression and other complex approaches. On a global scale, given its use by the World Health Organization (WHO) and other agencies, the method of direct standardization is one of the most important epidemiological techniques for controlling confounding by age and sex in the analysis stage.

8.3.1 Direct standardization

Before reading on, do the exercise in Box 8.3, based on Table 8.4. Then, compare your results with Appendix Table A8.1. Remember, the fundamental measures are, at least arguably, the age- and sex-specific rates.

Table 8.4 shows three groups with different age structures. Group A is not untypical of demographically stable industrialized countries, with similar numbers of people in the three decades. Group B is clearly an unusual age structure. This could be the age structure of hospital specialist doctors, or university academic staff. This could also be the population age structure after war, decimation by a disease such as AIDS, or the result of the major industry closing down, for example, in a mining town, leading to emigration of the young. Group C could be the population of soldiers, university students, doctors in the training grades, or the population in a new suburb with low-cost homes for families. These three populations will be used for several exercises that follow.

The age-specific rates (Appendix Table A8.1 will allow you to check your calculations) are identical in the three groups and they rise with age. The actual, overall (crude) rates differ markedly. Why? Group B has high overall rates because it has a comparatively older population. The larger number of older people is weighting (exerting influence upon) the summary rate. The size of the population in each age group influences the overall rates. While the actual, overall (crude) rates are accurately describing the experience in each of the three groups, they mislead us into thinking there are differences between them, because the influences exerted by the population structure differ. These differences cause confounding, and age is the confounding factor.

There are two major techniques for standardizing the rates to nullify the effects of the differing age structures and make overall comparisons possible—direct and indirect. In the direct method,

Box 8.3 Interpreting age-specific and actual overall (crude) rates

What kind of groups might have these age structures shown in Table 8.4? Calculate the age-specific and actual (crude rates) yourself, based on the data in Table 8.3 (the results are in the Appendix Table A8.1). Consider the age-specific and actual overall rates in Table 8.3. Comment on the age structure, and the effect this has on the overall (crude) rate, which varies in groups A, B, and C. Why does this effect occur? Do these three groups have the same disease rates or not?

Table 8.4 Groups size and cases: calculation of age-specific and actual overall (crude) rates in three populations of varying size (results for last column are in Appendix Table A8.1)

Age group	Population structure and size	Cases	Rate (as %) to be completed by the reader
Group A			
21–30	1000	50	
31–40	1000	100	
41–50	1000	150	
Actual overall (crude) rate	3000	300	
Group B			
21–30	500	25	
31–40	1500	150	
41–50	3000	450	
Actual overall (crude) rate	5000	625	
Group C			
21–30	5000	250	
31–40	1000	100	
41–50	200	30	
Actual overall (crude) rate	6200	380	

the age-specific rates from the study population are applied to a standard population structure. The source of the population structure is not of importance to the technique, as it will work with any structure. However, for global studies most people use the World Population Structure of the WHO (structures are also available at WHO region level) and for national studies, national census population structures. There are, however, consequences for the actual resulting rate, though not for the relative comparison between rates.

Table 8.5 (part a) shows the results of doing this standardization with a relatively young population as the standard. Before reading on, do the exercise in Box 8.4, including completing Table 8.5 (part b). Then compare your results with Appendix Table A8.2. The calculation is straightforward but note that when applying the rate from one population (say X) to another (say Y), the question is: how many cases would occur in population Y if it had the same rate as X? The footnote in Table 8.5 gives an example of how to do this.

The identical age-specific rates in groups A, B, and C obtained from Table 8.4 lead to the same number of cases expected in the standard population of Table 8.4 (a) and therefore, an identical overall (standardized) rate (7.5%). Here the standard population structure supplies the weights and these are, therefore, the same in all comparison groups. The overall standardized rates in Table 8.5 (part a), however, differ from those in Table 8.5 (part b). Compare your results for Table 8.5 (part b) with those in Appendix Table A8.2 (b).

The use of a young standard population leads to a low standardized rate (7.5%), and an old standard population to a high rate (13.9%). This explains why the standardized rate of CHD in the United States of America rose greatly (see end of section 8.3) when a modern, older age structure replaced the younger, 1940s age structure.

Table 8.5 Standardization with the direct method: effect of young and old standard populations (readers are invited to complete part (b))

Standard population structure	Standard population size	Applying age-specific rates from groups in Table 8.3 to standard population: cases expected		
		Group A	Group B	Group C
(a) A young population structure				
21–30	3000	150*	150	150
31–40	1500	150	150	150
41–50	500	75	75	75
Overall	5000	375	375	375
Overall standard rate = 375/5000 = 7.5% for groups A, B, and C				
(b) An older population structure				
21–30	200			
31–40	1000			
41–50	5000			
Overall	6200			
Overall standard rate =				

*Example: from Table 8.4 we see that the rate in the age group 21–30 in groups A, B, and C is 5%. In the young standard population (a) there are 3000 people. We expect, therefore, that 5% of them (3000) will develop the disease, i.e. 150 people.

The problem is that the overall standardized results of 7.5 per cent in Table 8.5 (part a) and of 13.9 per cent in Table 8.5 (part b) are not real, and differ from the actual, and true overall (crude) rates in Table 8.4. These are subtle but fundamental issues that you need to reflect on carefully. The method has allowed comparability but it has substituted fictitious figures for the reality. This is considered a necessary and worthwhile price. Table 8.5 shows, as do the age-specific rates in Table 8.4, that the differences apparent in the overall crude rates were a result of confounding by age.

The age-standardized rates can be compared by dividing one by another to create a relative risk, as shown in section 8.4. There is a technical, but unnecessary term for such a relative risk—that is, comparative mortality (or morbidity as appropriate) figure. Simply relative risk is better.

Box 8.4 Effect of directly standardizing on overall rates

First calculate the cases expected when you apply the age-specific rates in Table 8.4 to the older standard population (b) in Table 8.5. Follow the same approach as for Table 8.5(a). Consider the age structure of the standard structure populations, and the age-specific and overall rates in Table 8.5. What is the relationship between the overall standardized rates in Table 8.5 and those in Table 8.4? Why are the overall standardized rates now the same in groups A, B, and C? What is the influence of a relatively young and a relatively old standard population on the standardized rates? Where is the influence (weighting) on the overall rates coming from?

8.3.2 **Indirect standardization: calculation of the SMR**

The second approach to adjustment is called indirect standardization. Here, the standard population supplies disease rates, and not the population structure as in the direct method. These rates are applied to our own study's population structure to answer the question: how many cases would have occurred if the study population had the same disease rates as in the standard population? (Note: substitute the words disease rates with population structure and you have the equivalent question for the direct method.) The observed number of cases is divided by the expected number of cases giving the standardized morbidity (or mortality) ratio, which is usually multiplied by 100 and interpreted as a percentage and widely known as the SMR.

Table 8.6 shows a set of rates in the standard population, and these are high, while those in Table 8.7 are low. The original (crude) overall rates (Table 8.4 and Table A8.1 in Appendix 8.1) and, likewise, standardized rates in the three populations A, B, and C differ. Why? Before reading on do the exercise in Box 8.5. Then, compare your results with Appendix Table A8.3. In this exercise we will continue with the groups, population structure, and age-specific rates introduced in Table 8.4. An example of how to apply the standard age-specific rate is shown on a footnote in the table. The total observed is in Table 8.4. You get the expected number by adding the cases expected in the three age groups, as shown in the footnote.

The general expectation of a method of age standardization would be that, as in the case of direct standardization, it would remove the effect of confounding by age. It is a surprise that this

Table 8.6 Standardization with the indirect method

Standard population (high) rates

Age group	Population	Cases	Rate (%)
21–30	40 000	4000	10
31–40	50 000	7500	15
41–50	60 000	12 000	20
Total	150 000	23 500	15.7

	Group A		Group B		Group C	
	Population	Cases expected	Population	Cases expected	Population	Cases expected
21–30	1000	100*	500	50	5000	500
31–40	1000	150	1500	225	1000	150
41–50	1000	200	3000	600	200	40
Total	3000	450	5000	875	6200	690
Observed/ expected (standardized morbidity/mortality ratio, SMR)		$\frac{300**}{450} = 66\%$		$\frac{625}{875} = 71\%$		$\frac{380}{690} = 55.1\%$

*Example: The rate is 10% in the standard population above. We have 1000 people in this age group. If they had the same rate as the standard population then 10% would get the outcome, i.e. 100.

**Observed from Table 8.4—no. of cases in total.

Table 8.7 Standardization with the indirect method. Rates in standard population, cases expected, and SMR to be completed by reader

Standard population (low) rates

Age group	Population	Cases	Rate (%)
21–30	40 000	2000	
31–40	50 000	3750	
41–50	60 000	6000	
Total	150 000	11 500	

	Group A		Group B		Group C	
	Population	Cases expected	Population	Cases expected	Population	Cases expected
21–30	1000		500		5000	
31–40	1000		1500		1000	
41–50	1000		3000		200	
Total	3000		5000		6200	

Observed*/expected (standardized morbidity/mortality ratio, SMR).

*Observed from Table 8.4—no. of cases in total which is the same as the observed in Table 8.6.

does not happen. The reason it is surprising is that the method is widely used and interpreted as if it does so, and that it is an alternative to the direct method. The standardized mortality ratios differ because the standard rates are weighted differentially by the different population structures in groups A, B, and C. This is entirely analogous with the weighting effects in Table 8.4 shown in the overall (crude) rates. Rates adjusted by the indirect method are, to re-emphasize, weighted in relation to the age and sex structure of the population under study.

The summary output from such adjustment is the SMR. This means that SMRs from several study populations cannot be compared with each other. The exception is when the population structures in different groups are the same or very similar, but then the SMR is not needed—the overall (crude) rates can be compared. Only SMR comparisons between the study population and the chosen standard population are, strictly speaking, valid. This principle is often breached,

Box 8.5 Calculating and interpreting indirectly standardized rates

Reflect carefully on Table 8.6 and the calculation of cases expected and the resulting SMR.

Follow the same approach to do the calculations on Table 8.7, before comparing your results with Appendix Table A8.3.

Why are the SMRs for Groups A, B, and C different when the same standard rates in Table 8.6 are applied? Why are the standardized mortality ratios higher in Table 8.7 compared to 8.6?

Box 8.6 Interpreting SMRs in Table 8.3

- ◆ What is the correct interpretation of the all-ages SMR in area ABC and area S?
- ◆ Is it correct, strictly speaking, for the two SMRs (217 and 173) to be compared directly?
- ◆ In practice, why might this comparison be acceptable?
- ◆ What about the age-specific comparison (0–64, 65–74, and 75+ years)? Answer the questions above for these more specific comparisons.

sometimes knowingly but usually unknowingly. The benefit of the SMR is the production of a number that allows comparison with a reference population. Where comparisons are to be made between several populations, strictly, either age-specific rates, or those adjusted by the direct method should be examined. Reconsider Table 8.3, bearing in mind that the SMRs were calculated using the age-specific mortality rates of England and Wales applied to the population structures of the geographical areas ABC and S. Now do the exercise in Box 8.6 before reading on.

The SMR of 217 shows that the number of cases observed in area ABC was 2.17 greater than the number expected, if this area had the same age-specific death rates as in England and Wales. Area S had 1.73 times the expected number. As we do not know the population structure of areas ABC and S, strictly speaking we cannot directly compare ABC with S. If the population structures were the same, then there is no purpose in indirect standardization. The all-cause, all-age actual (crude) rates could then be compared without any confounding by age. As areas ABC and S are only 20 miles apart in the north-east of England, we would expect (and can demonstrate) only small differences in age structure. In practice, therefore, direct comparisons, inferring that area ABC has a higher SMR than area S, are reasonably safe. Readers will learn that such direct comparisons of SMRs are commonplace, and when population structures are very different, they are seriously misleading. Knowing the context of the research helps safeguard against serious errors. This explains why SMRs are common in national studies comparing regions, but not in international studies where age structures vary greatly.

The authors also calculated SMRs within age groups. At first glance, that is odd. There may, however, be age differences within age groups especially when these are broadly defined. This step excludes residual confounding caused by age differences within age groups. It is conceivable that in the age group 65–74 in area ABC, people have an average age of 71 years, while those in other areas have an average age of 69 years. This could make a big difference for an age-sensitive outcome such as cancer. We are on sounder ground in making direct comparison of the age-specific SMRs, especially if these can be in tight age ranges, for example, 60–65 years or even 60–61 years. In this instance, the SMR was used in knowledge of its limits.

The procedure of standardization can be extended to include sex and further variables, but the principles are the same as for age. In practice, when adjustment is needed for more than age and sex, regression analysis is usually performed. The results are very similar. Regression methods are briefly introduced in section 8.15. Regression methods have not replaced standardization methods and it is worth reflecting why not. Unlike regression methods, standardization is easily learnt and applied (even using a simple calculator or spreadsheet) and the results are intuitive and easy to interpret. As I have described, however, there are nuances and pitfalls even here.

8.4 Relative measures: relative risk

The phrase relative risk (RR) is derived from the fact that we are relating the risk of disease in those with the risk factor to those without. RR, as with the phrase risk factor, is often used generally where rates of any kind are compared. Ratios of incidence rates based on person–time denominators are often called RR, although rate ratio is accurate. Prevalence proportion ratio may be mislabelled RR. Usually, but not always, it is obvious that this is so. Similarly, odds ratios (section 8.5) are quite often labelled relative risks. (Some analysis packages, wrongly, label the outputs this way.) In this discussion, I base RR on cumulative incidence rates. The principles are the same for person–time incidence rates.

The RR is the most important summary measure of the size of the effect of the risk factor on disease rates and, hence, it quantifies the strength of the association (see Chapter 5). Correlation is another method of measuring association that has lesser utility in epidemiology (see section 8.15). Regression analysis can also calculate RR, rate ratios, and odds ratios. The formula for RR based on cumulative incidence rates is simple (see Table 8.8). The incidence rate (cumulative) is the prime measure of the probability of the outcome, that is, risk, in epidemiology. To see how the risk varies between populations (say, those with and without a particular risk factor) the incidence rates (age-specific, overall, or directly standardized) can simply be compared. Alternatively, and better, we can calculate the RR, which is the ratio of two incidence rates: that of the population of interest divided by that in a comparison (or control or reference) population.

The RR can be calculated from all studies providing incidence data: cohort studies, disease register studies with valid estimates of the denominator, trials and (very exceptionally) cross-sectional surveys (see Chapter 9). The RR can never be calculated from case–control studies (see Chapter 9), which do not give incidence data. As discussed in section 8.5, in some circumstances the odds ratio provides an acceptable estimate of the RR and sometimes an exact equivalent.

Interpreting the RR requires knowing the extent of error and bias in the incidence rates. Before reading on, do the exercise in Box 8.7.

The problems of interpreting relative risk lie in the measurement of disease incidence (Chapter 7). Differences between populations may reflect differences in the accuracy with which the diagnosis is made (numerator inaccuracy) or the population counted (denominator inaccuracy). For example, young people are less likely to consult for medical care, are more likely to be undercounted at census, and most likely to be lost to follow-up or be a non-responder in surveys. A different incidence of a disease in 15–24 year olds, compared to 25–34 year olds, may reflect such factors, rather than, say, effect of age.

The time periods for the measurements of incidence need to be comparable to avoid spurious differences arising from time trends. Data are often collected for large areas and presented for

Table 8.8 Incidence rate (cumulative), relative risk (RR), odds ratio (OR), and 2 × 2 tables

Risk factor/exposure	Clinical outcome		
	Diseased	**Not diseased**	**Total**
Present (exposed)	a	b	$a + b$
Absent (not exposed)	c	d	$c + d$
Total	**$a + c$**	**$b + d$**	**$a + b + c + d$**

(a) Incidence rate in those with the risk factor = $a/a + b$. (With the baseline population as the denominator.)
    Incidence rate in those without the risk factor = $c/c + d$.

(b) $RR = \dfrac{\text{incidence rate in those with risk factor}}{\text{Incidence rate in those without risk factor}}$ (8.4)

(c) $OR = \text{cross product ratio} = \dfrac{a \times d}{c \times b}$ (8.5)

Box 8.7 False estimates of relative risk

Consider why the relative risk might provide a false picture of the effect of the risk factor on disease and hence the strength of the association. As an example, consider a relative risk for a disease calculated in the age group 15–24 years compared to 25–34 year olds.

---

small areas. This process may create errors by incorrectly counting cases and populations in the smaller areas. These and other factors need to be checked before interpreting RR. Now do the exercise in Box 8.8 before reading on.

The RR of lung cancer in the polluted city is:

$$\frac{\text{Incidence rate in A}}{\text{Incidence rate in B}} = \frac{20/100\ 000}{10/100\ 000} = \frac{20}{10} = 2$$

The RR of lung cancer in city B compared with A is:

$$\frac{\text{Incidence rate in B}}{\text{Incidence rate in A}} = \frac{10/100\ 000}{20/100\ 000} = \frac{10}{20} = 0.50$$

We do not know the precision of the estimates. The precision can be assessed by calculating confidence intervals around the point estimate (see section 9.11 for an introduction, but the reader should consult a statistics textbook on how to do this).

The obvious and worrying explanation is that the pollution in town A causes lung cancer, and doubles the risk. Before reaching this conclusion, however, the investigator needs to ask questions such as these:

◆ Is the age distribution of the populations being compared similar? Lung cancer is more common in older people and it may be that town A has more older people. The solutions to this potential problem are to base RR calculations on age-specific rates or use age-standardized rates (section 8.3).

Box 8.8 Calculating and interpreting relative risk

Imagine that the cumulative incidence of lung cancer is compared in two cities, one with polluted air (A), the other not (B). In the polluted city there were 20 cases in a population of 100 000 over one year; in the other city there were 10 cases in a population of 100 000. Assume accuracy in the numerators and denominators.

◆ What is the relative risk of lung cancer in the polluted city (A)?

◆ What is the relative risk of lung cancer in the less polluted city (B)?

◆ Do we know the precision of this estimate of relative risk?

◆ What is the most obvious and worrying explanation for the higher relative risk in the polluted city?

◆ What alternative explanations (and technical approaches to testing them) will you consider before concluding that there is a real association between pollution and lung cancer?

- Are the prevalences of the known causal and protective factors for lung cancer different in town A from those in town B? If town A has a higher prevalence of smoking or other causal factors (or less exposure to protective factors such as a high fruit and vegetable consumption) then the increased RR may not be attributable to pollution. The solution is to do prevalence of risk factor studies in cities A and B on the major causal and protective factors.
- The induction period for occurrence of lung cancer is measured in decades. Were the differential pollution levels also present 20, 30, 40, and even 50 years ago? Were the risk exposure patterns several decades ago, when the disease was induced, similar to those in the present? (Data on exposure patterns in the distant past may not be available.)
- Were there differences in health care in the two cities?

Health-care differences between towns A and B are unlikely to explain the differences in lung cancer incidence unless the services prevent disease, that is, tobacco and pollution control campaigns delivered or influenced by health-care systems in town B may have been more effective than in town A. If the study had been of lung cancer mortality, rather than incidence, however, differences in diagnostic acumen leading to earlier detection of disease in town B, or better and more effective treatment in town B, are potential explanations.

Once these kinds of explanations are considered and due adjustments for confounding and other factors are made, the investigator can consider the RR as a fair measure of the strength of the association and can apply frameworks for causal thinking to judge whether pollution is the probable cause of the higher RR in town A (see Chapter 5). The methods by which adjustments to the RR are made, except by standardization of the incidence rates as already discussed, are beyond the scope of this book. The commonest approach is to use regression methods, which can include a number of interacting and confounding factors in a mathematical model (see also section 8.15 on correlation and regression). Another important and growing area in epidemiology is the quantitative adjustment of summary measures of risks to take account of errors and biases.

8.5 **The odds ratio**

The odds ratio (OR) is a more complex number than the RR and even though it is not as important, it merits more detailed explanation. The OR is popular in current epidemiological practice, and is invaluable in case–control studies (see section 9.5). However, it is used in many other contexts. This is most probably because multiple logistic regression modelling is common, and the output of that is usually expressed as an OR. It is also very commonly used in meta-analysis.

The odds ratio is simply one set of odds divided by another. The odds are the chances in favour of one side in relation to the second side. In epidemiology, usually the odds are the chances of being exposed (or diseased) as opposed to not being exposed (or diseased). In a standard 2 × 2 table (Table 8.8) the odds of exposure to the risk factor for the group with the disease are then $a \div c$ and for the group without disease, $b \div d$. The OR for exposure in those with and without disease is simply the odds $a \div c$, divided by the odds $b \div d$. Similarly, the odds of disease in those exposed to the risk factor are $a \div b$, and for those not exposed, $c \div d$. The OR here is $a \div b$ divided by $c \div d$.

These formulae can be expressed as:

$$\text{Exposure odds ratio} = \frac{a}{c} \div \frac{b}{d} \text{ and disease odds ratio} = \frac{a}{b} \div \frac{c}{d} \qquad (8.6)$$

Arithmetically, it is easier to multiply than divide two fractions, so to simplify this formula we use the arithmetical rule that division by a fraction is equivalent to multiplication by the inverse of the fraction; for example, division by 1/3 equals multiplication by 3/1. So, the odds ratio can be expressed as:

$$\text{Exposure odds ratio} = \frac{a}{c} \times \frac{d}{b} \text{ and disease odds ratio} = \frac{a}{b} \times \frac{d}{c} \qquad (8.7)$$

This equation (8.7), usually expressed as $\frac{a \times d}{b \times c}$ is arithmetically the same, and is known as the cross-product ratio. It is exactly the same for the exposure OR and disease OR. Product is another word for multiplication, so the phrase cross-product ratio is descriptive of the criss-cross multiplication in a 2×2 table (Table 8.8). As it is so easy, it has become the standard way of calculating the OR. To demonstrate the cross, you can draw lines from a to d and from c to b.

The drawback of the cross-product ratio is that the epidemiological idea behind the OR is lost. The epidemiological idea is simple: if a disease is associated with an exposure, then the odds of exposure in the diseased group will be higher than the corresponding odds in the non-diseased group and the OR will exceed one. If there is no association, the odds will be the same and the OR will be 1. If the exposure is protective against disease, the OR will be less than one. This idea fits in with the basic question behind a case–control study, that is, whether the risk factor is more common in cases than controls (Chapter 9). For a cohort study (see Chapter 9), the corresponding idea is that if an exposure is associated with a disease then the odds of disease in the exposed group will be higher than in the non-exposed group, so the disease OR will exceed one.

The odds ratio is a means of summarizing differences in odds, just as RR summarized differences in incidence rates. Before reading on, do the exercise in Box 8.9.

If a disease is caused by an exposure, the cases of the disease will have more exposure than controls. So, in the first study in Box 8.9 (a case–control study), the odds of exposure, lack of exercise,

Box 8.9 Disease, relative risk, and odds ratios

Imagine that a disease is caused by lack of exercise (risk factor exposure).

You compare the exercise habits of 1000 cases of this disease with 1000 otherwise similar people who are disease free. Now set out your data as in Table 8.8 as far as you can. Which group will have the higher odds of not taking exercise? Will the odds ratio of not taking exercise be more or less than one? (You do not need any more data to answer this.)

Now, imagine you follow up 1000 people over time who do take exercise and 1000 who do not, and count the number of cases over time. Set these data out as in Table 8.8 as far as you can. Which group will have the higher odds of becoming diseased? (Again, you do not need any more data to answer this.)

In the second example—in what circumstances will the OR approximate the RR? Why? Based on Table 8.8, try to figure this out for yourself before reading on. You may find this exercise easier if you put some figures into a table laid out as in Table 8.8. For example, you may wish to vary the number in a, b, c, and d to see what happens. You could start with 20 per cent of the diseased group taking no exercise and 10 per cent of the non-diseased group in the first part. In the second part, assume 10 per cent of the exercise group get the disease and 20 per cent of the no-exercise group do. Then, double these percentages and reconsider.

Box 8.10 Calculating odds ratios

A study of a disease compared cases with non-cases, and found that 25/100 cases smoked cigarettes compared with 10/100 of the non-cases.

- Develop a 2 × 2 table to display the data.
- Calculate the odds of exposure in cases and non-cases.
- Calculate the odds ratio using equations (8.7) and (8.8) given earlier.
- How does the difference between the two prevalence proportions of cigarette smoking (25% vs. 10%, i.e. ratio is 2.5) compare with the odds ratio?
- Which is the more accurate way of assessing the differences between the two groups, the odds ratio, or the comparison of prevalence proportions?
- Which gives the better feel for the degree of association between the disease and exposure, prevalence proportions ratio, or odds ratio?

will be higher in cases and the OR will exceed one. In the second study, which is a cohort study, the exercise group will have the lower odds of disease.

In the second study, for both the odds ratio and the RR, the numerators (a and c, as in Table 8.8) are identical. The denominators are different, that is, b and d, respectively, in the OR, and $a + b$ and $c + d$, respectively, in the relative risk. When b is similar to $a + b$, and d is similar to $c + d$, the OR and RR will be similar. This happens when the disease is rare, that is, when a and c are small in relation to b and d. Before reading on, do the exercise in Box 8.10.

Table 8.9 shows the data and the results for the calculation of ORs for the exercise in Box 8.10. The first calculation (exposure odds) follows the epidemiological logic, but it gives the same answer as the alternative formula for the cross-product ratio, which is easier to calculate.

In epidemiology, one of the key goals is to compare the health experience of one group with another, so our measures should give a feel for the degree of difference between groups. Here we

Table 8.9 OR relating to the exercise in Box 8.10

Risk factor/exposure	Disease group	
	Case	Control
Smoked cigarettes	25(a)	10(b)
Did not smoke cigarettes	75(c)	90(d)
The odds of exposure in:		
case group: $a \div c = 25 \div 75 = 1/3$;		
control group: $b \div d = 10 \div 90 = 1/9$.		

The odds ratio:

$$OR = \frac{a \div c}{b \div d} = \frac{25 \div 75}{10 \div 90} = \frac{1/3}{1/9} = 3.0$$

or, using the cross product ratio,

$$OR = \frac{a \times d}{b \times d} = \frac{25 \times 90}{10 \times 75} = \frac{2250}{750} = 3.0$$

Box 8.11 Varying prevalence of exposure: impact on odds ratio and its validity as an indicator of differences between populations

- What happens to the difference between the picture provided by the prevalence ratio and the odds ratio if the percentages exposed in the disease group were 15 per cent and in the control group six per cent (scenario 1)?

- What happens if the percentages were 50 per cent in the diseased group and 20 per cent in the control group (scenario 2)?

In both these scenarios, as in Box 8.9, the prevalence in the disease group is 2.5 times that in the control group.

---

see a 2.5-fold difference in the prevalence proportions (25% vs. 10%) change to a threefold difference in OR. Clearly, the two approaches are giving different results. Before reading on, try the exercise in Box 8.11.

The odds ratio approximates the prevalence proportion ratio when the exposure is infrequent, but not when it is common, as shown in Table 8.10. When $a:c$ (odds) is similar to $a/a + c$ (prevalence proportion) and $b:d$ (odds) is similar to $b/b + d$ (prevalence proportion) the OR and prevalence proportion ratio approximate each other. This happens when the prevalence is low. Before reading on do the exercise in Box 8.12, which concerns incidence. This exercise will introduce one of the strengths of the OR.

The results are given in Table 8.11. The OR is higher than the prevalence ratio in both instances, and the difference is greater when the prevalence is higher. The OR is extremely popular despite its disadvantages, for four main reasons. First, in some circumstances it approximates well, and in others is exactly the same as the RR. Second, in case–control studies where RR cannot be calculated at all, it provides an estimate of this. Third, the odds have desirable mathematical properties permitting easy manipulation in mathematical models and statistical computations, as, for example,

Table 8.10 OR in relation to cigarette smoking in Box 8.11: effect of changing prevalence

	Case	Control
Scenario 1		
Cigarette smoking	15	6
No smoking	85	94

$$OR = \frac{15 \times 94}{85 \times 6} = \frac{1410}{510} = 2.76$$

	Case	Control
Scenario 2		
Cigarette smoking	50	20
No smoking	50	80

$$OR = \frac{50 \times 80}{50 \times 20} = \frac{4000}{1000} = 4.0$$

Box 8.12 Effect of changing incidence on odds ratio

Imagine that an exposure to a causal factor triples the incidence of a disease, that is, the relative risk is three. This disease has a baseline five-year incidence of five per cent (in the non-exposed group). Imagine also that the baseline incidence is double in people with diabetes mellitus, that is, 10 per cent, and that the relative risk associated with exposure is the same (i.e. 3). You follow up 100 non-diabetic and 100 diabetic subjects with the exposure, and an equivalent number without the exposure. The study lasts five years. Work with five-year cumulative incidence and a constant denominator of 100 for simplicity of calculation.

Create two 2 × 2 tables to show the data for people with and without diabetes and calculate the OR of disease in the exposed group in relation to those not exposed. Compare the odds ratio with the RR of three.

Now calculate the RR and OR for not being diseased (b:a or b(a + b)) rather than being diseased. Compare the RRs and ORs.

in multiple logistic regression. For example, in epidemiology we are usually focused on the disease or other adverse outcome. If, however, non-occurrence of disease is of equal interest the OR provides a symmetrical result while the RR does not, as shown in association with the exercise in Box 8.12.

From the preceding data on people without diabetes in Table 8.11, the RR for being diseased is 3.00.

The relative risk of not being diseased (0.89) is not the reciprocal of 3, which is 1/3. The equivalent OR (0.298) is the reciprocal of 3.35. The OR has this arithmetical advantage. Furthermore, the OR can be calculated from all major study designs which is not true for RR.

Table 8.11 RR and OR associated with an exposure in people with and without diabetes mellitus: cumulative five-year disease incidence at baseline = five per cent in non-exposed and RR = 3 (five-year follow-up)

	People without diabetes		People with diabetes	
	Diseased	**Not diseased**	**Diseased**	**Not diseased**
Exposed	15	85	30	70
Not exposed	5	95	10	90

$$RR = \frac{15/100}{5/100} = 3.00 \qquad RR = \frac{30/100}{10/100} = 3.0$$

$$OR = \frac{15/85}{5/95} = \frac{15 \times 95}{5 \times 85} = 3.35 \qquad OR = \frac{30/70}{10/90} = \frac{30 \times 90}{10 \times 70} = 3.86$$

The RR for not being diseased is:

$$\frac{b}{a+b} \div \frac{d}{c+d} = \frac{85/100}{95/100} = 0.89$$

The OR for not being diseased is:

$$\frac{85 \times 5}{95 \times 15} = \frac{425}{1425} = 0.298$$

There has been a long debate on the merits and problems with ORs. It remains unresolved. Epidemiologists need to be aware that misinterpretation of ORs is common. Many writers, wrongly, interpret the OR as a true measure of the most relevant ratio (i.e. relative risk). Statistical packages may label the output of OR analysis as RR, creating a trap for the investigator. Some researchers, wrongly, use relative risk as a general term for any ratio comparing groups. Odds ratios are not comparable across times, populations, and between places if the exposure levels and incidence rates differ substantially. If we are interested, for example, in the size of the association between smoking and lung cancer in men and women, the ORs are not comparable across sexes if the underlying smoking prevalence and disease outcome differs in men and women. The odds ratio from a study done in London is likely to differ from one in Tokyo, simply because the exposure status in the control group differs even when the relative risk is identical (the point is illustrated in Table 8.11, though the example is diabetes mellitus).

Odds ratios give a fair estimate of the following:

- The prevalence proportion ratio when the prevalence of exposure is low. (There is no epidemiological reason to calculate ORs in cross-sectional and other studies, which mostly provide prevalence data—suitable models other than logistic regression are available.)
- Relative risk in a cohort study or trial when the disease incidence is low in the control group, usually taken as less than 10–20 per cent, which is usually true, except in very long-term studies. (There is no epidemiological reason to calculate ORs in cohort studies and trials except for tradition and comparability with previous studies, which may have reported odds ratios, especially as ORs are very popular in meta-analysis software.)

- The relative risk in a case–control study when the exposure in the control group represents the population from which cases derive (and, in some other designs, when the disease is care). (See also section 9.5.) In some kinds of case–control studies, where the control group is a sample of the population from which cases accrue, the OR is identical to, not an approximation of, the RR but this can usually only be demonstrated in case–control studies embedded in cohort studies.

As with relative risk, the OR is only valuable if the study is well executed.

In cross-sectional studies, the prevalence of exposures is usually high (and the prevalence of disease is sometimes so) and the odds ratio may be a poor estimator of prevalence proportion ratio. Statistical methods for adjusting the OR so it more closely approximates the RR or prevalence ratio are available, but are too rarely used.

8.6 Measurements to assess the impact of a risk factor in at-risk groups and whole populations: attributable risk and related measures

As discussed in Chapter 5, knowledge of the causes of diseases is the surest route to their prevention and control. In a few diseases there is a unique, known causal factor, for example, nutritional disorders such as scurvy, infections such as measles, and environmental diseases such as asbestosis. All cases of such diseases are attributable, by definition, to one cause. By removing asbestos from the environment, we can eliminate asbestosis, by ensuring vitamin C in the diet we prevent scurvy, and by removing the measles virus we eliminate measles. Cases of diseases that clinically mimic scurvy, asbestosis, and measles will, by definition, be a result of different causes and be different diseases.

Often, however, removal of the causes is impossible because we do not know what they are, or it is too difficult or costly, or the causes are multiple and complex. The best way of discovering

Box 8.13 Epidemiological information to choose between priorities

Several hundred factors have been associated with coronary heart disease (CHD). That said, the following modifiable risk factors have been established as important:

- high levels of some lipids in the blood, particularly low-density lipoprotein (LDL) cholesterol;
- high blood pressure;
- smoking cigarettes or other tobacco products;
- low levels of physical activity;
- obesity;
- diabetes mellitus.

Imagine that there are insufficient resources to tackle all six of these risk factors. We may wish to focus on one or two of them at least initially What epidemiological information would help us to choose between them to reduce CHD in a population?

the effect of removing a risk factor is to intervene to reduce it, or eliminate it and observe what impact this has. Unfortunately, interventions of this kind are rare and even with the best of interventions the impact on the risk factor is small (sometimes none at all). We may have to content ourselves with an answer to the hypothetical question: if we could remove the risk factor, what would happen?

Indirect methods to estimate the hypothetical effect of reducing the causal factor are needed, especially in public health but also for advising individual patients. For most chronic diseases, there are several risk factors. Stroke, ischaemic heart disease, and cancers such as those of the breast and the colorectal tract are such diseases. The extra problem that now arises is choosing between alternative actions, for there is always limited time, money, energy, and expertise. We need ways of helping to make choices by predicting the possible consequences.

Attributable risk provides a way of developing the epidemiological basis for such decisions. An extension of the concept—population-attributable risk—is discussed in section 8.6.2. (Attributable fraction/proportion and population-attributable fraction/proportion are among several synonyms for this concept.) Before reading on, reflect on the exercise in Box 8.13, which makes us think about the issues from these first principles.

Some of our information needs are as follows:

- Solid evidence that each of these risk factors is a component of the causal pathway and not merely artefactually or statistically associated with the disease. Actions directed at non-causal associations will not reduce disease. Such data usually come from case–control studies, cohort studies, and trials (Chapter 9), together with supporting information from the laboratory and clinical sciences, to provide understanding of the biological basis of the risk factor disease relationship. We need to specify the causal model, possibly using a directed acyclic graph, which we are using to judge the evidence (Chapter 5).
- Knowledge of the frequency of each risk factor in the population, usually measured as the prevalence proportion overall and in subgroups (Chapter 7). If a risk factor is rare then action to reduce it even further will have little effect on the incidence of the disease in the population.

For controlling coronary heart disease in the UK, for example, diabetes will be a more important risk factor in South Asian and African and African Caribbean-origin populations than in European-origin populations, simply because diabetes is about three to four times more common in these populations. Genetic causes of very high cholesterol levels are important causes of CHD, but thankfully, are rare so our public health strategy would not focus on them (though clinical strategies may do). Population-based strategies will focus on common risk factors.

♦ A precise estimate of the additional risk of disease that each risk factor imposes on our population. If the relative risk of CHD among those with diabetes was 1.1 (a 10% increase) the impact of controlling diabetes would be much smaller than if the RR was 3 (a 200% increase). Population-based strategies will focus on common risk factors associated with higher relative risks.

♦ An understanding of the actions that are (or might be) effective in reducing the prevalence of the risk factor and their costs (this latter subject, health economics, is beyond the scope of this book but see section 8.10). If we have no evidence then this points to the need for research to discover effective interventions, or improve the performance of those we currently have.

♦ Assuming a reduction in the prevalence of the risk factor, the expected reduction in disease outcome (this calculation is the attributable risk). The formulae to calculate attributable risks are shown in Tables 8.12 and 8.13 and are discussed in sections 8.6.1 and 8.6.2.

8.6.1 Attributable risk: estimating benefits of changing exposure in the at-risk group

The question being answered by attributable risk is—how many cases would have been avoided if a particular risk factor had been absent or less common? Another way of framing the same

Table 8.12 Formulae for attributable risk (synonym: attributable fraction or proportion)

Attributable risk (AR) answers the question: What proportion of the risk in those exposed is attributable to risk factor X?	
$AR = \dfrac{\text{Risk in exposed -background risk}}{\text{Risk in exposed}}$	(8.8)
$= \dfrac{\text{Incidence in exposed } (I_e) - \text{Incidence in unexposed } (I_u)}{\text{Incidence in exposed } (I_e)} = \dfrac{I_e - I_u}{I_e}$	(8.9)
$= \dfrac{RR_e - RR_u}{RR_e}$	(8.10)
$= \dfrac{RR - 1}{RR}$	(8.11)
When RR can be estimated by $OR = \dfrac{OR - 1}{OR}$	(8.12)
To express AR as a percentage we multiple the fractions by 100.	

AR, attributable risk; *RR*, relative risk; *I*, incidence; *e*, exposed; *u*, unexposed; *OR*, odds ratio.

Table 8.13 Formulae for population-attributable risk (PAR) (synonym: population-attributable fraction or proportion) to answer the question: what proportion of the incidence in the population as a whole is attributable to risk factor X?

$PAR = \dfrac{\text{Risk in total polulation} - \text{Risk in unexposed population}}{\text{Risk in total population}}$	(8.13)
$= \dfrac{\text{Incidence in total population} - \text{incidence in unexposed population}}{\text{Incidence in total population}} = \dfrac{I_p - I_u}{I_p}$	(8.14)
Or an alternative formula based on relative risk and prevalence data.	
$PAR = \dfrac{P_e(RR-1)}{1+P_e(RR-1)}$	(8.15)
Or an alternative formula based on OR and prevalence date $= \dfrac{P_e(OR-1)}{1+P_e(OR-1)}$	(8.16)

I, incidence; *p*, population; *u*, unexposed population; *e*, exposed population; *P*, prevalence of risk factor (P_e = proportion of population exposed); *RR*, relative risk; *OR*, odds ratio.

question is, what proportion of disease incidence in those exposed to the risk factor is attributable to that particular risk factor? In shorthand, what is the attributable risk associated with a risk factor?

The answer is conceptually simple. From the total number of cases observed, subtract the number that would have occurred anyway, if no cases had the risk factor. This number can never be known as a fact, but it can be estimated from the control, unexposed, group. These remaining excess cases represent those attributable to the risk factor. It is more elegant to express this excess risk as a percentage of the total cases, rather than just a count of cases.

Table 8.12 shows five formulae (these are easy to understand when applied to a practical example, as will be done below). In equation 1, the background risk (estimated from the control group) is subtracted from the risk in the exposed (study) group and expressed as a fraction of the risk in the exposed group. The difference in the two risks is the excess risk. Equation 2 simply substitutes incidence rates for risk.

Attributable risk (AR) is, therefore, the excess risk expressed as a fraction of total risk in the exposed group. The excess risk can be derived as the RR in the exposed group minus the RR in the unexposed group, which is, by definition, one. The total risk in this exposed group is reflected in the relative risk. The benefit of this formula is that when the OR is an accurate estimate of RR, it can be used to provide AR even without incidence data.

Before reading on, do the exercise in Box 8.14 to get accustomed to these straightforward calculations.

Box 8.14 Calculating attributable risk

Calculate the attributable risk associated with smoking based on equations (8.10) and (8.12) given in Table 8.12 and the data in Table 8.14. Now do the same for smoking and coronary heart disease. The answers are given in appendix 8.3 Table A8.4.

Table 8.14 Relative, excess, and attributable risk: study of lung cancer and coronary heart disease in heavy smokers and non-smokers (readers to complete the table—answers in Table A8.4)

	Annual death rates per 100 000	
	Lung cancer	**Coronary heart disease**
Heavy smokers	166	599
Non-smokers	7	422
Relative risk (RR)	23.7	1.4
Excess no. of cases caused by smoking based on incidence formula	166 − 7 = 159	592 − 422 = 177
Excess risk	159/100 000	177/100 000
Attributable risk given as a percentage of all risk; based on incidence (equation 8.10 in Table 8.12)		
Attributable risk based on relative risk formula given as a percentage; based on RR (equation 8.12 in Table 8.12)		

Source: data from Doll R and Bradford Hill A. Lung cancer and other causes of death in relation to smoking. *British Medical Journal*, Volume 2, Issue 5001, pp. 1071-1081, Copyright © 1956 BMJ Publishing Group Ltd.

So, from the study data in Table 8.14, among heavy smokers the excess risk of lung cancer associated with smoking is 166–7 = 159 cases = 159/100 000 persons annually (Doll and Bradford Hill 1956). We can express this as AR by using equation 8.10 in Table 8.12 with the total rate as the denominator, and the excess risk in the exposed group as the numerator, as shown in the Appendix Table A8.4 (159/166 × 100 = 95.8%). This percentage is identical to that obtained using relative risk (equation 8.12 in Table 8.12). We are claiming, therefore, that among heavy smokers 95.8 per cent of the lung cancer cases were attributable to smoking. By implication, if the cause could be removed, in heavy smokers the disease would be reduced by up to 95.8 per cent and 159 lives would be saved per 100 000 of the population of heavy smokers. The attributable risk for CHD was 29.5 per cent, as shown in Appendix Table A8.4.

It is worth noting that the excess risk is dependent on the actual incidence rate. Table 8.14 shows that even though the relative risk of CHD in heavy smokers was 1.42, the excess number of deaths (177) was greater than that for lung cancer (159), where the relative risk was 23.7. The public health impact of stopping smoking, at least in this population, is potentially even greater via CHD prevention than with lung cancer prevention.

Since the removal of the causes may be the goal of preventive health programmes, AR estimates their potential benefits. The concept of AR is a powerful tool in public health practice but we should critically appraise the underlying assumptions. Before reading on, you may wish to reflect on the questions in Box 8.15.

The foremost assumption is that the risk factor is a causal one. If not, the calculation of AR is merely an arithmetical exercise, which makes false promises. To re-emphasize, the calculation is hypothetical and assumes the association between smoking and these diseases is causal and not wholly or partially arising from other factors. (At best, it answers the question: if the association eventually turns out to be causal, what is the AR?) The second assumption is that the incidence

---

Box 8.15 Further reflection on the assumptions underpinning the attributable risks

Before we accept the result of the calculation, let us ask:

- ◆ What causal assumption is there and what are the implications of non-causality?
- ◆ Can attributable risks from elsewhere be applied to our local populations? Will they have the same implications in cases prevented?
- ◆ What allowance should we make for imprecision and error in our estimates.
- ◆ If exposure to a risk factor disease causes B, can we assume that stopping A, perhaps after some years of exposure, will stop disease B?
- ◆ What will be the role of susceptibility (interacting factors) in our estimates?

---

data apply elsewhere to other populations. It may be that in other populations, the relative risk is the same, but the incidence of lung cancer in the unexposed population is lower, say 3.5 per 100 000. Then, the incidence in the exposed populations would be 83 per 100 000 (3.5 × 23. 7, i.e. baseline incidence times relative risk), and the excess risk 79.5 per 100 000. When expressed as a percentage, the AR would remain at 95.8 per cent, but the potential for lives saved by the intervention is substantially less at 79.5 lives per 100 000 of the population. This will have a big impact on the cost per life saved.

The third assumption is that the study is valid and accurate. The true incidence rates and relative risk may not be the same as the point estimates, even if only because of random error, so allowance needs to be made in calculating AR. The precision of these estimates can be reflected in confidence intervals, though these only reflect sampling imprecision and not other errors. Therefore, calculations should use various incidence rates, relative risks, and estimate costs and impacts within the ranges given by the confidence intervals.

There is also a need to understand the natural history of disease and causal model to achieve the predicted benefit. How does smoking operate as a carcinogen? What are the causal mechanisms? Is there a threshold effect? Will smokers benefit from stopping or has the carcinogenic damage been done already? Without this understanding, we cannot properly interpret the AR or offer rational advice to smokers. If the damage is irreversible, or only partly reversible, the potential lives saved according to the attributable risk may not be achievable. Another consideration is whether smoking interacts with other factors to cause lung cancer or whether it acts alone. If it acts alone, then an intervention to reduce smoking will achieve the promise indicated by the attributable risk. If, however, there are other interacting factors, the effect may be greater or less than predicted. To take a well-known example, smoking and asbestos interact in the causation of lung cancer and increase the incidence rate greatly (Chapter 5). Stopping smoking in a community of shipbuilders previously exposed to asbestos may yield benefits far greater than predicted from a study based on British doctors, as in the data in Table 8.14.

8.6.2 Population-attributable risk: estimating the benefits of reducing exposure in the population as a whole

From a public health perspective, we are interested in the benefits of an intervention to the whole community, not just those with the risk factor. The question of interest is, what proportion of the disease experience in the population (not just the exposed population) is attributable to a particular exposure? This clearly depends on how common the exposure is. If a community had no or very little exposure to smoking, as in Sikh women living in the Punjab, India (and in many parts of the world), then cases of lung cancer in that population must be caused mainly, if not wholly, by other factors.

The measure that answers this question is known as the population-attributable risk (or fraction or proportion). The formulae are shown in Table 8.13. Essentially, equations 8.14 and 8.15 are similar to that for attributable risk except that the risk factor prevalence or disease incidence is not in the exposed group but in the entire population (or a random sample of the entire population). As such incidence studies are rare, and population-attributable risk is often calculated by combining data from representative cross-sectional studies providing prevalence of exposures, and relative risks from cohort studies or case–control studies, usually from selected populations as in equation 8.16 and its equivalent for odds ratios when the OR approximates the RR (equation 8.17). The attributable risk is, effectively, being influenced (weighted) by the prevalence of the exposure in equations 8.16 and 8.17.

Population-attributable risk can overturn perceptions and conclusions derived from studying RRs. The population-attributable risk rises as the excess risk, the RR, and the prevalence of exposure rise. In contrast, RR is unaffected by change in the prevalence of exposure.

The population-attributable risk can help to answer questions such as: if a choice needs to be made on which exposure to reduce, which will have the bigger impact on disease incidence? Try the exercise in Box 8.16.

Table 8.15 shows the result. Given the assumptions, the population-attributable risk calculation supports a programme to increase exercise uptake. Clearly, this is a simplistic example. Nonetheless, the calculation makes the expectation of risk reduction explicit.

Both population-attributable risk and attributable risk are theoretical exercises which provide estimates to help pose and debate options. To assess the benefits in practice, trials need to be done (Chapter 9). In the absence of such trials, the validity of population-attributable risk/attributable risk estimates remains questionable. This kind of reasoning is under continuing development, with formulae now available for many other similar kinds of calculation.

Box 8.16 Choosing between options for public health campaigns

Let us say that a sum of £100 000 (about $150,000) is available for a health promotion programme to reduce coronary heart disease mortality. We can spend it on either reducing smoking *or* increasing the level of exercise. Assuming that the relative risk associated with both risk factors that changes of prevalence are equally permanent, and that the cardioprotective effect occurs quickly, which choice will give a better return in lives saved?

First make a judgement on which of the two preventive programmes you prefer.

Now consider which is more common, smoking or lack of exercise? Does this change your opinion?

Calculate population-attributable risk using equation 8.16 in Table 8.13 with prevalence of smoking of 20, 30, 40, and 50 per cent and prevalence of lack of exercise 60, 70, and 80 per cent. (These are realistic prevalences in the context of industrialized countries.) Has the result altered or substantiated your earlier judgement?

Table 8.15 PAR* for smoking and not taking exercise

	PAR (%)
Prevalence of smoking (%)	
20	16.7
30	23.1
40	28.6
50	33.3
Prevalence of not taking exercise (%)	
60	37.5
70	41.2
80	44.4

*Formula: $\dfrac{P_e \times (RR - 1)}{1 + P_e \times (RR - 1)} \times 100$

e.g. for first row

$$PAR = \frac{0.20 \times (2 - 1)}{1 + (0.20 \times (2 - 1))} \times 100 = \frac{0.2}{1.2} \times 100 = 16.7\%$$

8.7 Presentation and interpretation of epidemiological data in applied settings: health needs assessment

The interpretation of epidemiological findings, and of the picture or pattern that is painted by them, is greatly influenced by the mode of presentation of data. If practical decisions are to be made, then providing the same data in several formats is essential. Two principles nearly always hold: (1) give the actual figures, especially the numbers of cases, in addition to the summaries arising from statistical manipulation; and (2) present absolute and relative rates. Pressures of publication space and the writer's time, both acting against following these principles, should be resisted. Table 8.16 summarizes some of the requirements in presenting disease data in applied settings, for example, health needs assessment. Before reading on, do the exercise in Box 8.17.

The first column gives the disease or condition. The value of this is self-evident. What is not self-evident is that a label for a disease may differ across times and places and even between diagnosticians working in the same health service. As discussed earlier (Chapters 1 and 7), standardized

Table 8.16 A standard, empty table (showing the column headings) for organizing information for the assessment of disease pattern in applied settings

		Absolute measures		**Relative measures**	
Disease or condition (standard name and ICD or other code)	Number of cases and the size of the population studied	Rate or proportion (incidence or prevalence)	Rank position on number of cases or rate	PMR/ratio of adjusted rates SMR/relative risk/ odds ratio	Rank on relative measure

Box 8.17 Need for each data item as in Table 8.16

- ♦ What unique information or interpretation does each column supply?
- ♦ What difficulty would the absence of the information cause to the user of the information?
- ♦ What harm could arise from the misinterpretation arising from such omissions?

definitions applied by trained observers are necessary. The simplest way to provide a definition is to give the standard name of the disease or condition and give its International Classification of Diseases (ICD) code (or use another standardized coding systems). The ICD edition also needs to be given. Depending on the intended audience, the definition of the disease and even the common name might need to be given, for example, myocardial infarction (heart attack), ICD tenth edition codes I21 and I22.

Without definitions, the data have little lasting value, especially in terms of comparison. Worse, the data may be misinterpreted. For example, the label heart disease is not enough, and is open to erroneous interpretation, particularly in places where ischaemic heart disease arising from atherosclerosis is not dominant (e.g. where rheumatic heart disease is common).

The second column states the number of cases for each specific cause and the size of the population from which they arose. (The less satisfactory alternative is to give the total number of cases for all causes as the denominator and the percentage relating to each disease/condition.) This information has unique value to health-service planners and professionals delivering care, in deciding the staffing, accommodation, and supplies needed or used. The numbers also give the best idea of the scale of the health problem and hence help to develop a sense of priority. The diseases may be ranked as numbers to help assess priority. The numbers are also needed to assess whether the sample size is adequate, to permit alternative presentations and analyses of data, and to check for errors which are hidden by all summaries. Finally, this number is the only data item that every reader will understand.

The rate or proportion is the primary epidemiological tool to permit comparisons over time and between places and populations, but it does not have the immediacy of case numbers. That there were 5000 deaths from a particular disease in a community of 500 000 people last year gives a different, and much more direct and forceful impression than knowing that the death rate was 10 per 1000 per year, although one can be calculated from the other.

Age-specific and actual overall (crude) rates or proportions have the advantage that they can be easily understood and applied to different populations. When the rates are adjusted for confounding factors, the resulting rates have no reality and cannot be used directly for health-care planning. This is the penalty paid for increased comparability. Depending on the context, there may be a need for both actual overall (crude) and adjusted rates or proportions. The source of the population denominators used to construct rates needs to be recorded, preferably as a footnote to the table, or space permitting, somewhere in the paper or report. Unlike case numbers, population denominators are usually easily accessible and, if so, the URL or other reference point should be given.

PMR should only rarely be used. The directly adjusted rate is, partially, a relative measure of disease frequency and not, as at first sight, just an absolute one. It is the disease experience in relation to other populations also adjusted to the standard population. The standard population used in adjustment needs to be described by location and year. This and other relative measures, such as the SMR (indirectly adjusted rates), RR, and OR, can be used to refine the picture of needs using

Table 8.17 Deaths and SMRs* in male immigrants from the Indian subcontinent (aged 20 and over; total deaths = 4352)

Cause	Number of deaths	% of total	SMR
By rank order of number of deaths—actual/absolute approach			
Ischaemic heart disease	1533	35.2	115
Cerebrovascular disease	438	10.1	108
Bronchitis, emphysema, and asthma	223	5.1	77
Neoplasm of the trachea, bronchus, and lung	218	5.0	53
Other non-viral pneumonia	214	4.9	100
Total	**2626**	**60.3**	–
By rank order of SMR—relative approach			
Homicide	21	0.5	341
Liver and intrahepatic bile duct neoplasm	19	0.4	338
Tuberculosis	64	1.5	315
Diabetes mellitus	55	1.3	188
Neoplasm of buccal cavity and pharynx	28	0.6	178
Total	**187**	**4.3**	–

*Standardized mortality ratios, compared with the male population of England and Wales, which was by definition 100.

Adapted with permission from Senior PA and Bhopal R. Ethnicity as a variable in epidemiological research. *British Medical Journal*, Volume 309, Issue 6950, pp. 327-330, Copyright (c) 1994 BMJ Publishing Publishing Group Ltd.

Source: data from Marmot MG, Adelstein AM, and Bulusu L. *Immigrant mortality in England and Wales 1970-78: causes of death by country of birth. (OPCS studies on medical and population subjects No. 47)*, London: HMSO, Copyright © 1984 Crown Copyright.

the power of analysis of similarities and differences. Finally, the diseases/conditions can be ranked on these relative measures. Such rankings aid interpretation and evaluation of the importance of different diseases/conditions, particularly for future research to explain differences.

Relative measures help generate hypotheses to explain differences. The problem is that attention tends to be focused on differences at the expense of similarities, and more attention is given to diseases that are relatively common, even though they may be less important as a cause of illness and death, than those which are relatively less common. These points are illustrated in Table 8.17. The list of diseases/conditions highlighted by an analysis focused on absolute (actual) frequency is quite different from that highlighted by the relative approach. Table 8.18 lists the main epidemiological measures of disease frequency as absolute, adjusted, or relative. Among the many other measures for applied settings are life years lost and numbers needed to treat, both discussed next.

8.8 Avoidable morbidity and mortality and life years lost

Death and much sickness, disability, and disease are unavoidable, so the idea of avoidable mortality or morbidity can be confusing. Avoidable mortality (or morbidity) is the idea that there is potential to avoid death (or morbidity) from specified causes if the best possible public health and health-care actions are taken. For death, however, at best we can delay it, so we

Table 8.18 Actual, adjusted, and relative measures

Actual/absolute measures	Adjusted measures, which are relative but not explicitly so	Relative measures
Numbers of cases	Weighted/adjusted numbers	Proportional morbidity or mortality ratio
– Overall, actual (crude) rate – Specific rates/proportions by age, sex, class, etc.		Standardized morbidity or mortality ratio
Percentages of cases	Weighted/adjusted percentages	Prevalence proportion ratio
Proportional mortality/morbidity		Relative risk/rate
	Weighted/adjusted rates and proportions	Odds ratio
Attributable and population-attributable risks		Hazard ratio*
Life expectancy		
Life years lost		
Numbers needed to treat		

*see glossary.

should say avoidable premature mortality. For example, death from appendicitis is avoidable given early diagnosis and treatment, and some morbidity ought to be avoidable (e.g. rupturing of the appendix). The specific lists of the causes of avoidable mortality and morbidity are chosen on their potential for prevention or cure, so they change with advances in knowledge and services.

The named avoidable causes of death tend to be those where an effective preventive and therapeutic intervention has been developed. The research challenge for these conditions is to implement (and evaluate) effective services. For non-avoidable conditions, the challenge is to develop new interventions and, usually, this will need causal understanding. Lists of these conditions are periodically updated. Services can be partially evaluated by seeing whether these conditions are, in practice, prevented, controlled, and cured. The data tend to be complex but the life-years lost approach does help to produce summary numbers.

Calculating how many years of life would potentially be saved if all avoidable deaths were averted (years of life lost, or YOLL) measures the impact of avoidable mortality in a population, assesses the potential benefits of actions to reduce avoidable mortality, and by comparing with the reality it provides a test of the health-care system.

The age at which death would have occurred naturally if the avoidable cause of death had not occurred, the key data item, is unknown so it is estimated. Can you think of how we might estimate it?

Usually, the expected age at death is set at the average life expectancy in the population. For example, assuming the life expectancy was 75 years, a 74-year-old woman dying of lung cancer would be said to have lost one year of life. In fact, life expectancy for a person who has reached the age of 74 is about 10 years, so in truth about 10 years of life were potentially lost. It would be more accurate, though not so simple, to calculate the anticipated life expectancy of every dead individual based on the population average at that age. However, mostly the simpler approach of a single cut-off is used.

Sometimes a lower age cut-off (65 years usually) is taken as a measure of premature mortality. Clearly, the idea of premature death is arbitrary and refers simply to chronological age. Deaths over this age, however, may be premature if the health status of the deceased was good, while some persons below 65 years may be riddled with disease and their deaths may be timely. Again, usually the pragmatic approach of a single cut-off is used.

The years of lost life approach gives emphasis to deaths in the relatively young. Given that we use an expectation of life figure of 75 years, a death at the age of 10 years would yield a years of life lost figure of 65 years, the same as 13 deaths at the age of 70 ($13 \times (75 - 70)$). Clearly, there is no moral, social, legal, or religious set of values to justify equivalence of these yields. Yet here is a rationale for, and echo of, the fact that societies usually hold the prevention and delay of death in childhood as a higher priority than prevention and delay of death in older ages.

Years of life lost can change the perceived importance of problems, which seem relatively unimportant in the light of disease rates. For example, injury has emerged from the shadows of its competitor conditions partly because of the powerful impact of years of life lost analysis (see Chapter 10, section 10.2, on priority setting).

The years of life lost approach provides a single way of judging the priority to be given to each cause of mortality. The concept provides a means of comparing the performance of the health-care system with the best possible and can be used to set targets. For example, it would be reasonable to say that the organization of the health-care system as a whole should mean that patients with appendicitis are sufficiently well-informed that they seek advice early, and that doctors are able to make the diagnosis and operate well in advance to prevent deaths. The setting of targets relating to avoidable mortality and evaluation of their achievement provides a means of health-care audit.

The years of life lost approach can be refined further by incorporating disability and quality of life, as discussed in section 8.10. Before doing so let us look at Lee's analysis of 10 health-status measures.

8.9 Comparison of age-specific and summary measures of health status: perceptions and interpretation

Lee explored age-specific mortality rates for pneumonia and suicide in Taiwan, 1995, using 10 summary measures, including years of life lost. Table 8.19 shows age-specific population size, number of deaths, and rates. Before reading on, do the exercise in Box 8.18.

There were more deaths from pneumonia (3070) than from suicide (1618). Pneumonia deaths occurred mainly in the age groups over 55 years and the number of deaths rose with age, except in the 85-years-plus group. By contrast, most deaths from suicide were in the 20–74 age group with the peak number in the 25–44 age group. The age-specific rates generally confirm the picture derived from case numbers for pneumonia but show that the highest rates were in the 85-years-plus group. For suicide, age-specific rates indicate an increasing problem with age, the greater number of deaths in the 25–44 age group simply being a function of larger population size. The differentials in the rates for pneumonia are huge; for example, the 80–84-year-olds have a RR of pneumonia mortality about 1255 times that in the 20–24 age group. By contrast, the equivalent relative risk for suicide is 6.7. There is a great deal of important information in these age-specific case numbers and age-specific rates that is completely lost in most summary measures, and yet this kind of information is rarely published. This said, summary measures add important new insights.

Table 8.19 Population size and mortality due to pneumonia and suicide in Taiwan, 1995

Age	Population	Pneumonia death	Mortality[a]	Suicide death	Mortality[a]
0–4	1 596 058	59	3.70	0	0.00
5–9	1 608 446	14	0.87	0	0.00
10–14	1 918 327	11	0.57	12	0.63
15–19	1 988 479	11	0.55	44	2.21
20–24	1 790 146	6	0.34	105	5.87
25–29	1 886 651	18	0.95	163	8.64
30–34	1 959 013	31	1.58	165	8.42
35–39	1 846 480	27	1.46	145	7.85
40–44	1 632 355	36	2.21	154	9.43
45–49	1 060 675	29	2.73	92	8.67
50–54	866 026	65	7.51	102	11.78
55–59	799 674	90	11.25	114	15.86
60–64	718 617	167	23.24	114	15.86
65–69	655 406	266	40.59	125	19.07
70–74	457 317	431	94.25	131	28.65
75–79	263 482	583	221.27	66	25.05
80–84	149 406	638	427.02	59	39.49
85+	71 094	588	827.07	27	37.98
Total*		**3070**		**1618**	

[a]Per 100 000 population.*Added by this author, i.e. RSB.

Reproduced with permission from Lee W-C. The meaning and use of the cumulative rate of potential life lost. *International Journal of Epidemiology*, Volume 27, Issue 6, pp. 1053–1056, Copyright © 1998 International Epidemiological Association/Oxford University Press.

What happens to this picture when summary measures are used? Lee used ten summary measures, but for simplicity there are four here. Table 8.20 shows that both the crude rate and the age-standardized rate show pneumonia deaths to be about twice as common as suicide mortality. The cumulative rate is much greater for pneumonia. The years of life lost (YPLL) are much lower for pneumonia than for suicide. The point is that the perception of the relative burden of disease depends on the choice and mode of data presentation. Table 8.21 summarizes the qualities of these measures, as a stepping stone to more advanced studies for readers interested in this kind of applied epidemiology.

Box 8.18 Summarizing data on age-specific rates

Summarize the results of Table 8.19, in terms of the pattern of deaths by cause and age group. Now do the same for Table 8.20.

Table 8.20 Comparison of various health-status measures in quantifying the impacts of pneumonia death and suicide in Taiwan, 1995

Measure[a]	Pneumonia	Suicide	*Ratio of pneumonia/ suicide
Crude rate	14.44[b]	7.61[b]	1.9
ASR	14.55[b]	7.06[b]	2.1
CR	0.0834	0.0122	6.8
YPLL	20 208	43 500	0.5

[a]ASR, age-standardized rate; CR, cumulative rate; YPLL, years of potential life lost.

[b]Per 100 000 population; *Column added by the author.

Reproduced with permission from Lee W-C. The meaning and use of the cumulative rate of potential life lost. *International Journal of Epidemiology*, Volume 27, Issue 6, pp. 1053–1056, Copyright © 1998 International Epidemiological Association/Oxford University Press.

8.10 Disability-adjusted life years and quality-adjusted life years

The underlying idea behind disability-adjusted life years (DALYs) and quality-adjusted life years (QALYs) is that life expectancy free of disability or impairment is of greater value than the same life expectancy with such problems. A year of life with a disability or illness such as stroke, diabetes, or multiple sclerosis is, therefore, worth less to an individual than a year of life without. This is a controversial idea. On the one hand, most of us prefer a life without disease, impairment, or disability; on the other, we are devaluing our lives when we do have such problems. The logical, but morally and ethically dubious, extension of this idea is that a year of life of a disabled or sick person is worth less than that of another person free of such disability or sickness. At the individual level, many contemporary societies have human rights laws and policies that prevent the application of this latter idea. These ideas underlying DALYs and QALYs do not fit with our views and laws on equality, so we should restrict them to populations.

In population settings, these measures provide a means of gauging the burden of disease. In making choices between health-care interventions, and by implication the populations to be served, these concepts have provided a way of presenting information, spurring debate, prioritizing, and targeting services and, fortunately, not for discriminating between individuals. It is,

Table 8.21 The properties of some health-status measures as summarized by Lee

Measures[a]	Between-group comparison	Need for an external standard	Value judgement on death	Lifetime projected risk	Individual-level interpretation
Crude rate	No	No	No	No	No
ASR	Yes	Yes	No	No	No
CR	Yes	No	No	Yes	Yes
YPLL	No	No	Yes	No	No

[a]ASR, age-standardized rate; CR, cumulative rate; YPLL, years of potential life lost;

Reproduced with permission from Lee W-C. The meaning and use of the cumulative rate of potential life lost. *International Journal of Epidemiology*, Volume 27, Issue 6, pp. 1053–1056, Copyright © 1998 International Epidemiological Association/Oxford University Press.

however, true that when population level priorities are set individuals are affected, albeit indirectly, as we will see.

The key question is this: how much less is a year of life with a particular disability (or other relevant problem or health state) worth than a year free of that disability? In the quality-adjusted life-year approach the answer is derived by asking people, usually those with the disability and their relatives, and also others without a disability. This type of questioning yields a so-called utility value for particular health states, usually expressed on a scale of 0 to 1. Such surveys show that some states, like irreversible coma, may be judged to be worse than death. A year of life in coma, for example, may have no value (or even a negative one). In contrast, a year of life with a minor disability, say correctable short-sightedness, may have little or no negative impact on perceived quality of life.

The QALY provides a means of adjusting the value of life expectancy, and hence years of life lost, taking into account the utility value associated with disability. Clearly, however, the adjustments are based on subjective judgements which depend on who is asked, by whom, when, and how. The judgements are unlikely to be lasting, as social values change and advances in management of disease occur. The QALY has proved to be particularly useful in health economics, where it has provided a general outcome against which costs can be considered (cost–utility studies).

Disability-adjusted life years are similar in concept to quality-adjusted life years. The main difference is that disability is used directly to value the life years lost or gained, and not indirectly using the perceived effect on value of life as in the QALY. The life years lost for each individual are, as discussed, based on life expectancy minus years actually lived. To this value is added the loss caused by disability. The losses are given different values for different conditions. For example, for angina the loss (weight) used in the Global Burden of Disease Project (see Murray and Lopez 1997) was 0.095, for congestive heart failure it was 0.171 and for acute myocardial infarction it was 0.395. These weights are based on a process of consultation with patients and health professionals. Assuming that cases of acute myocardial infarction are disabled for 3 months (0.25 of a year), on average, then 100 cases would contribute 9.8 years of DALY (100 cases × 0.25 years × 0.395 (weight) = 9.8). Some will go on to develop angina (9.5 DALY per 100 cases of angina per year) and heart failure (17.1 DALY per 100 cases per year). The value of these morbidity weights is critical. The weights were changed in the Global Burden of Disease (GBD) Project between 1994 and 1996. Mental disorders moved from third to first ranking cause of DALYs lost after the change.

The DALY calculations can be refined by including a discount rate, age weighting, sensitivity testing using different disability weightings, and restriction of analysis to avoidable causes of death and disease. The discounting argument hinges on the view that a health benefit now is worth more than a health benefit in the future. Not surprisingly, discounting features heavily in health economics. The argument is that as for money, a pound (or dollar) now is worth more than a pound made available in five years' time. So, a disability-adjusted life year lost or gained is weighted in accord with the discount rate (3% in the GBD Project). Saving one life at age 0 would result in 80 life years saved using the World Bank standard life table (which uses a life expectancy of 80 years at birth, and about 85.17 once 75 years are achieved), and saving the life of a 75-year-old saves 10.17 years. Without discounting, however, the infant life is worth about eight lives at 75 years. With discounting this is not the case, because the short-term benefits gained by 10 people aged 75 years are assumed by the method to exceed the very long-term benefits to be gained by the one infant.

In the GBD Project, DALYs at age 25 were valued highest and those in infancy and old age lowest. Age weighting is a controversial matter that openly accepts a stance that is ageist in being biased against the young and old.

The quality-adjusted life years and disability-adjusted life years are summary measures suitable for policy analysis. Others have been developed that follow similar principles, for example, the health-adjusted life year (HALY). A summary measure that is particularly useful for clinicians and patients is the number needed to treat or prevent.

8.11 **Number needed to treat or to prevent, and the number of events prevented in your population**

The accurate perception of risks and benefits is vital to making decisions, particularly where the patient must give informed consent. Research shows that the public and professionals alike find it very hard to grasp the meaning of most measures we use in epidemiology and other medical sciences. Numbers and percentages are among the few measures that most people find easy. The number needed to treat (NNT) is a measure that combines directness with simplicity. It simply states the number of people who need to be treated for one patient to benefit. Conceptually, the same measure could be applied to preventive measures (numbers needed to prevent, or NNP) but this is done less often, quite possibly because the number is usually staggeringly high.

The calculation of an accurate NNT needs incidence rates for outcomes, from a well-conducted trial (Chapter 9). So if in a reliable trial we found:

- Cumulative incidence rate of outcome per year in the untreated group = 30/1000 and
- incidence of outcome per year in the treated group = 25/1000 then

- the reduction in risk $= \dfrac{30-25}{1000}$ per year and $\dfrac{5}{1000}$

- NNT = 1000/5 = 200.

In this trial, five people in every thousand benefit, at 0.5 per cent. In other words, one in 200 benefit, or alternatively, 200 need to be treated for one to benefit. The reduction in risk is known as the absolute risk reduction (and it is similar in concept to excess risk). The NNT is the reciprocal of the absolute risk reduction. Before reading on, reflect on the exercise in Box 8.19.

The physician can explain to the patient that the annual risk (incidence) of disease will decline from 30/1000, or 3 per cent, to 25/1000, or 2.5 per cent. While the rates may not be easily understood, the percentages will be. The absolute risk reduction can simply be stated as 5/1000 or 0.5 per cent per year (the excess risk is 5/1000). These all suggest modest benefits. These are all measures of absolute risk. While these measures are straightforward, it is hard for patients to see what they mean for them, except that the benefits are small.

Box 8.19 NNT in relation to other summary measures

Compare the directness and value of this information with alternatives, for example, stating the two incidences possibly as percentages, the excess risk, the attributable risk, the relative risk, or the odds ratio.

The relative risk here (the treated group is exposed and the one of interest so is in the numerator) is

$$\frac{25/1000}{30/1000} = 0.83.$$

The odds ratio is essentially the same here.

The relative risk (and OR) imply a 17 per cent reduction in risk, a seemingly large benefit. Patients may be impressed. Essentially, there is a substantial benefit on a very low baseline risk, for the risk of the adverse outcome is very low even in the absence of treatment. This is another example of relative and absolute measures leading to very different perceptions. Drug companies and those running preventive services, including screening, like relative measures because they are usually more encouraging.

The NNT tells the patient that for every 200 people treated, one will benefit. By comparison with the other measures, this one requires no technical knowledge or sophistication, or intuition in mathematics. Of course, this does not answer the question for the patients as to whether it is worth taking this treatment but at least they have the information in a clear way. This NNT is only slightly higher than that for statins to prevent heart disease in healthy people of about 50 years without a family history of the problem. So, given the increasing guidance in favour of these drugs, millions of people will be using NNTs to help make their decisions.

The NNT based on results in a trial, of course, may not apply to real health-care settings, simply because trials enrol highly selected patients. The NNT, nonetheless, usually provides a more sobering assessment of benefits than the relative risk or the odds ratio. Policy-makers and clinicians have been quick to apply NNTs to therapies but not to preventive actions. This may reflect a fear that public support may be lost by this approach, for the NNP tends to be large. The NNP and NNT can be calculated from cohort and case register studies providing incidence data, but such figures are not as reliable as those from a good trial (Chapter 9).

Gemmell and colleagues (2005) have been working on a new set of population impact measures to help public health policy decisions. One of these extends the NNT idea to the population. The number of events prevented in a population (NEPP) is defined as 'the number of events prevented by the intervention in your population over a defined time period'. So these kinds of ideas are being developed for public health practice.

8.12 **Describing the health status of a population**

One of the vital contributions of epidemiology is the portrayal of the health status of a population. The first challenge is to define health. Based on the WHO definition, health is not merely the absence of disease or infirmity but a state of physical, mental, and social well-being. To be healthy it is necessary to be alive, functioning, and to have a sense of well-being. Before reading on do the exercise in Box 8.20.

Your data for the Minister of Health will probably comprise a mix of health and disease measures, but less obviously, it ought to include both qualitative and quantitive information. Qualitative information may include the public's and professionals' values, beliefs and attitudes in relation to health and disease. Quantitative measures will be both self-reported such as on smoking, alcohol, and exercise habits, and directly measured such as height, weight, visual acuity, blood pressure, and cholesterol. In this chapter, I have concentrated on categorical data but continuous data are also important. A relatively brief section on handling such data, and the role of correlation and regression analysis is in section 8.15.

Box 8.20 Describing health status: choice of measures

Imagine you are asked to describe, as comprehensively as possible, the health status of your population to a new Minister of Health. The minister has no previous background in the health field. What kinds of measures would you choose to portray the health of your population?

Consider not only the specific types of data, but also the qualities of the data you would seek out.

There may be information on actual health-related events, such as recent mortality and morbidity rates, and life expectancy. You might impress the minister by emphasizing the potential for avoidable deaths and disease, and the reduction of lives lost. The minister might understand the priority areas as reflected in DALYs. It would be impressive to show trends, emphasizing both those conditions which have reduced and are being controlled and those which are increasing. As comparing health status between time periods and between populations and places is likely to be important in developing and interpreting the profile, the minister will need to be reassured that the validity and quality of measurement is high. Do not mislead the minister by implying, tempting though it is, that the reductions can be attributed to government, unless it is true (unlikely). The minister is likely to be impressed by, and grasp, numbers of cases and percentages rather than more complex measures. However, it is imperative that you explain that more of some diseases of old age, for example, cancers and dementia, is a good sign—it means people are living long enough to get them. Providing age-standardized rates or percentages (perhaps as graphs) would show what is happening when you take the ageing of the population into account.

You may emphasize differences in subpopulations, for example, by demonstrating inequalities (disparities) in health status.

The portrait of health would be incomplete without an indication of the health-care facilities and services and the effects of such services on the population's health. These might be described as structures (number of doctors, nurses, hospitals, etc.), processes (consultation and hospitalization rates, etc.), and outcomes (effect on morbidity, mortality, avoidable mortality, and well-being). The influences of some public health and clinical services might be described in terms of the cost to gain a QALY. Governments, rightly, are very interested in costs in relation to benefits. You may demonstrate that there is inequity (or unfairness and inequality) in service delivery and how that impacts on the health of the population. These points are captured in Boxes 8.21, 8.22,, and Table 8.22.

The question of why the patterns and changes arise is almost inevitable. This requires relating the determinants of health status such as age, sex, social, and economic status, ethnicity, and health-related behaviours, to the measures of health status, and through study of the relationships, deriving conclusions about cause and effect. To complete the description of health status, therefore, the minister should be informed on these matters too.

Population-based data tend to be rich in information on death rates, and poor on function and well-being.

In summary, the health minister might reasonably expect your report to include some specific information on:

♦ the population and its demographic and socio-economic characteristics, generally;
♦ life expectancy, years of life lost, disease states, and causes of disability and infirmity;

Box 8.21 Creating a health portrait: some attributes of required health-status data

- Health and disease are both measured
- Qualitative and quantitative aspects of population health are included
- Self-reported and measured (e.g. weight) variables are provided
- Actual death rates and anticipated disease trends, as well as age-adjusted rates and trends
- Health-service structure, number of doctors and nurses, processes (e.g. consultations), and outcomes (e.g. death)
- Effects and costs of health care is related to health status

- measures of physical well-being;
- measures of mental and social well-being;
- measures of functioning;
- measures relating to health services;
- explanation of variations and particularly those that could be considered unjust or that are avoidable—usually called inequalities, inequities, or disparities;
- trends in these above points.

Given the importance of epidemiological data suggesting inequalities, inequities, and disparities, especially in health policy and public health, the next section focuses on the tricky issue of whether these should be measured in absolute or relative terms.

8.13 The relationship between absolute and relative risks: a conundrum for public health action on inequalities, inequities, and disparities in health

As disease risks change, we see a curious, unexpected yet arithmetically unalterable relationship that has profound implications for one of the foremost priorities in public health policy and

Box 8.22 General classification of some indices of health status or relevant health status

- Socio-economic circumstances
- Demographic structure of population, including sex, race, ethnicity, etc.
- Behavioural and other lifestyle aspects of the population
- Physiological/biochemical/anatomical/pathological/microbiological characteristics
- Genetic profile
- Psychological well-being
- Morbidity (i.e. illness, disease, impairment, etc.)
- Mortality
- Health-care facilities, policies, and systems in relation to costs and outcomes

Table 8.22 Specific examples of some health-status measurements

Biological function	Social function	Well-being	Disease and death	Health-service utilization
Physical measures such as height, weight, body shape, and obesity	Reproductive status of the population, e.g. fertility rates	Mental well-being, e.g. General Health Questionnaire	Mortality and morbidity rates, overall and by cause	Consultation activity
Physiological function, e.g. blood pressure, heart rate	Activities of daily living	Well-being, e.g. as self-reported	Life expectancy, as measured from current mortality rates	Effectiveness and cost-effectiveness of services
Biochemical status, e.g. serum cholesterol, plasma glucose	Social networks	Attitudes to health and health-related behaviours	Predicted disease and life expectancy patterns	Equity of health-service use
Genetic profiles, e.g. prevalence of sickle cell trait or cystic fibrosis gene	Health-related behaviours		Disability: prevalence and severity	

practice; that is, reducing inequalities, disparities, and inequities in health. The best way to visualize this relationship is by doing the exercise in Box 8.23 before reading on.

Public health policy, in virtually all countries, emphasizes not only reduction in disease but reduction in inequalities in disease. Inequalities in disease (and death) arising from many causes are considered inappropriate in fair societies. Yet, inequalities are pervasive. When these inequalities are clearly linked to social, economic, and environmental circumstances most people agree they are unjust. In Table 8.23, we see a pleasing reduction in the cumulative incidence rate in both populations A and B. We also see there is a gap between them but it is not getting bigger. When you calculate the relative risk, however, the gap has grown from 1.20 to 1.40 (see Appendix 8.4 Table A8.5). This simple example illustrates a powerful principle: as inequalities decline in absolute terms, they increase in relative terms. The only way to keep the relative inequality stable or to reduce it is for a faster decline in absolute risk in the worse off population. Almost invariably, public health aims for a reduction in relative inequalities, but this is almost never achieved. However, absolute risks usually show there have been benefits to all populations' health. This is a good reason for showing both absolute and relative measures in these circumstances.

Box 8.23 Relationship between absolute and relative risks

Examine the data in Table 8.23 and reflect on the pattern you see. Comment on the change in absolute risks particularly on the difference between the populations. Now calculate the relative risks. Comment on how these change. Reflect on the public health policy implications of the two kinds of data. (The numerical results are in the Appendix 8.4 Table A8.5).

Table 8.23 Absolute and relative risks over time in two populations

Time	Disease cumulative incidence rate per 1000 per year		Relative risk (B/A)
	Population A	**Population B**	
1960	100	120	
1970	90	110	
1980	80	100	
1990	70	90	
2000	60	80	
2010	50	70	

8.14 The construction and development of health-status indicators

Having chosen an aspect of health—whether life expectancy, death rates, or fertility—we need to define how the indicator is to be constructed and calculated. The general principles are those underlying the calculation of incidence rates and prevalence proportions, but the practice varies for each indicator, usually being reflected by the availability of data, as illustrated next with life expectancy and maternal mortality.

Table 8.24 exemplifies the construction of some key health indicators. Life expectancy at birth, or at a specified age, is not based on a theoretical expectation for the individual or the actual living

Table 8.24 Examples of the construction of some indices

Indices	Defining and operationalizing the index
Life expectancy	Years of life in a population expected on basis of current mortality rates by population structure ÷ total population
Maternal mortality rate	Deaths from puerperal causes during pregnancy or within 42 days ÷ live births
Stillbirth (synonym, fetal death) rate	Stillbirths ÷ total births
Neonatal mortality rate	Deaths in 28 days ÷ live births
Perinatal mortality rate	Stillbirths + 1st week deaths ÷ total births
Postneonatal rate	From 28 days to first year deaths ÷ live births
Infant mortality rate	Deaths at <1 year ÷ live births
Birth rate	Live births ÷ population
Fertility rate	Live births ÷ women aged 15–44 years
Abortion rate	Number of abortions ÷ women aged 15–44 years
Consultation rate	Number of consultations ÷ registered population
Hospitalization rate	Discharges and deaths in hospital ÷ population
Death rates	As discussed earlier in Chapter 7

population, but the years of life lived as calculated from the most recently available mortality rates in the population. Life expectancy is calculated from life tables (discussion of these is beyond the scope of this book). In most societies, therefore, life expectancy estimates are underestimates, because mortality rates will drop in future. (This has had serious repercussions for the pensions industry, which has under-estimated life expectancy gains.) This improvement, however, is not a certainty as the experience of dropping life expectancy in some Eastern European countries and Russia (due to economic difficulties) and some African countries (due to AIDS) has shown. Knowing the life expectancy permits us to estimate the potential years of life lost by an individual (as discussed in section 8.8). The point is that a workable, albeit imperfect, solution is found to estimate that which cannot be known.

The maternal mortality rate is another excellent example of how pragmatic decisions are made. We are actually interested in deaths in women associated with any aspect of childbirth. The first challenge, therefore, is to define those causes of death that are associated with childbirth. Rather than create a long list of specific causes, the puerperal causes definition is a pragmatic general one: any cause related to or aggravated by the pregnancy or its management, but not from accidental or incidental causes. This leaves a judgement that is made by the health professional and the coder of the death certificate. The next question is whether there is to be a time limit. According to the WHO definition, a maternal death needs to occur during pregnancy or within 42 days of the termination of pregnancy. The denominator for this rate ought to be all pregnancies. This figure cannot be estimated accurately so the definition, again pragmatically, uses live births. The principle illustrated here is that definitions need to work in widely varying circumstances, to permit comparable data, say from rural China and from inner London. This requires absolute clarity (e.g. as in the time limit of 42 days) and the use of readily available data; for example, number of live births rather than, say, pregnancies or the number of women registered at antenatal clinics.

The resulting fraction in such calculations is multiplied to create a whole number, and is calculated for an appropriate time period. Most such indices are expressed per 1000, 10 000 or 100 000 and per year. (By custom and practice, most of these indices are called rates even when they are, strictly, proportions.)

In most indices relating to health events around birth the number of births is used rather than population size. Sometimes the denominator is all births, sometimes live births. The reader has no option but to learn the definitions, or look them up, though there is some logic behind the choices. The stillbirth rate, for example, includes live and stillborn in the denominator, the neonatal mortality rate does not. The numerator of stillbirth includes stillborn, so the denominator does too. The numerator for neonatal mortality excludes the stillborn, so the denominator excludes them too.

Sometimes definitions cannot be agreed internationally, either for legal or other reasons or because the availability of data differs too greatly. The WHO definition of perinatal mortality uses live births in the denominator, whereas most industrialized nations use all births, dead or alive. Clearly, live births are easier to count accurately than all births.

Definitions are subject to periodic review and revision. There are, as the reader can see, intricacies and controversies behind apparently simple definitions of commonly used indices. The term *rate* is used generically, even though some of those in Table 8.24 do not conform to the principles discussed in Chapter 7. These are time-honoured phrases that are ingrained in clinical, public health, and epidemiological practice, and are unlikely to change in the foreseeable future.

8.15 Handling continuous data using correlation and regression: contributions to description of health status and causal thinking

So far, we have concentrated on categorical data, but continuous data are important to both description of health states and analysis of associations, and methods of analysing such data make a large contribution to epidemiology. For example, describing the average height of the population and how it has changed over the last 100 years, and how it varies by sex, ethnic or racial group, and social and economic status, is very informative. When we also have the weight of the individuals measured, we can calculate an index of overweight and obesity, that is, body mass index (BMI). These simple measures are very important for tracking changes in population health. Continuous measures can also be important in thinking about causal relationships.

Correlation is another word for association (or a link). Correlation, as with association, is not necessarily causation. In statistics correlation refers to a particular form of analysis of linear relationships between quantitative variables, mostly used for continuous measures. The relationship can be shown in a graph, of the type known as a scattergram (or scatter diagram) as in Figure 8.1. Here, for each person, the value for variable 1 (say height) and variable 2 (say weight) is represented by one dot. It is evident in Figure X that there is an association (Figure Y). The relationship can be calculated and summarized by a number known as a correlation coefficient (called r). The relationship can also be described by drawing the line that best fits the picture seen between the two variables. The line for the fictitious data here is drawn by eye, but there are mathematical methods for doing this (least squares). If there was no association, the dots would be scattered randomly but they are not. The correlation coefficient varies between 0 (no association, when the dots are random) and –1 or 1 (perfect association, when the dots form a straight line in a downwards or upwards direction, respectively).

We do not use correlation as an indicator of the strength of the association in epidemiology. The reason is that we are not primarily interested in whether two variables are associated, but by the amount of increase associated with a change in one of the two. (The relative risk is the classical example of this.)

The closely aligned methods of regression analysis, however, meet this epidemiological need. The question being answered here is: by how much is a change in variable 1 associated with a change in variable 2? The scatterplot is thus created, as in Figure 8.1. The regression line is calculated, using the same method as for correlation (so-called least squares method), as is the summary output known as the regression coefficient (r). The regression coefficient is the statistical

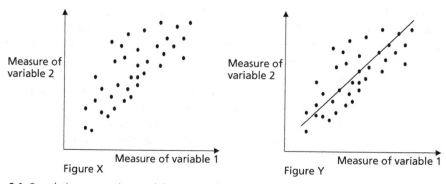

Fig. 8.1 Correlation, regression, and the scatterplot.

estimate of how much a unit of change in variable 1 is associated with variable 2. This is analogous to dose–response based on relative risks. The techniques of regression can cope with both continuous and categorical data, and permit the incorporation of numerous other variables (covariates or cofactors). The interactive and confounding effects of these cofactors can be explored.

Regression methods currently dominate analysis of epidemiological data where the objective is to explore associations. Although the terminology used may imply causal inference (predict, explain, independent effects, and other similar terms) this is misleading. They only produce estimates of the strength of the association and extent of variation in the data explained statistically. These estimates need to be considered in the frameworks of causal reasoning in exactly the same way as any other summary measures of association, for example, the odds ratio or relative risk. Regression techniques can be applied to categorical and quantitative variables, whether of exposure or outcome.

8.16 **Conclusion**

Chapters 7 and 8 are practical ones outlining some of the common and basic techniques in epidemiology. These techniques were not developed in an atheoretical vacuum. Clearly, epidemiological purposes, theories, and study designs underpin measurement, and presentation and interpretation of data. To a surprising extent, however, the capacity to measure and analyse data also alters our theories and study designs. Practical matters such as ease of analysis, and the availability of computers and computer software, also alter our choice of measures and mode of presentation. In the exemplar panel (Exemplar 8.1) I show how the Scottish Health and Ethnicity Study refined its methods over time. Computers and analytic software made the study possible. For example, our sample was of 4.62 million people. It would have been practically impossible to adjust the denominator to use the life-years approach (rather than an estimated denominator for the cumulative incidence approach) without the power of computerized data linkage of millions of records from different databases. This, in turn, has an effect on the interpretation of data and the conclusions, and on the arising recommendations. The interpretation of data, more than most aspects of epidemiology, is influenced by investigators' philosophy on the nature of knowledge (epistemology) and by the theories they hold.

Most epidemiologists adhere consciously or subconsciously to the doctrine of positivism, that is, the philosophic system that is based on facts, acquired by empirical observations, and logic. Anecdote, opinion, intuition, experience, and even observations made informally are not easily admitted as evidence. In this book, and in Chapters 3, 4, 7, and 8 specifically, I have emphasized that facts do not exist in a vacuum, but are extracted by analysis and interpretation from data that are invariably flawed. These 'facts' are contestable, and not surprisingly epidemiologists are renowned, even notorious, for their capacity for critique (see Chapter 10, sections 10.10–10.13).

These general points could be illustrated with many examples but let us consider just two, one reflecting a measure—the odds ratio—the other an approach—relative and absolute risk.

The odds ratio has had a profound impact on epidemiology. Its use in epidemiology can be traced to a paper by J. Cornfield in 1951. The appeal of the odds ratio at that time was its capacity to yield an estimate of the relative risk from case–control studies (Chapter 9). With increasing understanding of when this estimate was an accurate one, came a change in the design of case–control studies with an emphasis on studying incident cases and on ensuring controls were representative of the population providing the cases. The mode of analysis (odds ratio), therefore, altered the theoretical understanding and design of case–control studies. Yet there is no need to analyse a case–control study using an odds ratio. Landmark case–control studies on adenocarcinoma of the vagina (Herbst *et al.*) published in 1971, and on smoking and carcinoma of the lung (Doll and Bradford Hill) published in 1950 did not, for example, report odds ratios. Presently, the case–control study and the odds ratio are inextricably intertwined.

The odds ratio has now become a dominant summary measure in a range of studies, despite its drawbacks, because its mathematical properties make analysis easy (e.g. in a logistic regression model). It is not a coincidence that epidemiology has been powerfully influenced, undoubtedly for the better, by statisticians. In previous editions of this book, I predicted that this use of the odds ratio is likely to change as the drawbacks are more widely debated and other models are incorporated into standard statistical computing packages. This has happened, for example, with more use of the Poisson which models counts, rather than the logistic regression model, which models odds.

Different ways of presenting the same data have a major impact on the perception of risk, and in particular, relative and absolute risks portray dramatically different priorities giving different perspectives on the health needs of populations. Usually, relative measures of risk are more useful in causal enquiry, while absolute measures (including simple numbers) are better in health planning and policy. The tensions inherent in the choice of whether to present data using a relative or absolute risk approach go to the core of epidemiology. What is epidemiology for? Is it a science aiming for causal understanding? If so, the 'compare and contrast' mode of analysis is the time-honoured way of generating hypotheses and the relative risk approach is right. If, however, epidemiology is equally (or even predominantly) concerned with feeding into public health policy, needs assessment, clinical care, and health planning, then the burden of disease as measured by absolute risk is of critical importance. The relative risk approach tends to dominate. Ideally, investigators should report both relative and absolute risk, hence achieving a dual purpose. This simple advice is usually resisted because it creates extra work, makes the messages harder to convey, and takes up scarce publication space. More than that, most epidemiologists are more comfortable with the relative risk approach. With online publication, there is no reason for not giving both kinds of data, and publication guidelines are increasingly recommending this.

The example in Table 8.17 of the mortality of Indian subcontinent-born men illustrates the vastly different perspectives offered by relative and absolute approaches. It also raises a question about how researchers see the world. Why did the original investigators not report their data in this way? Why, so often in race and ethnicity research, is the reference or standard population a 'White' one? Why is the health of the 'White' population not compared with the minority ethnic groups using the latter as the reference population? The answers are not simply technical ones. One explanation is that there is an ethnocentric approach, whereby the population that is dominant in status (and possibly numbers) is automatically assigned as the standard because investigators (most of whom come from or are trained in such populations) see the world through the eyes of this population.

The measurement and portrayal of population health is a dynamic and creative aspect of epidemiology with much scope for innovation. Lee's (1998) and Gemmell *et al.'s* (2005) work referred to in this chapter illustrate this well. The challenges of creating simple, understandable, and valid summary measures of health states are formidable. There is the practical task, at the interphase of epidemiology and public health, of putting measures together to create a profile of the community's health, and using this to help improve it. In Chapter 7 I emphasized the even greater challenge of collecting data to get valid numerators and denominators measures. That is not just a role for epidemiologists, but they must provide leadership.

Epidemiological data on diseases can be combined with other information such as socioeconomic circumstances, social values and attitudes to health, and behaviours relevant to health, to build up a community health profile. Combining data sets in this way helps to generate causal understanding of disease processes in populations and the means of developing interventions to improve public health. As epidemiology is a positivist discipline founded on empirical observation, mastery of quantitative data interpretation is vital to its proper practice.

Exemplar 8.1: The Scottish Health and Ethnicity Linkage Study (SHELS)

I introduced this study in Chapter 7 when discussing numerators, denominators, and incidence rates. Cohort studies are the richest source of data in epidemiology because they produce both cross-sectional and longitudinal outcome data. I now illustrate some of the principles and measures in this chapter using extracts of some published data. SHELS is actually a retrospective cohort (Chapter 9).

Myocardial infarction: numbers, directly standardized cumulative incidence rates, rate ratios, risk ratio, survival proportions (case fatality), and hazard rates

Background

In Chapter 7 I discussed the sources of, and possible accuracy of, numerator and denominator data in a pilot study of myocardial infarction (MI). We, the SHELS investigators, built on this to both verify the descriptive data and to test hypotheses (Bansal *et al.* 2011). Our hypotheses were:

1. Indians and Pakistanis would have the highest, and Chinese the lowest, incidence of first MI compared to the White Scottish population.

2. The better survival in South Asians demonstrated in the pilot study would be explained by decreased travel time to hospitals, as South Asians are more likely to live near them.

3. South Asians would have a lower uptake of cardiac interventions in line with studies elsewhere.

Methods

The methods were as described in Chapter 7. The analysis was in people ≥ 30 years of age. The numerator was the first of either MI death in the community or hospitalization, in the seven-year period 2001–2008 (excluding those hospitalized in the 10 years before April 2001 so these were apparently first events).

Travel times were off-peak road traffic time from postcode (zip code) of the patient's home to hospital attended, or in the case of death in the community, to the nearest hospital with appropriate facilities.

MI was defined as the relevant codes from ICD9 and 10 on the death record or hospitalization discharge record (see Exemplar 7.1).

Cardiac intervention, likewise, was defined as angioplasty (OPCS 4 code K49, K50.1 and K75) or coronary artery bypass graft (K40–K46) within 28 days of first MI.

In the analysis of incidence rates, the confounding variables adjusted for were age group (in decades) and individual-level educational level. In the analysis of survival to 28 days after MI, the variables adjusted for were age, education, travel time, and cardiac intervention. (The statistical models used go beyond the scope of this book but were Poisson regression for risk ratios and Cox regression for survival to 28 days.) The analyses were for men and women separately.

Results

There were 8510 episodes of first MI in our analysis. We examined the age stratified data in 10-year categories by sex and ethnic group, and ensured the patterns were as expected.

We presented our data on rates, rate ratios, and risk ratios in men and women and we calculated survival to 28 days and risk ratios for cardiac intervention uptake. The quantitative results are not central to this discussion.

Comment and interpretation relating to hypotheses

This example shows how a range of analyses can be done on simple numerator and denominator data both to illustrate the pattern of disease in a population and, with chosen co-variables, to test pre-specified hypotheses. To see how the results were interpreted in the light of the strengths and weaknesses, read the paper. In relation to the hypotheses: (i) Pakistanis, but not so clearly Indians, had higher rates than White Scottish people and Chinese had the lowest rates. (ii) The travel time hypothesis was not upheld. (iii) The lower uptake of cardiac interventions was not seen as hypothesized.

Gastrointestinal disorders: introducing rates based on person-years of observation

SHELS extended observations to 9 years, and among the outcomes examined were gastrointestinal disorders (Bhopal *et al.* 2014). Some changes were made to the analysis. First, we adopted the person-years denominator, adjusting it by censoring observations of time for case occurrence, request for medical notes from the Scottish NHS to be sent to other parts of the United Kingdom following migration, and deaths. (This explained in Chapter 7). In addition, we adjusted for age within a Poisson regression model without using the direct method of standardization, and we calculated person–time incidence rate ratios.

Place of death: proportional mortality ratios for place of death

In many analyses we calculated prevalence proportions, using the same kind of approaches to numerators and denominators as described for cumulative incidence and person–time incidence rates above.

In addition, we have calculated proportional mortality ratios for place of death by ethnic group (Sharpe *et al.* 2015).

The numerator is the number of deaths for cancer in hospital, home, and hospice by ethnic group (some merging of groups was done as numbers were small). The denominator was the total deaths from cancer by ethnic group.

Avoidable and preventable (collectively amenable) mortality

The SHELS project obtained lists of conditions agreed to be amenable to health-care interventions and preventive measure. This work is ongoing.

Concluding remarks

SHELS illustrates how there are many approaches to analysis and how the approaches are dynamic; that is, they evolve and change over time according to availability of data, changes in follow-up periods, the study questions, and analytical advances. The cohort design offers great flexibility in analysis, so setting the direction of analysis by an analysis plan is vital.

Summary

Basic epidemiological data on disease occurrence and population structure can be manipulated and presented in many ways. The choice should be guided by the purposes of the research and the likely application of the findings. Data manipulation, inevitably, both sharpens the findings in some ways and distorts them in others. Epidemiological summary measures, broadly, estimate absolute risks (e.g. numbers, rates, life expectancy, life years lost, numbers needed to treat) or relative ones (e.g. age-adjusted rates, PMRs, SMRs, relative risk, odds ratios).

Different ways of presenting the same data have a major impact on the perception of risk, and in particular relative and actual risks portray dramatically different perspectives on the health status of populations. Usually, relative measures of risk are more useful in causal enquiry while absolute measures are better in health planning and policy. Epidemiological studies should give both relative and absolute risk. These measures, usually in association with risk factor prevalence data, allow estimation of the risk attributable to a risk factor in those exposed and in the entire population. Inequalities, inequities, and disparities can often be shown to be declining on absolute measures but rarely on relative ones.

Avoidable mortality (and morbidity) refers to the potential to avoid death (or morbidity) from a number of specified causes if the best possible health-care actions were taken. Years-of-life-saved measures help to measure the impact of avoidable mortality in the population. Avoidable mortality helps us to focus on priorities for new research, apply epidemiological knowledge in public health, guide health-care actions, and assess effectiveness of health-care. The life years lost can be adjusted for quality of life (QALY) and disability (DALY) to give a more nuanced interpretation.

Epidemiological data on diseases can be combined with other information such as socio-economic circumstances, social values and attitudes, and behaviours relevant to health, to build up a community health profile. Combining data sets in this way generates causal understanding of disease processes in populations and the means of developing rational interventions to improve public health. Continuing advances in calculation of summary measures and interpretation are vital to the future success of epidemiology.

Sample questions

Question 1 Define relative risk and briefly outline its value in epidemiology.

Answer Relative risk is the ratio of the incidence rate (whether measured by the cumulative incidence or person–time incidence) in different groups, often those with the exposure of interest (risk factor) and those without.

Its value is in helping assess the strength of an association, part of the process of causal analysis, which in itself is important to weighing up the potential for the association arising from error, bias, and confounding, rather than being really causal.

The relative risk is a key component of outcome prediction models and in estimating the prospects for prevention through public health actions.

Question 2 A population register assessed the incidence of heart attacks (non-fatal and fatal events) by ethnic group in the UK population (Tables 8.25 and 8.26). The following data were obtained after one year follow-up:

Table 8.25 White ethnic group

Age group	Cases of heart attack	Total number of people in study
45–54	5	7500
55–64	24	6500
65–74	37	4500
75+	71	3200
Total	137	21 700

Table 8.26 Indian ethnic group

Age group	Cases of heart attack	Total number of people in study
45–54	3	1800
55–64	6	1500
65–74	8	800
75+	10	400
Total	27	4500

(i) Calculate the age-specific and overall (crude) incidence rates of heart attack per 1000 population for the White and Indian ethnic groups.

Answer (i) Incidence of heart attacks by ethnic group in the United Kingdom. Age-specific and overall (crude) incidence rates (Table 8.27).

Table 8.27 Age-specific and overall (crude) incidence rates

Age group	White	Indian
45–54	0.66	1.6
55–64	3.69	4.0
65–74	8.22	10.0
75+	22.19	25.00
Actual/Crude	6.31	6.00

(ii) Calculate the indirectly standardized rate—summarized as a standardized morbidity ratio (SMR) of heart attack for Indian ethnic groups using the White population rates as the reference population.

Expected:	45–54	1.19
	55–64	5.54
	65–74	6.58
	75+	8.88
Total expected		22.11 cases

$$\text{SMR} = \frac{\text{observed}}{\text{expected}} = \frac{27}{22.11} \; 1.22$$

Answer (ii) SMR for heart attack in the Indian group is 1.22; with the White population as the standard

(iii) Comment on the strengths and limitations of standardized and overall crude (actual) measures of disease incidence in (a) comparing populations and (b) planning services for one population (e.g. the Indian ethnic group).

Answer (iii) The overall actual (crude) measures are not good for comparing populations where there are differences in other important respects (e.g. age, or sex structure). Here, for example this measure wrongly suggests Indians have less heart attacks than White people. These kinds of data are, however, vital for planning services. For this we need to know the number of cases likely to be seen and their age and sex composition. Where there are large numbers of cases and people, then age-specific rates are excellent.

The standardized methods produce a summary that is not real world data—it is distorted by the procedure of weighting (here by age). Therefore, these summaries need to be used with care in planning health care, though they do help refine a sense of relative priority or need.

Standardized measures are excellent for permitting comparison where the differences in age structure (or sex or both) have been taken into account. This standardization means that age is not a confounding variable in that specific comparison.

Question 3 An examination of mortality data for disease A (Table 8.28) gave the following findings:

Table 8.28 Mortality rate for disease A

Year	Cases	Population (millions)
1961	73	4.9
1971	81	5.1
1981	87	5.2
1991	90	5.3

(i) Calculate the annual cumulative mortality rate per 100 000 population.

Answer (i)
See Table 8.29.

Table 8.29 Cumulative mortality rate for disease A

Year	Mortality rate
1961	73/4 900 000 × 100 000 = 1.49 per 100 000
1971	81/5 100 000 × 100 000 = 1.59 per 100 000
1981	87/5 200 000 × 100 000 = 1.67 per 100 000
1991	90/5 300 000 × 100 000 = 1.70 per 100 000

(ii) Based on the 1961 rate as the standard, calculate the mortality rate ratios for the other years.

Answer (ii)
See Table 8.30.

Table 8.30 Mortality rate ratios for disease A for three years using the 1961 mortality rate as the standard

1971 rate/1961 rate	1.59/1.49 = 1.07
1981 rate/1961 rate	1.67/1.49 = 1.12
1991 rate/1961 rate	1.70/1.49 = 1.14

(iii) Describe the mortality trend. What explanations can you think of for this change?

Answer Both the actual (absolute) and relative frequency measures suggest more people are dying from disease A over time, although the population size is also increasing. Therefore, concomitant changes in the population structure (e.g. increase in the number of old people in the population or immigration of people more susceptible to or already having disease A) are possible explanations of the increase in the mortality rate. On the other hand, it is also possible that an increase in case fatality occurred due to changes in the disease, for example, increased virulence if it is infectious in origin or decreased resistance to the disease explains the trend. There may have been changes in diagnostic procedures or recording of deaths resulting in more deaths being attributed to disease A. These explanations can be investigated.

Question 4 A cohort study assessed the cumulative incidence rate of stroke (non-fatal and fatal events) by ethnic group in the UK population (Tables 8.31 and 8.32). The following data were obtained after one year of follow-up:

Table 8.31 White ethnic group

Age group	Cases of stroke	Total number of people in study	Annual incidence rate per 1000
45–54	4	7000	0.6
55–64	19	6000	3.2
65–74	32	4500	7.1
75+	63	3500	18.0
Total	118	21 000	5.6

Table 8.32 Indian ethnic group

Age group	Cases of stroke	Total number of people in study	Annual incidence rate per 1000
45–54	2	1700	1.2
55–64	5	1300	3.8
65–74	6	700	8.6
75+	8	400	20.0
Total	21	4100	5.1

(i) Calculate the directly standardized incidence rates of stroke for the White and Indian ethnic groups using the 1976 European standard population as the external reference population (Table 8.33). (As an extra, you may wish to find the revised 2013 European standard population and re-do the calculation.)

Table 8.33 European standard population

Age group	1976 European standard population
45–54	140 000
55–64	110 000
65–74	70 000
75+	40 000
Total	360 000

Answer (i)
See Table 8.34.

Table 8.34 Expected incidence rates of stroke for the White and Indian ethnic groups using the 1976 European standard population as the external reference population

Age group	1976 European standard population	Expected cases of stroke: White	Expected cases of stroke: Indian
45–54	140 000	84[1]	168
55–64	110 000	352	418
65–74	70 000	497	602
75+	40 000	720	800
Total	360 000	1653	1988
Directly standardized		(1653/360 000) × 1000 = 4.6	5.5

[1] (0.6/1000) × 140 000 = 84 (the rate in that age group in the White population multiplied by the population in that age group in the standard population).

(ii) Compare the results of the overall (crude) rate and the directly standardized rate in the two ethnic groups. Comment on the strengths and limitations of these two measures in (a) understanding the causes of stroke and (b) planning health services for stroke.

Answer

(ii) Overall, crude rate ratios (Indian:White) 5.1:5.6 = 0.9.
Directly standardized rate ratios (Indian:White) 5.5:4.6 = 1.2.

The data show that the incidence of stroke is higher in each age group in UK residents of Indian ethnic group than in the White population. Despite this, because the Indian population has a substantially younger age structure than the White population, and the incidence of stroke increases with age, the Indian population has a lower overall (crude) rate of stroke than the White population. When the differences in age structure are accounted for by age standardization, the higher risk of stroke in the Indian population is reflected in a higher directly standardized disease rate.

In general, crude disease rates provide useful information for health-services planning, as they reflect the actual number of cases of disease the health service will have to provide care for. Standardized rates reflect the risk of disease after accounting for differences in population structure and hence provide more useful information for studying the causes of disease and which population subgroups are most at risk. Prioritizing health promotion interventions can be particularly challenging as a compromise between overall population health improvement and reduction in health inequalities often needs to be made (in this example, most cases of stroke occur in the majority White population but disease risk is higher in the Indian population, so which group should get priority?).

Question 5 What is the proportional mortality ratio? In what circumstances would you use it? What are its main limitations when comparing different populations?

Answer The proportional mortality ratio is a summary measure whereby the pattern of the causes of death in the study population is compared to a reference population. The formula is:

$$\frac{\text{Proportional mortality for disease X in study population}}{\text{Proportional mortality for disease X in reference population}}.$$

The proportional mortality is the proportion of deaths from disease X, where the denominator is usually all deaths. It can, however, be deaths from another cause. We might use this summary measure when a mortality rate cannot be calculated for lack of a population denominator.

The proportional mortality ratio cannot, on its own, tell us whether mortality from disease X is actually different from that in the reference population. This is because differences in other diseases will also alter the ratio. For example, the proportional mortality ratio for heart disease in the study population may be high because other causes of death—for example, cancer mortality—are lower than in the reference population.

Question 6 In a cohort study of university students examining the association between meditation or prayer and sickness absence as a health outcome, the response rate was 70 per cent: 5700 women who responded reported they meditated or prayed, while 12 300 did not. The outcome, sickness absence, was obtained from a questionnaire to students one year later. In the meditation/prayer group, 900 students recorded having at least one day off university. In those who did not report meditating or praying, 1350 women were recorded as having at least one day off university in the same time period.

(i) Place these data in an appropriate 2 × 2 table with all appropriate labels and numbers.

Answer (i)

See Table 8.35.

Table 8.35 Relationship between meditation, prayer, and sickness absence

	Sickness absence		
	Yes	**No**	**Totals**
(a) Prayed/meditated	900	4800	5700
(b) Did not pray/meditate	1350	10 950	12 300
	2250	15 750	18 000

(ii) Estimate the relative risk of sickness absence in those who do not meditate or pray (use the cumulative incidence rate for your calculations with the baseline population as the denominator).

Answer (ii)

$$RR = \frac{\text{Incidence rate in B}}{\text{Incidence rate in A}} = \frac{1350 \div 12\ 300}{900 \div 570} = \frac{10.98}{15.78} = 0.69.$$

Readers may find it better to do the next part after reading Chapter 9.

(iii) Do you think this kind of study is good for showing cause and effect? What problems make it difficult to interpret the results?

Answer (iii)

The cohort study is one of the classic and powerful ways of studying cause and effect. Nonetheless, the evidence arising needs to be interpreted very cautiously using frameworks for separating causal and non-causal association. One crucial issue is of timing—did the exposure truly precede the effect? Cohort studies are usually good on this matter. Nonetheless, problems arise in errors of measurement, recruitment and retention of population, confounding, and interpretation of the associations found. Studies based on incomplete data and on self-selected populations are problematic.

References

Bansal, N., Fischbacher, C., Bhopal R., Brown, H., Steiner, M., and Capewell, S. (2011) Ethnic inequalities in myocardial infarction incidence, interventions and survival in Scotland: the Scottish Health and Ethnicity Linkage Study (SHELS). *Journal of Epidemiology and Community Health*, **65**(Suppl 1), A225.

Bhopal, R.S., Cezard, G., Bansal, N., Ward, H.J.T., Bhala, N., on behalf of the SHELS researchers. (2014) Ethnic variations in five lower gastrointestinal diseases: Scottish Health and Ethnicity Linkage study. *British Medical Journal Open* [4:e006120].

Cornfield, J. (1951) A method of estimating comparative rates from clinical data. Applications to cancer of the lung, breast and cervix. *Journal of the National Cancer Institute*, **11**, 1269–75.

Doll, R. and Bradford Hill, A. (1956) Lung cancer and other causes of death in relation to smoking. *British Medical Journal*, **2**, 1071–81.

Doll, R. and Hill, A.B. (1950) Smoking and carcinoma of the lung: preliminary report. *British Medical Journal*, **2**, 739–48.

Gemmell, I., Heller, R.F., McElduff, P., *et al.* (2005) Population impact of stricter adherence to recommendations for pharmacological and lifestyle interventions over one year in patients with coronary heart disease. *Journal of Epidemiology and Community Health*, **59**, 1041–6.

Herbst, A., Ulfelder, H., and Poskanzer, D. (1971) Adenocarcinoma of the vagina: Association of maternal stilbestrol therapy with tumour appearance in young women. *New England Journal of Medicine*, **284**, 878–81.

Lee, W. (1998) The meaning and use of the cumulative rate of potential life lost. *International Journal of Epidemiology*, **27**, 1053–6.

Marmot, M.G., Adelstein, A.M., and Bulusu, L. (1984) *Immigrant Mortality in England and Wales 1970–78*. London, UK: HMSO.

Murray, C.J.L. and Lopez, A.D. (1997) Mortality by cause for eight regions of the world: Global burden of disease study. *Lancet*, **349**, 1269–76.

Pless-Mulloli T., Phillimore, P., Moffatt, S., Bhopal, R., Foy, C., Dunn, C., and Tate, J. (1998) Lung cancer, proximity to industry, and poverty in northeast England. *Environmental Health Perspectives*, **106**, 189–96.

Roman, E., Beral, V., Inskip, H., McDowall, M., and Adelstein, A.A. (1984) A comparison of standardized proportional mortality ratios. *Statistics in Medicine*, **3**, 7–14.

Sharpe, K.H, Cezard, G., Bansal, N., and Bhopal, R.S. (2015) Policy for home or hospice as the preferred place of death from cancer: Scottish Health and Ethnicity Linkage Study population cohort shows challenges across all ethnic groups in Scotland. *British Medical Journal Supportive & Palliative Care*, **5**, 443–51.

Appendix 8.1

Table A8.1 Population size, and cases: calculation of age-specific and actual overall (crude) rates in three groups of varying size (completing Table 8.4 in main text)

Age group	Population structure and size	Cases	Rate (as %)
Group A			
21–30	1000	50	5
31–40	1000	100	10
41–50	1000	150	15
Actual overall (crude) rate	3000	300	10
Group B			
21–30	500	25	5
31–40	1500	150	10
41–50	3000	450	15
Actual overall (crude) rate	5000	625	12.5
Group C			
21–30	5000	250	5
31–40	1000	100	10
41–50	200	30	15
Actual overall (crude) rate	6200	380	6.1

Table A8.2 Standardizing with the direct method: effect of young and old standard populations (completing Table 8.5 in main text)

Standard population	Group size	Applying age-specific rates from Table 8.4 to standard population: cases expected		
		Group A	Group B	Group C
(a) A young population structure				
21–30	3000	150*	150	150
31–40	1500	150	150	150
41–50	500	75	75	75
Overall	5000	375	375	375
Overall standard rate = 375/5000 =		7.5%	7.5%	7.5%

Table A8.2 Continued

Standard population	Group size	Applying age-specific rates from Table 8.4 to standard population: cases expected		
		Group A	Group B	Group C
(b) An older population structure				
21–30	200	10	10	10
31–40	1000	100	100	100
41–50	5000	750	750	750
Overall	6200	860	860	860
Overall standardized adjusted rate = 860/6200 =		13.9%	13.9%	13.9%

*Example: from Table 8.4 we see that the rate in the age group 21–30 in populations A, B, and C is 5%. In the young standard population (a) there are 3000 people. We expect, therefore, that 5% of them will develop the disease, i.e. 150 people.

Table A8.3 Standardization with the indirect method (completing Table 8.7 in main text)

Standard population (low rates)

Age group	Population	Cases	Rate (%)
21–30	40 000	2000	5
31–40	50 000	3750	7.5
41–50	60 000	6000	10
Total	150 000	11 500	7.7

	Population A		Population B		Population C	
	Population	Cases expected	Population	Cases expected	Population	Cases expected
21–30	1000	50	500	25	5000	250
31–40	1000	75	1500	113	1000	75
41–50	1000	100	3000	300	200	20
Total	3000	225	5000	438	6200	345
Observed*/expected (standardized morbidity/ mortality ratio, SMR)	$\frac{300}{225} \times 100$ $= 133$		$\frac{625}{438} \times 100$ $= 143$		$\frac{380}{345} \times 100$ $= 110$	

*Observed from Table 8.4—no. of cases in total.

Appendix 8.2

Formula relating SMR to PMR:

$$\text{SMR (for a specific cause)} = \frac{\text{All cause SMR} \times \text{PMR (for a specific cause)}}{100} \qquad (8.17)$$

When SMR can be calculated only for all causes this formula might be useful. It is, however, rarely used.

Appendix 8.3

Table A8.4 Relative, excess, and attributable risk: study of lung cancer and coronary heart disease in heavy smokers and non-smokers

	Annual death rates per 100 000	
	Lung cancer	Coronary heart disease
Heavy smokers	166	599
Non-smokers	7	422
Relative risk (RR)	23.7	1.4
Excess no. of cases caused by smoking based on incidence formula	1661 – 7 = 159	591 – 422 = 177
Excess risk	159/100 000	177/100 000
Attributable risk given as a percentage of all risk; based on incidence	$\frac{159}{166} = 95.8\%$	$\frac{177}{599} = 29.5\%$
Attributable risk based on relative risk formula given as a percentage; based on RR	$\frac{23.7 - 1}{23.7} = 93.8\%$	$\frac{1.42 - 1}{1.42} = 29.5\%$

Source: data from Doll R and Bradford Hill A. Lung cancer and other causes of death in relation to smoking. *British Medical Journal*, Volume 2, Issue 5001, pp. 1071–1081, Copyright © 1956 BMJ Publishing Group Ltd.

Appendix 8.4

Table A8.5 Absolute and relative risks over time in two populations

Time	Disease rate cumulative incidence 1000 per year		Relative risk (B/A)
	Population A	Population B	
1960	100	120	1.20
1970	90	110	1.22
1980	80	100	1.25
1990	70	90	1.29
2000	60	80	1.33
2010	50	70	1.40

Chapter 9

Epidemiological study designs and principles of data analysis: A conceptually integrated suite of methods and techniques

Objectives

On completion of the chapter you should understand that:

◆ the three key purposes underlying all epidemiological studies are studying disease causation and/or measuring the burden of disease and/or predicting disease patterns;

◆ epidemiological studies are unified by their common purposes, by their utilization of the survey and registry methods, and their foundation on defined populations;

◆ all study designs potentially contribute to disease prevention, health policy and planning, and clinical practice;

◆ a clinical case series (or register) study is of a coherent set of cases compiled by one or a few clinicians;

◆ a population case series (or registry) study is of a set of cases in a defined population and time and lays the foundation for description of disease by place, time, and characteristics of populations (sometimes wrongly called the ecological design);

◆ a case–control study compares a group of cases with a comparison, control group from the same population to generate and test causal hypotheses, through the analysis of associations;

◆ a cross-sectional study measures prevalence in a sample of individuals in a population in a defined time period, mainly to explore the burden of disease and risk factors, but also to generate associations and hence hypotheses;

◆ a cohort study follows up populations over time to observe changes in health status, to measure disease incidence, and to examine associations between risk factors and health outcomes;

◆ a trial examines the consequences of an intervention on one or more study groups;

◆ a natural experiment is akin to a trial but one where the intervention is imposed by nature, not the investigators. Mendelian randomization studies are one example of this;

◆ ecological studies are of environmental variables;

◆ in practice, the 'ecological design' is, usually, a mode of analysis based on variables being studied in relation to places rather than individuals—usually the data come from a population case series (or registry study);

◆ there are conceptual and practical interrelationships between study designs;

♦ the size of the study and the analysis should meet the prior aims, which are usually either to measure the frequency of the risk factors and disease outcomes, or to study the associations between them;

♦ the analysis should be efficient, accurate, and unbiased.

9.1 Introduction: interdependence of study design in epidemiology, and the importance of the base population

The first eight chapters have considered what epidemiology is and what it wants to achieve. This complex population health science intends to describe and understand the burden and causes of ill health in populations (Chapters 1, 2, and 5). It does this by aiming for accurate and unbiased quantitative data on risk factors and disease outcomes (Chapters 3, 4, and 7) and often the relations between them in contrasting groups (Chapter 8). It wants to apply this information in clinical and public health practice, for example, by early detection of disease by screening (Chapter 6). Now that we have a sound understanding of our aims, it is time to look at the means (or tools) at our disposal to achieve these aims. These tools are the study designs; however, study designs are not epidemiology itself. Indeed, epidemiology existed before these methods were invented and will do so when new ones supersede the current ones. Furthermore, often the methods have been shared with or borrowed from other disciplines. Nonetheless, whatever their origins, epidemiology has become the champion of the study designs and methods considered here. Historically they have developed separately, but because of their common goals and shared conceptual basis they can be considered as a suite, or family.

There is a growing number of apparently disparate study designs in epidemiology, and the labels used to describe them are numerous. However, underlying these there are five basic designs based on individual data, as listed in Box 9.1 and summarized in Table 9.1, which outline some of their characteristics and overlapping purposes. Confusion about these five designs is common, and is partly caused by the varying use of terms, the existence of many synonyms, and the development and invention of new terms and designs. Therefore, understanding the ideas underlying the designs is very important.

There are modifications of these five study designs to suit different purposes. For example, there are retrospective and prospective cohort studies, there are case series studies based on clinical records and population-based registers, and many forms of case–control studies (including case only) and trials. It is important, therefore, to understand the ideas which underlie study designs, particularly in terms of purpose, form, analysis, interpretation, and basis in the concept of population.

Box 9.1 Five core epidemiological designs for studies based on individuals

♦ Case series (based on clinical and population registers)
♦ Cross-sectional
♦ Case–control
♦ Cohort (prospective and retrospective)
♦ Trial (or experiment)

Table 9.1 Epidemiological designs and applications: an overview of the underlying ideas and purposes of five designs

Study design	Essential idea	Some research purposes
1. Case series and population case series based on registers holding clinical information (increasingly electronic clinical records are yielding such data)	Count cases (numerator) and relate to population and time data (denominator) when possible to produce rates and analyse patterns Look at characteristics of cases for clues on causal hypotheses Use clinical information	Study signs, symptoms, and laboratory investigations data and create disease definitions Surveillance of mortality/morbidity rates Seek associations Generate/test hypotheses Source of cases or foundation for other studies
2. Cross-sectional, usually based on surveys	Study health and disease states in a sample of the population at a defined place and time Measure burden of disease and its possible causes, i.e. risk factors	Measure prevalence (very rarely incidence) of disease and related factors Seek associations between disease and related factors Generate/test hypotheses Repeat studies (on different samples but in same source population) to measure change and evaluate interventions Starting point of a cohort study
3. Case–control	Look for differences and similarities, usually in possible causal factors between a series of cases and a control group	Seek associations Generate/test hypotheses Assess strength of association (using odds ratio)
4. Cohort (retrospective and prospective)	Follow-up populations over time, relating information on risk factor patterns and health states at baseline, to the outcomes of interest	Provide prevalence data especially in the baseline stage Study natural history of disease Measure incidence of disease Link disease outcomes to possible disease causes, i.e. seek associations Generate/test hypotheses Assess strength of association (relative risk)
5. Trial (or experiment)	Intervene with some measure designed to improve health, then follow-up people to see the effect*	Confirm understanding of causes Study how to influence natural history of disease Evaluate the effects (side effects and benefits) and costs of health interventions

*Measures designed to worsen health or to make no difference would be ethically unacceptable, though this may commonly be done (with ethical or regulatory approval) on animals and rarely in humans. Sadly, harmful experimentation has been a feature of medical sciences, including epidemiology.

The common goal of epidemiological studies is contributing to understanding the frequency, pattern, and causes of disease in populations and they are usually analysed to provide one or more of the measures considered in Chapters 7 and 8. They are also united by their reliance on the survey method. This is an investigation in which information is systematically collected, but without using the experimental method (and experiments are excluded). Epidemiological studies are all rooted in the concept of population, in that knowledge of the relation between the people studied and the population from which they originate is essential for interpretation, generalization, and application of data.

Vital questions in interpreting studies, therefore, include these: where and when was the study done (as populations differ by place, and change over time)? Of which population is the study group a subset? What are the characteristics of the study and source populations? In particular, what are the risk factor patterns relevant to the outcome; for example, a study of obesity and myocardial infarction (MI) may be interpreted differently in populations where smoking is common compared to where it is rare. Are the findings generalizable to the whole of the population in the community, or to communities elsewhere? These questions will be reconsidered in the context of critical appraisal of epidemiological papers in Chapter 10. The underlying source population or, more technically base population, then, is the starting point of epidemiology.

All epidemiological studies permit comparisons of disease experience in terms of one or more of the triad of time, place, and person (Chapter 2, section 2.1). They contribute to measuring the burden of disease or risk factors and study the relationship of disease and risk factors, though to a greatly varying extent. This integration is not only theoretical but is also practical, as demonstrated by the way one study design may lead to another, the relatively minor modifications needed to switch the study design, and the way they complement each other, particularly in adding to the weight of evidence in causal analysis (all discussed next). One of the epidemiological guidelines for causality is consistency, which requires evidence from more than one study, preferably using different study designs (Chapter 5), so this complementary aspect of designs is invaluable. The lessons and principles from one design are usually transferable to another.

The epidemiological literature refers to an ecological (sometimes with inverted commas as 'ecological' to reflect the author's doubts) study design, but here most such work is considered as a mode of analysis. This issue is briefly discussed in the section after the basic five designs are explained. First we consider the value of several simpler classifications of study design that are sometimes used instead of specific labels.

9.2 **Classifications of study design: five general approaches**

Three commonly used classifications that you will need to know are: (1) descriptive and analytic studies, (2) retrospective and prospective studies, and (3) observational and experimental studies. The other two in table 9.2 have been added by me as possibly helpful.

Table 9.2 shows the traditional view on whether the five study designs in Box 9.1 are descriptive or analytic. The term *descriptive* implies a study that focuses on information about the pattern of disease or risk factors but not on the underlying causes. This does not, however, preclude them from examining associations and contributing to causal thinking. Usually, however, they will generate hypotheses for further examination using analytic designs. The term *analytic* applies to studies that are exploring hypotheses about causes of those diseases but, by inference, are not primarily concerned with elucidating patterns. Insights about hypothesis on the causation of disease are, however, inherent in the pattern of disease and risk factors in all epidemiological studies. The pattern is used both to generate and to test hypotheses. Equally, description is

Table 9.2 The five core study designs in relation to five of possible classifications

Design	Descriptive/ analytic	Retrospective/ prospective	Observational/ experimental	Beginning with disease/ risk factor of disease	Specific comparison group/no such group needed
Case series (clinical and population)	Descriptive	Retrospective	Observational	Disease	Not needed
Cross-sectional	Descriptive	Retrospective	Observational	Both simultaneously	Not needed
Case–control	Analytic	Retrospective	Observational	Disease	Needed
Cohort (prospective and retrospective)	Analytic	Prospective and retrospective	Observational	Usually risk factors	Needed (though it is usually integral to the study population)
Trial (experiment)	Analytic	Prospective	Experimental	Usually disease, but sometimes causes of disease	Needed

a necessary step in analysis of all studies. All epidemiological studies may be simultaneously descriptive and analytic in the sense of exploring hypotheses. One of the finest examples of causal thinking in epidemiology is the investigation by Semmelweis of childbed fever, where descriptive data were the foundation for a causal hypothesis (Chapter 5, Table 5.1). Equally, cohort studies may be used to provide, in the main, descriptive data on disease incidence, and not be concerned with hypothesis testing.

Retrospective studies are concerned with data in the past, and the prospective ones with data in the future (Table 9.2). The terms retrospective and prospective have been used synonymously with case–control and cohort studies, respectively, and readers may still occasionally see this use. The distinction between retrospective and prospective studies is inaccurate, for case–control studies may enrol subjects prospectively and cohort studies may enrol subjects retrospectively (see later) and both do, of course, collect data on risk factors in the past. This classification should be abandoned except to describe two forms of cohort study: prospective and retrospective.

The observational study is one where the investigator observes the natural course of events (Table 9.2). The experimental study is one where the course of events is deliberately altered. Most epidemiology is observational, for experiments are the exception. This classification is, therefore, of little practical help except that the biases and challenges inherent in descriptive studies are different from those of trials, as we will see (e.g. Table 9.5). The line of critical thinking for the reader of a descriptive study will focus on different matters (e.g. confounding) to that in a trial (e.g. randomization and blinding). These three classifications mentioned here are mostly needed to understand the epidemiological writings which use them.

Some alternative classifications may help readers. One important distinction lies with the presence or absence of disease at the beginning of a study (Table 9.2). Studies where the disease has already occurred focus on the risk factors that led to it or influenced its course. Studies where the risk factor is present but no disease has yet occurred focus on the occurrence of disease and other outcomes.

Another classification is between studies which incorporate a specific comparison group and those which do not (Table 9.2). Those with comparison groups are generally designed for testing hypotheses about disease causation. In epidemiology, we depend heavily on comparing and contrasting, comparing like-with-like, and ensuring that the principles we derive can be repeated and generalized across geographical areas and time periods. The use of a comparison population helps to achieve all this. (The comparison group is substituting for our ideal counterfactual findings.)

The five core study designs are now explained using the concepts of population (Chapter 2) and the natural history of disease (Chapter 6).

9.3 Case series: clinical and population-based register and administrative system studies

9.3.1 Overview

Table 9.1 gives a brief summary of these kinds of study and Table 9.2 indicates how they fit the five classifications. As you read you may wish to reflect on the questions on strengths and weaknesses of designs in Box 9.10, but do not read the answers in Table 9.5 until later.

The case reports are detailed summaries of patients' problems, usually focused on one disease. They are usually on one or a few cases, and are an essential learning tool of clinical practice. Case reports of rare disorders and, especially, previously unknown ones, can help develop ideas on case definitions and even ideas on causation and treatment. They are not, however, either research studies or epidemiological studies. When collected together (as a case series), however, case reports do shed light on the health of populations and are the simplest of study designs.

The clinical case series is usually a coherent and consecutive set of cases of a disease (or similar problem) from either the practice of one or more health-care professionals, or a defined health-care setting such as a hospital or family practice. Clinical case series are usually put together by clinicians on a topic of their interest. A case series is, effectively, a detailed local register of cases. These studies can occasionally be very large, especially when they are compiled by specialist associations through pooling resources.

The cases can be analysed to aid clinical practice and clinical research, and explored in an epidemiological way by seeking commonalities and differences in characteristics of cases. My work on Legionnaires' disease, for example, described in Table 3.3 and Figure 3.7, was done by me building on a clinical case series compiled by a laboratory clinician (my close collaborator the late Dr Ronald Fallon). One of the great classics of epidemiology is the hypothesis generated by the ophthalmologist Norman McAlister Gregg after his observation in 1941 of a series of 13 of his own cases of congenital cataract, and seven of his colleagues'. He devised and tested a hypothesis on why there should be so many cases of an extremely rare condition that year. The result was a new understanding of how a mild virus infection (German measles) in early pregnancy could seriously damage the fetus, and a worldwide rubella immunization programme to prevent it. In modern research there is an ethos favouring large, expensive studies, preferably trials or cohort studies. This ethos should not let the value of other kinds of work be overlooked.

The case series is a powerful weapon in medical practice and research, and in epidemiology—perhaps even indispensable. Clinical case series are of value in epidemiology, at least, for studying symptoms and signs and creating case definitions, and are important for clinical education, audit, and research. They are usually the first step in the study of newly discovered diseases or

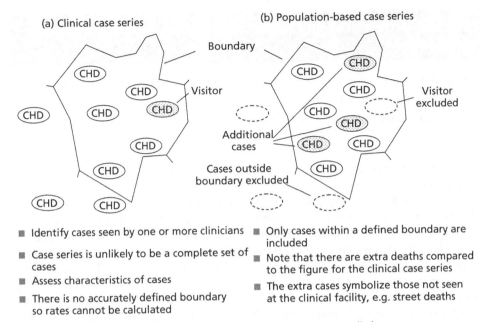

(a) Clinical case series

(b) Population-based case series

- Identify cases seen by one or more clinicians
- Case series is unlikely to be a complete set of cases
- Assess characteristics of cases
- There is no accurately defined boundary so rates cannot be calculated

- Only cases within a defined boundary are included
- Note that there are extra deaths compared to the figure for the clinical case series
- The extra cases symbolize those not seen at the clinical facility, e.g. street deaths

Fig. 9.1 Concept of clinical and population-based case series (registry studies).

other health problems, but they have also been adopted for long-term study of major common diseases including diabetes (e.g. Scottish Diabetes Register) and heart disease (e.g. GRACE, the Global Registry of Acute Coronary Events and MINAP, the Myocardial Ischaemia National Audit Project). The GRACE registry involves 30 countries, 241 hospitals, and more than 100 000 patients.

Figure 9.1(a) illustrates the concept of a clinical case series using coronary heart disease (CHD) deaths. Typically, a hospital clinician or group of clinicians would examine the case notes of all the cases seen, extract data, and analyse them to learn about the disease. As Figure 9.1(a) illustrates, some of the cases may, and indeed are likely to, live outside the defined geographical boundary and may well include patients from overseas. People living in the area, but not under the care of these particular clinicians, would not be included, and usually incidence rates or prevalence proportions cannot be calculated because the population corresponding to the list of cases cannot be defined well. In these circumstances, either some estimation of denominators will be needed, or proportional morbidity methods can be used (Chapter 8, section 8.2).

When a clinical case series is complete for a defined geographical area for which the population is known, and people outside that area are excluded, it is, effectively, a population-based case series consisting of a population register of cases. Figure 9.1(b) illustrates a population case series. There are two main differences from Figure 9.1(a). First, only cases within a defined geographical area are included and, second, extra cases that would not be in a clinical case series (e.g. street deaths, coroners' cases, etc.) are included. Effectively, a population case series is a collection of the cases seen by all clinicians serving a particular area, and also people living in the area but not seen by clinicians at all, or seen by clinicians working in distant parts. Ideally, temporary migrants and overseas visitors (and these may be overseas patients) should be excluded. Ideally, and this is difficult, local people becoming ill or dying when away from the area should be included. In essence, if a case arose from the denominator population it should be included if possible. In short, the list of diagnosed cases should be complete for a geographical area and particular time period.

Box 9.2 Differences and similarities in clinical and population case series

♦ Is there, conceptually, a difference between a clinical case series and a population one?
♦ What are the differences?
♦ In what circumstances are clinical and population case series identical?

To achieve this usually requires a well-administered system of data collection or a rigorous case-finding study, and usually both.

The biggest and epidemiologically most important sources of population case series are registers of serious diseases or deaths, and administrative systems recording health-service utilization (e.g. hospital admissions). These registers are usually compiled for administrative and legal reasons but are widely used by statisticians and epidemiologists. These types of studies are sometimes called registry studies. These data sets typically hold basic identification data and diagnostic data. However, with computerization of health records, cheaper computers and software, linkage of registers, and increasing demands of policy-makers and planners, the amount of information available is rising steeply. In many nations, the vision is of linkage-based detailed information systems (health and non-health) including much of the content of electronic clinical records. This vision, if (or perhaps more accurately when) enacted will create retrospective and prospective cohort studies of tens, perhaps hundreds of millions of people. Such data sets are already becoming dominant sources of epidemiological data. Reflect on the questions in Box 9.2 before reading on.

Conceptually there is no difference between these two types of data sets but the clinical case series is likely to be much more detailed. The main practical difference between the clinical and the population case series is that the former is likely to be incomplete. The cases will come from an undefined area and the source or base population from which they come may not be known accurately. The exception to this occurs when the clinician(s) compiling the series provides all the care to the population in a defined catchment area or has collected information on all cases diagnosed by other clinicians (including pathologists doing post-mortems) within that area. In these circumstances, clinical and population case series will be the same. This is unlikely to occur except for rare and distinctive diseases, or for rural areas with small populations and a single health-care provider. The difficulties of compiling a complete case series were discussed in Chapter 7 (section 7.4) in relation to counting the numerator for incidence rates. Reflect on the question in Box 9.3 before reading on.

Figure 9.2 shows a case series of patients with suspected and overt coronary heart disease. Clinical case series often include the dead. The cases are, therefore, at a variety of stages in their natural history and the spectrum of symptoms, signs, and severity is likely to be broad. By delving into the past circumstances of these patients, including examination of past medical records, and

Box 9.3 Case series and the natural history and spectrum of disease

How does the case series (clinical and population) contribute to our understanding of the natural history and spectrum of disease?

by continuing to observe them until death (and necropsy as appropriate), clinicians and epidemiologists can build up a piecemeal picture of the natural history and spectrum of a disease. The population case series is a systematic extension of this series which includes additional cases, such as those dying without being seen by the clinicians. Such cases will add breadth to the understanding of the spectrum and natural history of disease. For example, sudden death in the home setting from a first myocardial infarction will not appear in the hospital doctor's case series, but will in the population-based case series and will be particularly valuable if linked to post-mortem data. The hospital-based clinical case series might conclude that most people with myocardial infarction survive, but the population case series is likely to be contradictory—in fact, about 30 per cent of all people with a first heart attack die within 30 days, many of them never reaching hospital. The epidemiological approach seeks to turn clinical case series into population-based ones—a perspective that clinicians are increasingly sharing.

Making full use of case series data needs information on the source population both to permit calculation of rates, and to develop an understanding of the context in which the disease occurs. The choice, from the base population, of the population at risk for calculating rates needs an understanding of the biology of the disease and the purpose of the analysis. For example, for the dementia of Alzheimer's disease, the population at risk might reasonably be restricted to those over 65 years of age.

The population case series is the primary means of understanding the distribution of disease in large, national, and even international populations and to the study of variations over time, between places, and by population characteristics. (Readers will find this kind of work is often referred to as descriptive epidemiology (correctly) or ecological studies (wrongly).) Generally, these studies are done to describe rather than test generate hypotheses. Nonetheless, their label as descriptive studies downplays their potential. Furthermore, the case series designs can provide the key to sound case–control and cohort studies and trials (as we shall see).

9.3.2 **Design and development of a case series**

The design of a case series is conceptually simple. The investigator defines a disease or health problem to be studied and sets up a system for capturing data on the health status of, and related factors in, consecutive cases. The database may be as simple as this: reference number, diagnosis, or International Classification of Disease (ICD) diagnosis code, age, sex, alive or dead. Clinicians and clinician researchers could do this easily (given that a computerized health environment such a clinical case series could be generated easily). Obtaining these kind of data for populations defined by geographic area is, by contrast, a huge challenge. The difficulties of developing population case

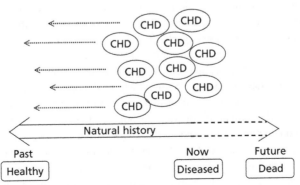

Fig. 9.2 Natural history and spectrum of disease in case series.

series are so great that many countries have no valid national data even for mortality. For example, India has a well-developed health service and service infrastructure with an established decennial census, but does not have comprehensive national mortality data. (Verbal autopsies, periodic surveys, and local data are substitutes.)

To make sense of case series data in an epidemiological sense, the key requirements are:

1. the diagnosis or, for mortality, the cause of death

2. the date when the disease or death occurred (time)

3. the place where the person lived, worked, etc. (place)

4. the social and economic characteristics of the person (person)

5. the opportunity to collect additional data from medical records (possibly by electronic data linkage) or the person directly if still alive (hence the value of a reference number that potentially gives access to personal details such as name, address, etc).

6. the size and characteristics of the source population from which the cases arose.

It is important, but not immediately obvious, that the need for item 6 favours collecting data around census years, or other years when population data are most accurate. Where case series data are collected continuously, there will be a case for analysing data around the census years. In some countries, there are no reliable population data so this principle is of no value. In others, there is an ongoing population register and if that is equally accurate at all times, the principle is unnecessary. Given such registers become inaccurate and may be corrected periodically, this provides an optimum time for such studies.

The date and time of death, for example, is recorded on the UK death certificate. The death data can thereby be analysed in relation to the time of day, day of week, month, season and, over the long term, by year, decade, or even century. When the death is not witnessed forensic methods can be used to judge the time and cause of death. Information on the main residence is also usually available on the death certificate. This can be used to find the postcode (zip code), map grid reference number, enumeration district (census tract in the United States), local government area, health authority area, region or state, and country. The home address is also vital to exclude from the analysis the deaths of visitors (a procedure which may not be routinely applied). Workplace address is important for many diseases but is not usually recorded in population case series, but will be in case series of occupational medicine clinicians. This information allows comparisons by place.

In geographical epidemiology, particularly in small area comparisons, the exact address is critical information in deciding whether the case is within the geographical area of interest. Computerized information systems usually record postcode (zip code), not address. Except in national studies, there are difficult decisions to be made on people living near the boundaries of the study area. Decisions on which small area a person lives in can be critically important, especially in investigations of rare disease (e.g. childhood leukaemia).

Population denominator data are usually only available on a predetermined grouped basis, that is, the number of people living in a particular area. In small area studies, the geographical boundary required for a study may not match that for which the denominator data are available. In this case, map grid references based on the full postcode or full address may be used to re-assign location to the areas where denominators are available, but even then errors are inevitable, depending on the precision of the method of conversion. If individuals' data are available in the denominator database, matching methods may lead to a linkage between numerators and denominators. This data set would no longer be a population case series but a retrospective cohort study. An example was described as an exemplar in Chapters 7 and 8, that is, the Scottish Health and Ethnicity Linkage Study.

In compiling a case series, data on some characteristics are easily obtained, such as sex and date of birth. For most other characteristics, obtaining reliable and valid information is a problem, for example, on race, ethnicity, religion, occupation, income, or socio-economic position. The problem of inaccurate information on the diagnosis was discussed in Chapter 7 (section 7.4). The veracity of diagnoses needs to be checked by validity studies of diagnoses in the database. Effectively the work done in making the diagnosis, and listing the cases, is treated as for a screening test and compared to a more definitive (gold standard) data set (usually the fuller medical record).

Where clinical diagnoses of death are not available, 'verbal autopsies' may be done where relatives are quizzed about the circumstances of death and this information is used to code the cause of death. Extra work will be needed to supplement the basic database.

The population case series register is unlikely to hold information on the natural history of disease although some cases may have repeated entries/records over long time periods that can be linked up. This is particularly true of primary care (general practice, family medicine) case series where the full medical records may provide extra details. However, case series data can be linked to other health data either in the past or in the future; for example, mortality data can be linked to hospital admissions including at birth and childhood, cancer registrations and other records to obtain information on both exposures and diseases. The cases may also be contacted for additional information on their lifestyles, socio-economic circumstances, family history, and so on. In effect, this type of action turns a case series design into a cohort design (described later).

9.3.3 Analysis of case series

Ideally, case series data are analysed using incidence rates, and this is normal when there is a denominator (Chapter 7). There are at least three circumstances, in particular, where rates are not used. First, in the study of spatial clustering of disease, techniques of point pattern analysis based on the grid reference, created from an exact address or postcode (zip code), may be preferred. The level of expected clustering may be assessed using a second case series of another disease as a control. Clearly, the chosen control disease will be one not expected to show spatial clustering. The second circumstance is when the population is stable as is usually the case for studies of short time periods, as in an examination of the number of deaths by hour of the day, or day of the week. The analysis here is on the count of cases. Even if denominator data were available for such short time periods (improbable) it would be unwise to use them, for the errors in measurement of the denominator would outweigh any advantage. The third case is when there is no suitable denominator, for example, in case series derived in occupational settings, where accurate information on the population at risk is unavailable, or the study is of a sub-population, for example, an ethnic group which has not been identified in a census or a population register. The partial solution usually adopted is to use proportional mortality/morbidity ratios, as explained in Chapter 8 (section 8.2).

Rates derived from population case series sometimes pose serious problems of interpretation. Many clinicians are likely to be contributing to the data set. In the case of national statistics, there may be tens of thousands involved. Even for a register of a common disease in a single city, there may be several dozen clinicians involved. The investigator, therefore, may have little control over the quality of numerator data, particularly in the case definitions applied and variations in diagnostic methods. The case series may cross time periods when accurate denominator data are not available, and this is usually so, except in and around the census year. Awareness of the problem, training of clinicians and coders, use of agreed disease classifications such as the ICD, and basing studies around the census year are partial solutions. Above all, however, epidemiologists' awareness and thoughtful interpretation of such data is essential.

Table 9.3 Sources of data for case series (register) studies: examples

Clinical case series	Population-based case series
Disease registers created by individual doctors or groups of doctors, e.g. chronic disease registers	Death registers
	Cancer registers
Disease registers created by specialist associations by pooling specialist experience, e.g. nationally MINAP, internationally, the GRACE registry.	Hospitalization registers
	Notification of infectious disease registers
	Prescriptions databases (if patient identification data are present)
	Child health surveillance registers

Population-based case series have great advantages to counter their disadvantages; for example, data sets may be complete over long periods of time (for deaths even more than 100 years), there may be huge numbers of cases, and there are likely to be comparable case series in different regions in one country and internationally. Much important epidemiology centres around such data, which are the key to health-service administration, health and public health policy and strategy development, burden of disease studies, and the spur to hypothesis generation and occasionally also testing.

Table 9.3 lists some major sources of clinical and population-based case series.

9.3.4 Unique merits of and insights from case series: large-scale studies, and ecological and atomistic fallacies

Studies based on population case series permit two, arguably unique, forms of epidemiological analysis and insight. Reflect on what these might be using the question in Box 9.4 before reading on.

First, they can provide a truly national and even international population perspective on disease. A dream of mine is a global register of the health of every person in the world that would be used to monitor health, deliver care, and undertake research. The mobile phone is likely to make the dream a reality and future population case series may be on hundreds of millions or even billions of people. Second, the disease patterns can be related to aspects of society or the environment that affect the population but have no sensible measure at the individual level (see also Chapter 2, section 2.5). These kinds of studies need huge national, even international data sets. Some indicators of the social, economic, and physical environment are not calculable at an individual level (e.g. income equality); do not exhibit individual variation within a geographical area (e.g. ozone concentration at ground level and the thickness of the ozone layer in the Earth's atmosphere); or are not available in the required accuracy in large data sets (e.g. income). For

Box 9.4 Making use of indicators with little variation at national or regional level and with no valid individual measures

How might epidemiology study the potential role in disease causation of factors that vary little between individuals within a region or nation? For example, factors such as fluoride content of the water, the hardness or softness of water supplies, or weather? These kinds of factors sometimes have no valid or possible measure at individual level.

Box 9.5 Applying individual data to populations and vice versa

- Reflect on whether observations on individuals are always applicable to populations and vice versa.
- Can you think of examples of when this is so and when it is not?
- Why do you think this happens?

---

example, studies have related international rates of multiple sclerosis to the latitude of the country, mortality rates to income inequality in a region or country, and infant mortality rates to the gross national product.

Sometimes health status or exposure data are available for an aggregate population but not for each individual separately. In these cases, the relations between these aggregate measures are studied. For example, we may know the fluoride content of the water in the health authority areas of a country but not the fluoride intake of individuals. We may also know the amount of expenditure on oral health, and from that the payments made for fillings, teeth extraction, and so on, but not the oral health status of each individual. These two data sets could be studied to seek associations. This type of study, based on aggregate data, is often referred to as an 'ecological' or correlation design.

The viewpoint that case series studies (whether based on individuals or aggregate data) are descriptive, observational, and as a result weak, is inappropriate. These studies are the bedrock of epidemiology and are gaining strength in the modern era of 'big data', and also of relative austerity, recovering from the 2008 economic crisis. In this era, low cost studies are desired and electronically linked health databases are seen as one promising direction.

One prominent criticism of studies based on populations studied in aggregate is known as the ecological fallacy. The ecological fallacy is commonly referred to but not so for the atomistic fallacy. Try the exercise in Box 9.5. These two fallacies and the exercise in Box 9.5 are further discussed in section 9.9. The weakness of case series studies lies in the quality of data, and is not inherent in the study design. These studies offer some unique opportunities and perspectives on the pattern and causes of disease in populations, and provide a solid platform from which to explore the pathways to disease causation. Sometimes, they provide the only way to explore causality in human populations when we need to integrate causes at various levels of social organization and environment. The reason for that is pragmatic, however, not theoretical. For this kind of work, data are needed on millions of people over large geographical areas. Currently, only population case series can provide this. (This may change as the large biobank type studies become available although many of them are not tied to clearly defined geographical settings.) Virtually all epidemiologists will use, perhaps compile and analyse, case series data in their work. Further issues relating to analysis of data from these studies are in section 9.11.

Many of the points in this section, for example, on quality of the diagnostic data, are transferable to all the designs.

9.4 Cross-sectional studies

9.4.1 Overview

As stated in section 9.3.1, Table 9.1 gives a brief summary of this study design and Table 9.2 shows how it fits into five classifications. As recommended, you may wish to reflect on the questions relating to the strengths and weaknesses of these studies in Box 9.10. Do not, however, look at the answers in Table 9.5 until later. A cross-section is the shape that results from cutting right through an object. In doing so we expose and study a part of it.

A cross-sectional study exposes and studies disease and risk factor patterns in, preferably, a representative part of the population, in a narrowly defined time period. The data are usually collected by one or more of the following methods: questionnaire, interview, examination, and blood and other tests. Medical records may also be accessed by permission of the study participants. The rarely used synonym, prevalence study, captures the key role of cross-sectional studies in epidemiology. The general term *survey* fits the cross-sectional study well. In addition to measuring prevalence, the cross-sectional study seeks associations between risk factors and diseases and helps generate and test hypotheses. By repetition in different time periods, it can be used to measure change, and hence evaluate interventions or describe trends. Its focus is simultaneously on disease, population characteristics, and risk factors. Comparisons between subgroups within the sample are usually made.

The study can be, but is usually not, designed with comparison groups. When this is done, it is mainly a case of adjusting the sample size of subgroups to ensure there are enough people to make the desired comparisons. The measurement methods may sometimes need to be adjusted too; for example, in a multilingual population the questions need to be designed to give comparable answers even after translation. The comparisons are usually based on differences in the prevalence of risk factors and diseases, and the association between risk factors and diseases in different subpopulations, for example, men versus women, or employed versus unemployed.

9.4.2 Design and development of a cross-sectional study

An ideal cross-sectional study is of a geographically defined, representative sample of the population studied in a narrow slice of time and space. Figures 9.3 and 9.4 illustrate the idea in relation to prevalence of CHD. A target population is defined (here, all ovals within the boundary in Fig. 9.3). A list is made or obtained of the target population (called a sampling frame). A sample of the population at a point in time is taken (here shaded ovals, though sometimes all people in the target population are studied). Measurements are made, preferably simultaneously, to identify people with the characteristic(s) of interest; in this case, CHD. Assuming that the shaded ovals are representative of the population within the boundary, the findings on the sample are generalizable to the whole target population. There are, of course, limitations of random statistical variation and the method of selection of the sample, so generalization will need to be cautious.

Sometimes results are generalized beyond the target populations. For example, if the prevalence of CHD is two per cent in Liverpool, England, can this information be used in Newcastle, England? The answer is, probably, yes. This result is, however, unlikely to be valid in Newcastle, Australia. We would need to ensure that the characteristics of the populations of the two cities are similar and then generalize with caution. If the population in Liverpool is of a different age, sex, and ethnic structure from that in Newcastle, England, the extrapolation should be avoided. The alternative to making such extrapolations is undertaking national studies, or locality-based studies, both of which are expensive and difficult endeavours. For this reason, extrapolation is done more commonly than scientific rigour would recommend.

Rarely, cross-sectional studies are of the whole population. The national population census is a cross-sectional study, albeit an extremely large one, and one where the cross-section is only in time and not space. (In some countries demographic data are held in a population register. This is not a cross-section, like a census, but the demographic equivalent of the population case series.) A survey of the blood pressure of all the patients registered with a particular doctor is also one of a whole (or target) population, albeit a small and narrowly defined one. Harland *et al.* (1997)

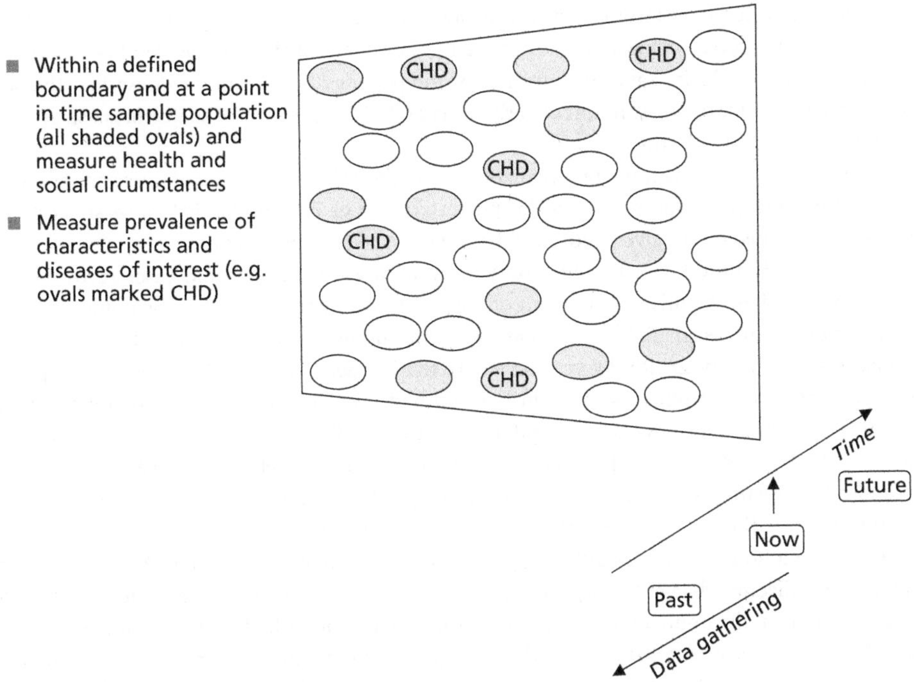

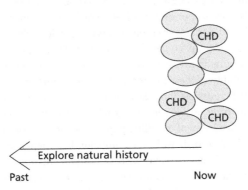

- Within a defined boundary and at a point in time sample population (all shaded ovals) and measure health and social circumstances

- Measure prevalence of characteristics and diseases of interest (e.g. ovals marked CHD)

Fig. 9.3 Population concept of a cross-sectional study in relation to time.

reported a study which attempted to measure the prevalence of diabetes and coronary risk factors of all Chinese-origin people in Newcastle, England; an example of a cross-sectional survey based on the whole target population, sometimes called a census sample. This is sometimes done when a sampling frame cannot be constructed, that is, the target population cannot be listed, so we try to find everyone.

Cross-sectional surveys are sometimes said to provide a snapshot of health. This is a simplistic but helpful analogy. The selection, compilation, and definition of the target population and the listing of the sampling frame usually conform to the snapshot analogy, that is, the people are present at a point in time. Measurement of risk factors and disease, however, is usually made over a

Fig. 9.4 Natural history of disease in cross-sectional studies.

period of time which varies from as little as a day to several months, though rarely several years. A rare example of a truly snapshot study is the measurement of the prevalence of bedsores in a Glasgow hospital on 21 January 1976. Ironically, the paper's title inaccurately describes this as a study of the incidence of pressure sores (Barbenel *et al.* 1977). This kind of snapshot is usually only possible in institutional settings.

In most studies, the measurements are made over a relatively short period of time such as a year. The merit of collecting data over a year (as portrayed in Figs 7.1 and 7.2) is that seasonal differences will be evened out to give a more valid annual measure of prevalence.

If there is a dynamic but balanced state with new cases arising and old cases recovering in equal numbers, then the mismeasurement of the point prevalence proportion by doing the study over a period of time is small. The mismeasurement of point prevalence is likely to be important for diseases which vary greatly by year or where the incidence is changing rapidly. The prevalence proportion of a problem such as in hospital bedsores, for example, may be much higher in winter than summer. Obviously, hospitals tend to be fuller in winter so there will be more patients. The kind of patients also changes in winter with more elderly people admitted with hip and other fractures—the kind of condition that predisposes to bedsores—so the prevalence proportion rises. The date on which the study was done is important. To gauge the true picture, repeat cross- sectional studies at different points of the year may be advisable. Alternatively, the strategies of collecting data at the beginning of and then over a year (period prevalence) or doing surveys in parts of the population across the year might also provide the better estimate (Figs 7.1 and 7.2). For the measurement of a rapidly changing phenomenon, such as the use of different kinds of illicit drugs in teenagers, the cross-sectional study would need to be conducted quickly (and repeated) to give useful results.

9.4.3 Analysis, value, and limitations of cross-sectional studies

The cross-sectional study design is excellent for measuring the population burden of both risk factors and disease using prevalence proportions, the most reliable summary measures obtained from such surveys. We considered the measurement of prevalence in Chapter 7 and prevalence proportions in subgroups can be compared as for the relative risk (Chapter 8), though the interpretation is a little more complex. There is no need to analyse cross-sectional studies using odds or odds ratios (though this is, unfortunately, common). As a denominator is always available, there is no need for proportional morbidity calculations.

In theory, when the data on past diseases from a cross-sectional study are accurate, the disease incidence can be estimated if non-response bias can be adjusted for and deaths are rare. In practice, collecting disease incidence using a cross-sectional design is a problem, mainly because study subjects' memory of diseases is poor and medical records may be incomplete. The possibility of estimating incidence should not, however, be dismissed, particularly for populations and topics that do not easily permit follow-up studies; for example, young people joining the workforce (18–25 years), migrants from rural to urban areas in the developing world, or ethnic minority groups in the inner city. The mobility of these groups is high and cohort or case series studies to collect incidence data may not be possible, not least for lack of accurate denominators. Some topics, such as the use of illegal drugs, experience of sexually transmitted disease, or sexual behaviour, are so sensitive that the possibility of enrolling populations for follow-up cohort studies is small and information in medical records will be incomplete. Experience shows that cross-sectional studies are feasible for these issues. We may wish to study the incidence of gonorrhoea in young men of 18–25 years. Reliable incidence data are not available because it is treated in both primary care settings and sexually transmitted diseases clinics. In a cross-sectional study, information on whether and when in the last year the people in the sample had a diagnosis of gonorrhoea could be elicited to estimate its incidence. As clinic records are incomplete, population census denominator data are unreliable, and the possibility of long-term follow-up of a representative sample of this population is small, the cross-sectional study offers a way of measuring incidence, albeit not an absolutely ideal one, which other studies cannot achieve. People can also be asked for permission to access other records so supplementary data may be obtained.

An example is shown in Table 9.4, which is from the study summarized in Table 4.8 and Exemplar 4.1. Here the incidence of consultation for asthma with a general practitioner (physician) has been calculated, as well as the prevalence of asthma. A cross-section of people was identified from the list of people registered with general practitioners held by district health authorities. Medical case records of this sample were examined. (Of course, we could have asked these people directly, but it is more convenient and easier to get the data from the record.) The study illustrates that cross-sectional studies can do more than measure prevalence. Later, we will reflect on the similarity between this design and a retrospective cohort study (section 9.6).

Data about the past medical history and other circumstances can be, and usually are, collected. This is illustrated in Figure 9.4 in relation to the natural history of disease. In a cross-sectional study of a sample of the general ('well') population, there will be people representing virtually all stages of health and disease, and the full range of exposures of interest. They will represent a wide spectrum of disease. Cross-sectional studies can only give indirect insights on the natural history.

People with severe disease, however, may be institutionalized, sometimes permanently, for example, in care homes, convalescence hospitals, or asylums for the psychiatric patients, and either not on the sampling list from which the sample was drawn or not available for study. For example, in a study to measure the prevalence of heart failure, people with the most severe disease may be missed because they are hospitalized long-term, or may even have died since the sample list was prepared. While it is usual practice to exclude the recently dead from cross-sectional studies, there is no principle at stake here. Data on dead people could be collected from clinical records or from acquaintances and family. For pragmatic reasons, the recently deceased are usually excluded. This leads to survivor bias in cross-sectional studies whereby the most severe, possibly fatal, variants of disease are missed. This imbalance can be partially corrected, as discussed next.

Other points related to analysis are in section 9.11.

Table 9.4 Reasons for consultation by area in a cross-section of people registered with general practitioners in three areas of north-east England (shown here as zones CA, CB, CC)

	Zone CA	**Zone CB**	**Zone CC**
Number of people	734	724	734
Incidence rate (cumulative) of consultations per patient-year	3.97	4.45	3.86
Incidence rate (cumulative) of asthma diagnoses per patient-year	0.04	0.05	0.06
Prevalence proportion per thousand patients for asthma	74	97	113

Adapted with permission from Bhopal RS, Moffatt S, Pless-Mulloli T, Phillimore PR, Foy C, Dunn CE, Tate JA. Does living near a constellation of petrochemical, steel, and other industries impair health?, *Occupational and Environmental Medicine*, Volume 55, pp. 812–822, Copyright © 1998 BMJ Publishing Group Ltd.

> ## Box 9.6 Differentiating between a case series and a cross-sectional study
>
> Reflect on the difference between a case series study and a cross-sectional study of diseased cases, basing your thinking on a particular problem such as heart failure or diabetes.

9.4.4 Cross-sectional studies in relation to the iceberg, spectrum, and natural history of disease

In studies of the apparently well people in the community, cross-sectional studies discover people with previously unknown disease, that is, they uncover the iceberg of disease. A simple example of this is of a cross-sectional study focused on obesity. It is likely that the pulse rate and blood pressure will also be measured. People with previously unknown problems with heart rhythm (e.g. atrial fibrillation) and high blood pressure will be identified. The full spectrum of disease can be described only by a combination of cross-sectional surveys of the apparently well population and of the diseased population, the latter more often obtained from clinical case series than from cross-sectional studies. Cross-sectional studies help to piece together the natural history of disease, particularly the early stages, by asking well people about their earlier lives—that is more difficult to do when people are seriously ill.

9.4.5 Cross-sectional studies in relation to case series, and potential for comparisons

The investigator may choose to restrict the sample, for example, by studying only people with disease. The sample may be taken from a register of people with diabetes for example, with the purpose of measuring, at a point in time, the prevalence of smoking in relation to diabetes and its complications. Such registers often include the recently dead and the full spectrum of disease. In doing this we have done a cross-sectional study within a case series or, even better when possible, within a population case series. Reflect on the exercise in Box 9.6 before reading on.

To recap, a case series studies a coherent group of cases (or potential cases, i.e. those consulting) accrued over a period of time, sometimes over the entire career of a clinician or life of a clinic or service. By comparison, the cross-sectional survey studies all or a sample of the patients under care at a specified and usually narrow interval of time. For example, studies of all patients ever seen at a diabetic clinic, or those seen consecutively over a year, are case series. The study of all or a sample of patients on the diabetes clinic's list at a point in time, perhaps to check the proportion taking medication, is a cross-sectional study. The distinction is subtle, and emphasizes the interrelationships between study designs.

The cross-sectional study can be of populations in different places, so comparisons can be made (as in Table 9.4). Studies can also compare people with different characteristics, for example, there may be a sample of women and another of men, or one of people belonging to a Chinese-origin population and another of the Indian population. Such studies are comparative cross-sectional studies. (But they are not case–control studies, which are discussed next.) If a new sample is taken a year later and the study is repeated, then that new work is a cross-sectional study. If, however, the same sample is used, then the work becomes a cohort study as discussed in section 9.6.

9.5 Case–control studies

9.5.1 Overview

As stated in section 9.3.1, Table 9.1 provides a brief summary of this design and Table 9.2 shows how it fits the five classifications. Reflect on the questions in Box 9.10, but do not, however, look at the answers in Table 9.5 yet.

The term *case–control study* is actually referring to a suite of studies with slightly different designs but the same underlying concept. In this account, as in practice these specific labels are not widely used, I use the single phrase to include the others; for example, case–cohort design, density case–control (both case-base studies). In Chapter 8 I noted that the odds ratio sometimes gives an exact estimate of the incidence rate ratio (relative risk or rate) and this is so for some designs. These are complex design and analysis issues and readers should consult more advanced texts for further information.

The case–control studies are comparative where people with the disease (or problem) of interest are compared with an appropriate control group. The meaning of the word *case* is close to its medical use to describe the characteristics and medical history of a patient. The comparison, control, referent, or reference group (all synonyms) supplies information about the expected risk factor profile in the population from which the case group is drawn. (The control group is a practical substitute for the counterfactual—discussed in Chapter 5—i.e. what would have happened to the cases if they could have relived their lives without the same exposure to the risk factor, here substituted by the control group.) The cases are compared with controls, associations between the disease and potential risk factors are measured (usually by the odds ratio—section 8.5), and through analysis of similarities and dissimilarities, hypotheses about disease causes are generated or tested.

9.5.2 **Design and analysis**

While they are sometimes used for hypothesis generating, case–control studies are best reserved for hypothesis testing. Therefore, hypotheses, research questions, and objectives should be specific enough to focus the inquiry. The case–control study is mostly used for advancing causal understanding so prior causal knowledge should be summarized, perhaps including causal diagrams (Chapter 5). We have already considered the main output of these studies, the odds ratio, in Chapter 8.

The next challenge, and usually one of the easier ones, is to find the cases. The cases can be obtained from a number of sources: a clinical case series; a population register of cases; the cases identified in the follow-up of a cohort study; and from those identified in a cross-sectional survey. The ideal set of cases would be new (incident) and early diagnoses, and representative of all cases in the target (base) population under study. The cases from a population case series register and cohort studies usually meet this ideal the best. The cases identified in a clinical case series are usually highly selected. The exceptions will be those rare diseases where the clinicians compiling the case series see most, if not all, the cases that occur in the target (base) population. Cases from a cross-sectional study are usually prevalent ones, though there will be incident cases in a period prevalence study. Prevalent cases are not ideal because they are selected from survivors, may have had the disease for a long time, and maybe they have thought long and hard about their past exposures to risk factors, quite possibly generating their own hypotheses and even false memories. So, a consecutive series of recently diagnosed cases is preferred.

The harder challenge is to select the control group. As for all comparative work the ideal, counterfactual control group (the same people and here same cases without the exposure of interest) is not achievable (see section 4.2.4). This concept, however, points to what we are looking for. Classically, the emphasis was placed on the control group being free of disease. This emphasis does not fit with the current concept of this design. The control group represents the population from which the cases arose. We should be sampling to try to achieve that.

There are three main approaches to selecting controls. First, we can define the control group at the starting point of the study. Imagine we recruit 300 children aged 5–12 years with newly diagnosed eczema between January 2008 and December 2009 from a primary care setting. We can define 300 (or more) controls in January 2008. Some of them may have, or in due course, be diagnosed with eczema but they could remain in the control group (although these cases could also be removed as it unlikely to make much difference—the investigator should tell us what they did, why, and what the consequences were). Controls can, perhaps confusingly, be in both the case and the control group for analysis. This case–control design is known more specifically as the case-base study. This design provides an odds ratio that is equivalent to the cumulative incidence rate ratio, that is, relative risk, and the rare disease assumption is not needed.

Secondly, as cases arise, we can find appropriate controls so they are recruited over the same timescale as cases, that is, concurrent sampling of controls. It is normal practice to find controls without the disease, but even this is not essential. This design provides an odds ratio that is equivalent to the person–time incidence rate ratio, again without the rare disease assumption.

The third approach is to find controls at the end of the study (i.e. Dec 2009). These will exclude cases as they are already in the study. In this design, the rare disease assumption in the calculation of the odds ratio applies.

Information is obtained on the social and medical history of cases and controls and on potential causal, mediating, effect-modifying and confounding factors. As the causal factors have already had their effect in causing disease in the case group, and the information required is recalled from the past, the case–control study was commonly, and still is sometimes, referred to as a retrospective study, but this is not a helpful term (see also section 9.2). It is important to emphasize that while key data are gathered in each person at one time (say 5 August 2015) the enquiries may, and probably will, range over a long period of time, perhaps even from birth or before; for example, asking about the mother's smoking habits during pregnancy. Even for the outcome of CHD, the enquiries will not just be about health status now but also signs, symptoms, and related tests in the past. A systematic method of collecting data e.g. the life grid approach may be helpful (Edwards *et al.* 2006).

The basic idea is shown in Figure 9.5. Even if this is not explicit, there is an assumption that the source population for cases and controls is known and is the same for both groups. If not, there is no way of interpreting and generalizing the results. Ideally, the cases are related to a defined known source population (all ovals in Fig. 9.5). If the aim of the study is to explore the causes of coronary heart disease (marked on Fig. 9.5 as CHD), then preferably a consecutive series of new cases would be identified. From the same population are drawn a set of control subjects, marked with the letter C in Figure 9.5. These control subjects should be chosen with no selection in relation to their pattern of exposure to the postulated causes, but should otherwise be similar to the cases. If, for example, the study was on exercise as one of the causes of CHD in post-menopausal women of about 50–75 years, then the control group should also be of women in this age group. Obviously, recruitment of men or children into the control group would be inefficient, and if they were included in the analysis, this would be highly misleading. This strategy is called restriction and it is helpful both for confounding (Table 4.4) and for maximizing the efficiency of the study. (There is an exception to this: in case–control studies examining the role of genetic variants that are not on the sex chromosomes, which are fixed at conception, these restrictive strategies are not needed—the same principle could potentially apply to other risk factors.)

In some studies, controls are recruited to match each case; for example, if a woman of 53 years was recruited as a case, the investigator would seek a woman as control of similar age (57 would be fine, but maybe not 72). This tight matching process is reducing the risk of confounding, here by age and sex. If a mix of ages is likely to arise anyway, the control group can be recruited without one-to-one matching, particularly in large studies. Matching cases and controls on several characteristics, such as sex, age, ethnicity, smoking status, and social class, is not advisable. Such complex matching procedures create difficulties in finding controls, require more complex statistical

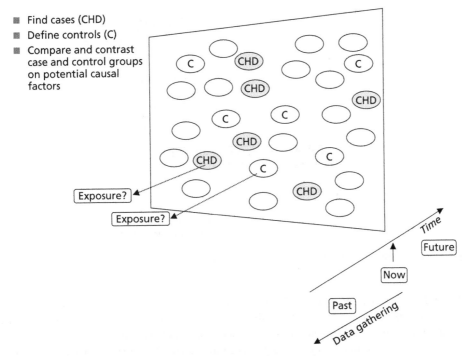

- Find cases (CHD)
- Define controls (C)
- Compare and contrast case and control groups on potential causal factors

Fig. 9.5 Population concept of a case–control study in relation to time.

analysis, and run the risk of overmatching. Overmatching leads to missed associations because the causal factors have been inadvertently matched for. For example, in the aforementioned study of CHD and exercise, if we matched women for smoking status, social class, and income, we may find no association between CHD occurrence and exercise habits, because exercise, smoking, social class, and income are linked. The matching process has created a selection bias, such that differences between cases and controls in exercise habits have been removed or reduced. To avoid this it is advisable to match on few variables.

Information is collected to confirm, objectively, the presence of disease in cases. In some, but not all, types of case–control study the absence of disease in controls is also confirmed (though, of course, controls may be at a prediagnostic phase of the disease's natural history). Information is collected on the past exposure to factors that may have caused the disease. This is shown in relation to the natural history of disease in Figure 9.6. Since CHD develops over years or decades (and risk factors may operate even *in utero*, or be transmitted by previous generations) the collection of information on the causal exposures will need to delve deep into the past, and inevitably, this will be fraught with difficulty. In interpreting associations and inferring causality, it is essential to establish that the cause preceded the effect. In relation to physical activity and CHD it is vital to check that some symptoms of early CHD (before a diagnosis is possible) did not alter exercise habits; for example, breathlessness on climbing stairs could inhibit exercise so the disease could have caused the change in the risk factor—a phenomenon called reverse causality.

The concept behind the analysis is clear: to find differences in exposure to the hypothesized causes in the past lives of cases as compared with controls. It is unusual for case–control studies to pay attention to similarities but these do provide important information that these factors do not seem to be important potential causes.

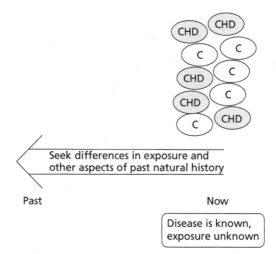

Fig. 9.6 Natural history of disease and case–control studies.

These differences can be quantified and summarized either as differences in the prevalence proportion of exposure as in the past, or more usually in modern times as the odds ratio, which estimates the relative risk (Chapter 8). An exposure that may have caused disease will be more common in cases than in controls giving an odds ratio greater than one, and one that may protect against disease will be less common, giving an odds ratio less than one. An odds ratio of one means there is no association. For exposures that are continuous measures, for example, mean serum cholesterol or time spent doing exercise, the average, or mean, value will be compared. It is tempting to convert these data to yes/no outcomes using cut-offs—for example, does this person take the recommended amount of exercise or not (currently 150 minutes per week in the United Kingdom). This kind of simplification should be resisted, as there is loss of information. Here, for potential causes the mean value will be higher in cases than controls and vice versa for protective factors. Other matters relating to analysis are in section 9.11.

9.5.3 Population base for case–control studies

The need for a population base for a case–control study is an especially interesting, and possibly not obvious, issue. Of the epidemiological designs, this one is most focused on establishing aetiology and least on measuring burden of disease or risk factors, which are by-products. So why should it be population-based? Surely, it may be argued, a finding of a difference between cases and controls is informing us about differences irrespective of whether the population base is known or not.

A classic study by Herbst *et al.* (1971) on the occurrence of the extremely rare disease of adenocarcinoma of the vagina in girls and young women illustrates the issues. The study demonstrated an association between the disease and use of a drug, diethylstilboestrol, by mothers of cases in the first 12 weeks of pregnancy; seven of eight cases were treated with the drug compared with none of the 32 controls. This result was statistically unlikely to occur by chance; an odds ratio was not calculated but if it had been, the result would be infinity. Might it be argued that the striking findings tell an underlying biological truth independent of the population base? Do the exercise in Box 9.7 before reading on.

There are both conceptual and pragmatic reasons why this apparently clear-cut study needs, and benefits from, a population base. We must know the geographical area and the time period

Box 9.7 Case–control studies and the source population (base): example of the study by Herbst *et al.*

◆ Why do we need an understanding of the source population (base) both to execute the study and interpret the findings?

◆ In what way would the study be impaired if the population base were unknown?

when the cases occurred to draw an appropriate control group. In fact, the cases were in the United States of America. If the cases of the rare adenocarcinoma of the vagina are from all over the country, and have been admitted to one or a few hospitals because of the reputations of the local surgeons, the control group also ought to be a USA-wide sample. Taking a local control group may mislead us. For example, if the local area physicians had a policy for not using diethyl-stilboestrol, while there was no such policy in the rest of the country, a local control group would lead to a spurious association; that is, the control group would have a low exposure to the risk factor under examination because of a local policy.

We also need to know whether the cases are typical of all cases to evaluate the public health importance of the findings. Do the findings of this study apply to this disease generally? If the selection of cases in the case–control study is not known, this question cannot be answered satisfactorily. We need to be particularly careful that the cases were not selected for reasons related to the exposure under study, for example, adenocarcinoma of the vagina in girls whose mothers had threatened miscarriage (the condition for which the drug was given). Even if, indeed especially if, such a hypothesis has been aired, the cases must not be selected with regard to it.

On a pragmatic note, the validity of the estimate of relative risk in a case–control study, the odds ratio, is based on the assumption that:

◆ the cases are a fair sample of the incident cases drawn from a known and defined population;

◆ the controls are drawn from the same defined population and would have been in the case group if they had had the disease under study;

◆ controls are selected in an unbiased way, for example, independently of exposure status; and

◆ in some, but not all, types of case–control studies that the disease is rare;

◆ in some designs that the exposure distribution in the source population is stable.

Case–control studies are, for these reasons, best conducted within a population framework. One source of cases and controls that meets these criteria is the population-based cohort study as discussed next. Case–control studies can be conceptualized as part of a theoretical population cohort, even when they are not part of an actual cohort. Additional issues relating to analysis are covered in section 9.11.

9.6 Cohort study

9.6.1 Overview

As mentioned before, Table 9.1 provides a brief summary of the design and Table 9.2 an analysis based on five classifications. Reflect on the questions in Box 9.10, but look at the answers in Table 9.5 later.

It is common to hear people, particularly clinicians, speak of 'their cohort', usually meaning a group of patients, irrespective of the study design. This is not what we mean in epidemiology

but it reflects that our technical terms have other meanings in normal language. In epidemiology the cohort is a group of people with something in common, usually an exposure or
involvement in a defined population group who are enrolled in a follow-up study. Merely being
associated with a group being cared for by a doctor or health-care facility does not warrant the
term cohort.

Currently, cohort studies are mainly used for hypothesis generation and testing. The cohort
study involves tracking the study population over a period of time, a feature reflected in three
other words for this design: follow-up, longitudinal, and prospective. Another, but dated, term
for this kind of design is a *panel study*. Curiously, as we shall discuss, we can do cohort studies
retrospectively too, so prospective study is a poor label.

As with the cross-sectional survey, the cohort study population may be a general one, or one
with characteristics of particular interest, for example, people with a defined lifestyle or even
a disease. The hallmark of this design is that health data are obtained on the same individuals
in a population on more than one occasion, not just once as in the cross-sectional study or the
case–control study. The idea is to study part of the natural history of risk factors or diseases in
individuals, and to relate one or more characteristics, exercise for example, to future outcomes
such as coronary heart disease (Figs 9.7 and 9.8 illustrate this point).

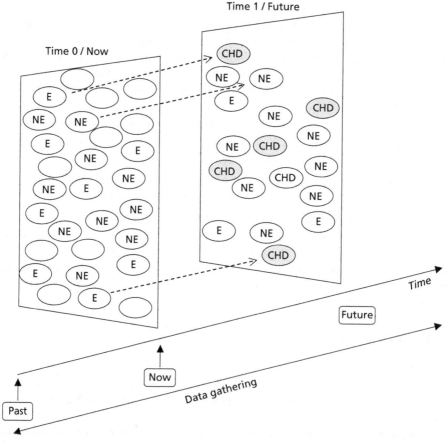

Fig. 9.7 Population concept of a cohort study in relation to time.

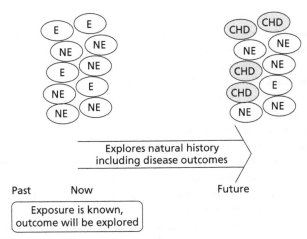

Fig. 9.8 Natural history of disease and cohort studies.

9.6.2 **Design, development, and analysis: prospective and retrospective cohort studies**

While it might seem sensible to choose our study populations on the basis of the presence or absence of the risk factor of interest, perhaps surprisingly, this is rarely done, with the exception of drug or other medical exposures. This, however, illustrates the ideal concept. More often, the cohort population is assembled, exposures measured, and study subgroups then defined. Conceptually, however, the ideal cohort study would recruit people with and without the risk factor.

In Figure 9.7 two groups are identified in the base population (all ovals): those who exercise (ovals marked E) and those who do not (NE). These two groups are followed up to ascertain the new cases of the outcome (CHD), thereby calculating a disease incidence rate. Data are collected after the point of construction of the sampling frame and assignment of exposure status. This applies to retrospective cohorts too. Figure 9.8 shows that cohort studies are future orientated in relation to the natural history of disease, while case–control and cross-sectional are past orientated. Cohort studies are better than other designs for studying natural history.

Comparison groups are usually identified within the cohort (e.g. people who smoke or do not smoke). This actually means that many exposures can be studied within the one cohort study. It is not uncommon for hundreds of variables to be studied simultaneously. In some such studies, hypotheses are not specified in advance and, as such, these cohort studies are hypothesis generating rather than hypothesis testing. Sometimes separate sub-cohorts by exposure are set up at the outset. In these, the study is usually exploring a specific hypothesis, which dictates the nature of the comparison group.

If a particular exposure or characteristic of interest is rare, then the identification of separate cohorts will be necessary. Enrichment of the study sample with people with such exposures, or so-called boosted sampling, will be necessary in these circumstances. Mostly, researchers expect to find enough people with the exposures of interest in their large cohort samples.

In causal research, cohort studies test the hypothesis that disease incidence differs in people with different characteristics (exposures) at baseline; that is, there is an association between exposure and outcome.

The cohort study begins by establishing baseline data, usually from a cross-sectional study (but not usually of a representative population-based sample), or less commonly by the extraction of baseline data from sources such as the census or a routine information system such as a birth register. In cross-sectional studies of prevalence, samples representative of the source population are essential but, perhaps surprisingly, this is not so important in cohort studies unless their primary purpose is to measure incidence rate. More often, they aim to measure the association between risk factors and outcomes. These associations tend to be quite robust and are not affected greatly by the population chosen; for example, the relationship between cholesterol and CHD is very similar across all populations.

The cohort can either be followed up directly with repeated surveys of the same population or the baseline data can be linked to health or other records, so providing information on outcomes of interest, usually disease-related but potentially also on changes in and associations between risk factors. The new cases of disease identified are incident cases and can be enrolled into a case–control study. Controls can also be identified from within the cohort, and this is often done as each case occurs. This is known as a nested case–control study. (See also section 9.5.2 on controls in case–control studies.) This is a very valuable option as case–control studies can provide similar statistical precision as a cohort study with only a fraction (10% or even less) of the sample size. This property and design also reflects the interrelationship between case–control and cohort studies.

Where medical records permit accurate assessment of both risk factors and disease outcomes, only possible when data are collected systematically (and preferably computerized), cohort studies may be possible without any new data collection. The label retrospective cohort study is then applied. Essentially, the cohort is identified from past records of exposure status and this is the vital step. Usually, the outcome data are also obtained from records but this information can be supplemented with direct questioning of those subjects who are alive, and can be traced. Once identified, the subjects can be followed up over time (prospectively) so using both currently available and future data on outcome. Figures 9.9 and 9.10 illustrate the concept of the retrospective cohort in the context of populations and the natural history of disease. In Chapters 7 and 8, the exemplar panels were based on the retrospective cohort study known as SHELS (Scottish Health and Ethnicity Linkage Study).

The conceptual difference between this design and the prospective cohort is minimal; a retrospective cohort is assembled from historical records on exposure status, the prospective cohort on exposure status in the present. You should seek out the differences between Figures 9.7 and 9.9. The great strength of the retrospective cohort is its low cost and speed, but it is limited by what data were collected and can be linked. By contrast, the prospective cohort study gives the investigators great freedom to specify and control data collection. The practical work to implement these studies is, however, very different. Before reading on, reflect on the question in Box 9.8.

This question in Box 9.8 is difficult. The study in Table 9.4 is, in my view, not a prospective cohort—we did not collect any information prospectively. It does, however, have similarities with a retrospective cohort study. Arguably, the feature that makes the study in Table 9.4 a cross-sectional study and not a retrospective cohort is the construction of the sampling frame using a contemporary list of people living in the area of interest and collecting information retrospectively. The information on health is retrospective from the point at which the sampling frame was prepared in the 1990s. If the investigators had constructed a list of people living in the same areas (zones A, B, and C) in, say, 1940, and looked at consultation patterns prospectively from that point, say 1941–1946, this would have been a retrospective cohort study. This exercise teaches us a new lesson and reinforces one made on several occasions. The new lesson is that assigning studies into a specific category of study design is not easy and is somewhat superficial, although academic journals sometimes insist on a design label. These labels are sometimes wrong so the readers should take care. The reinforced lesson is that study designs overlap and merge.

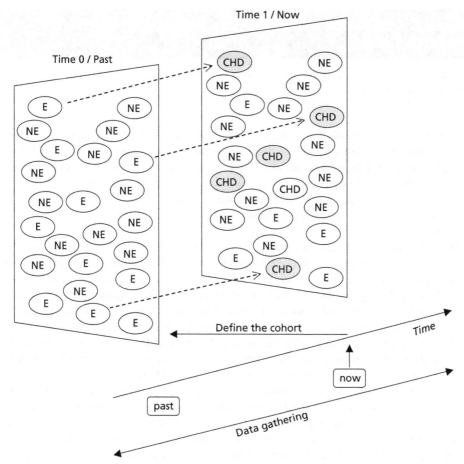

Fig. 9.9 Population concept of a retrospective cohort study in relation to time.

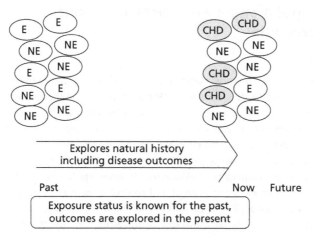

Fig. 9.10 Natural history of disease and retrospective cohort studies.

Box 9.8 Comparing a retrospective cohort with the study in Table 9.4

What is the essential feature that differentiates the cross-sectional study in Table 9.4 from a prospective cohort study?

Cohort studies are described as analytic (Table 9.2) but one of their main functions is to provide information on the incidence and the natural history of disease (to describe) and not just to explore or generate hypotheses, for which they are extremely useful too. If the cohort study is based on a defined and well-characterized population, the incidence rates can often be extrapolated beyond the study group to similar populations elsewhere. This is especially easy when the cohort is based on a representative population, which is, however, unusual except for retrospective cohorts.

The most important information from a cohort study, nonetheless, is on incidence rates. Unless the cohort group has been assembled and followed up over a short period of time, the amount of time people spend being observed will vary greatly. Over long follow-up periods, members will leave the study, develop the outcome and hence no longer be at risk, emigrate, or die. As explained in Chapter 7, the person–time incidence rate is the ideal way of handling such data. The ratio of the incidence rates in the exposed and non-exposed groups derived from the cohort study is the relative rate or risk, the primary basis for measuring the strength of an association, one of the keys to causal thinking in epidemiology. The calculation and interpretation of incidence rates was discussed in Chapter 7 and the relative rate and risk was discussed in Chapter 8. There are, however, many other kinds of analysis possible in cohort studies, for example, change in risk factors (blood pressure, cholesterol, weight, etc.) or disease severity. The time to occurrence of outcomes allows survival analysis. There is an unparalleled richness and flexibility in prospective cohort studies, especially when follow-up is from birth to death, and they are designed to be multigenerational. The exemplar for Chapter 1 was the Framingham Cohort Study and for Chapters 7 and 8 SHELS. You may wish to re-read these accounts. Cohort studies best exemplify the essence of the strategy of epidemiology and are, currently, the dominant force, even though trials are even more coveted as discussed next. Other matters relating to analysis are in section 9.11.

9.7 Trials: population-based clinical and public health experiments

9.7.1 Overview

As before, Tables 9.1 and 9.2 provide a brief summary and description of the design in relation to five classifications. Reflect on the questions in Box 9.10 and look at the answers in Table 9.6 later.

Trials are experiments and evaluations where an intervention, usually designed to improve health, has been applied to a population, and the outcome assessed at follow-up. It could reasonably be questioned whether trials, and other similar studies evaluating interventions, are part of epidemiology. Trials and experiments are the mainstay of the laboratory and clinical scientist, and their evolution has been advanced by statisticians. However, epidemiology includes in its definition the application of knowledge to prevent and control disease and improve health. Trials are important to this aspect of applied epidemiology by helping find effective interventions to this end. Epidemiology can certainly lay claim to a contribution towards the development of trials. Indirectly, trials also help us understand the causes of diseases. For example, if an intervention increasing exercise leads to less CHD, it is indirect evidence that low exercise levels might also cause CHD. Such studies may help us to understand disease causes, assess the effectiveness of interventions designed to influence the natural history of disease by improving prognosis, and weigh up the costs and benefits of changing services or treatments.

Trials are experiments, and may be described by various terms including intervention studies, clinical trials, and community trials. Experiment is a word that is viewed suspiciously by the public so is best avoided, though is a more accurate one than trial. The term 'trial' in medicine and public health is usually reserved for experiments that are not performed in the laboratory setting, and are on humans. The trial has a similar design as a cohort study with one vital difference—that the exposure status of the study population has been deliberately changed by the investigator (Figs 9.11 and 9.12). This has huge implications for the ethics of research, both in terms of consent, and for ensuring safety of participants.

Clinical and public health trials are costly, difficult, and important endeavours, which usually have a practical question to answer, mostly on whether a particular intervention is sufficiently effective to be introduced into clinical or public health practice. The majority of trials evaluate drugs, but in this account I prefer to emphasize studies on humans and epidemiological and public health, rather than the clinical/pharmaceutical, perspective. The principles are identical, though the practice is much harder for the former.

Trials that are to be applied need to be based on a study population with proper understanding of how it relates to the (target) population, which will be offered the intervention should it be

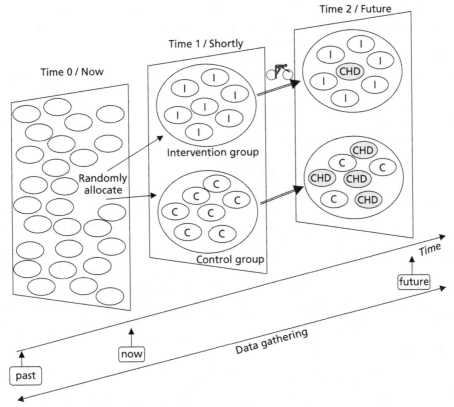

Fig. 9.11 Population concept of a trial in relation to time.

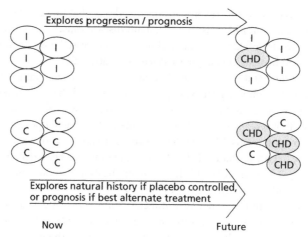

Fig. 9.12 Natural history of disease and trials.

shown to be successful. An intervention that works in a selected population may not fulfil its goals when put into public health or clinical practice in the general population.

Some trials are, however, designed solely to produce knowledge about cause, mechanism, and effect, the intention being to test the efficacy of the intervention in actual practice at a later date. For these trials, sometimes called proof of concept trials, with their limited purpose, understanding the relationship of the study population to the target population is not essential (but still advised). These proof of concept studies are often on paid volunteers and these are not the focus of this account. In this account, we will assume some intervention is ready for population-level evaluation. (This kind of trial is known as a phase III trial.)

In trials of actions aiming to prevent disease or death, the intervention may be either an active intervention, say enrolment into a diet and exercise programme, or the attempted manipulation of a natural way of life, such as reducing the consumption of salt. Such trials are more difficult to do than trials of treatment based on drugs, for they require complex interventions, usually of modest potential impact, in complex circumstances.

9.7.2 Design, development, and analysis

The essential and first requirement for a trial is a promising intervention but one where its effectiveness is still in doubt. Such interventions need not be new, for there is still much doubt about the value of many interventions that are in routine use. The intervention should not be so good, however, that a trial is completely unnecessary (i.e. that there is no need for evaluation).

The development of such interventions is a major research exercise that itself may cost hundreds of millions of pounds for drugs and millions of pounds for public health interventions. For example, in the Born in Bradford 1000 study, more than £2 million pounds (about $3m) was spent to lay the foundation of evidence, and test the feasibility of preventing overweight and obesity in infants. The work took five years, after which a feasible and promising intervention was identified (McEachan *et al.* 2016). The intervention has been modified and now funding is being sought for a full trial. Trials are not suitable for unsubstantiated ideas.

Let us assume that in our trial we want to reduce CHD by increasing exercise and that we have developed a promising exercise programme—the first step.

The second step is to define a study population suitable for answering the question, that is, people either with disease (for clinical trials), early stage disease (for screening trials), or without disease (for prevention trials). Ideally, this study population will be drawn from the target population, perhaps those who could potentially benefit, as shown in the ovals in the first box in Figure 9.11, which is a trial of exercise in the prevention of CHD. Unfortunately, usually trials are on highly selected, non-random groups of people, such that relating the results to the target group is nigh impossible. Most drug trials, for example, are done on the middle-aged groups without multiple health problems, whereas the target population in terms of their use is the elderly population with multiple health problems. We then divide the study population into two or more groups, the intervention group(s) and the control group(s). The way we divide them is critically important and discussed shortly. In the figure the intervention, symbolized by a cyclist, is an exercise programme.

The control group may be offered nothing or (better) the best known alternative but one that does not work through the same pathways (e.g. meditation classes), or an activity with no major expected effect on the outcome (e.g. participation in a pottery class). Trials should only be done to resolve reasonable uncertainty. There may be circumstances where the uncertainty is about the amount of an intervention that will be effective. In those circumstances, different amounts (doses) of the intervention may be used.

In the recently completed prevention of diabetes and obesity in South Asians trial (PODOSA), led by myself, the investigators agreed that the control group would be given basic information in a four-visit programme and that would be compared to a 15-visit intensive, personalized, interactive programme of dietary and exercise advice. This was deemed ethical and less than this for the control group was deemed unacceptable (Bhopal *et al.* 2014). The important thing is that, excepting the intervention, the two groups gain an equal amount of attention in the study. Otherwise, the changes seen might be attributable to differences in the amount of attention each group receives, not the intervention itself. The intervention group provides information on prognosis, the control group on the natural history (although this may be affected by the placebo or alternative intervention offered to this group). The control group is acting as a counterfactual contrast.

In the ideal trial, the study and control populations are at the same stage of the natural history of disease (Fig. 9.12), and are similar in the characteristics that affect disease outcomes, differing only in exposure to the intervention. This emphasis on comparability at the design stage, rather than adjustment of outcomes at the analysis of data stage, is a hallmark of modern day trials. Indeed, without this a trial would lack credibility and, for this reason other kinds of intervention studies, for example, with no control group, or a historical control based on what happened in the past without the intervention, are not considered here. The investigator who cannot include a control group—and there are sometimes good reason for that—will need to use other evaluation methods.

To minimize the chances that the intervention and control groups are different at baseline, and hence minimize confounding, the trial design should ensure that individuals in the study are assigned randomly to the groups. There are several ways of assigning study subjects randomly. As this is a critically important issue, increasingly, the randomization process is done by individuals or organizations (clinical trial units) who are independent of the running of the trial. This process solves the problem of finding the matching control group. This is the closest we get to the counterfactual comparison in epidemiology. If comparability is achieved, the groups are said to be exchangeable. Exchangeability cannot be assumed, and needs to be empirically demonstrated. In large trials, the laws of chance work to create two comparable groups through random allocation. This is a randomized, controlled trial.

Where there is no 'best known alternative', an intervention which is 'psychologically' of similar impact to the study intervention, but has no influence on the diseases process is used (a *placebo*, from the Latin word meaning 'to please'). This is a placebo-controlled, randomized trial. The placebo for the control is necessary because all interventions have general effects even though the intervention itself does not work in the specific way the investigators think it does. Although the word placebo implies that this general effect is a helpful one, this is not true. The effect may be harmful and might be more accurately described as a *nocebo* effect (from the Latin for 'I will harm'). These effects are powerful and probably underpin much of the success of good healers including physicians. The mechanisms for these effects are complex and psychological, including the recipients' expectations. If they expect relief they may get a placebo effect and if they expect harm, then a nocebo effect. In the modern era, as with randomization, a trial that does not account for such effects will not be credible.

These effects are not just important in research but also in practice. The commonest prescribed drugs in industrialized, wealthy countries are statins, given to prevent cardiovascular outcomes by reducing low density lipoprotein cholesterol. Trials indicate they are extremely safe and that side effects are rare, similar to a placebo. Yet, a high proportion of people stop them because they have problems. This may be well be an example of the nocebo effect. There is also a broader lesson about trials here—the real world implementation of the results and recommendations of trials may be quite different to that in the trial setting.

To prevent bias, the subject, the field investigator, and the subjects' health carer might not be told whether the subject receives the active intervention or the control intervention (they are so-called blind). This is a triple-blind, randomized, placebo-controlled trial (if the investigator and either the subject or the health carer do not know, this is 'double-blind'). Blinding is very difficult for many complex interventions. Even for drugs patients and their carers may recognize whether they are on the active or placebo pill even though these look identical. The active pill may have a specific side effect, say heartburn or nausea. Investigators should also be careful the placebo pill does not have an ingredient, such as lactose sugar, that is difficult for billions of people to digest.

For the trial in Figure 9.11, as is characteristic for trials of public health interventions, it would be impossible to disguise who is getting the intervention to increase exercise and who is getting the control intervention. Such trials are rarely placebo controlled. Those who know the allocation of groups should not, ideally, make the measures of outcomes to avoid bias. This may, however, be costly and difficult to arrange. In the PODOSA trial mentioned already in this chapter, the final trial outcomes (weight, waist, and circumference) were made by research nurses hired to do this one task (Bhopal *et al.* 2014). They were not told which group the person being measured was in. Sometimes daring solutions are applied, especially in trials of surgery, including real versus sham surgery where the person is cut open but sewn up without surgery. This illustrates the consensus on the importance of placebo effects in trials.

We now follow-up the study populations and count or measure the outcomes of interest; in the example in Figure 9.11, the number of cases of coronary heart disease and, in the PODOSA trial, the weight. Analysis is by comparing the outcomes, for example, incidence rates of outcome (Chapters 7 and 8), calculating relative risks (section 8.4) and numbers need to treat or prevent (8.11), the QALY (8.10), and other event-based measures that are beyond the scope of this book. Event-based outcome trials usually are both large and lengthy. Continuous measures such as blood pressure, cholesterol, weight etc., are much less demanding in these regards and are popular because they make trials more feasible. Most usually, however, the events that matter to people are illness, disease, and death.

In large randomized trials, confounding is usually unimportant, though any remaining differences between groups will usually be adjusted for statistically. The greater problem is loss to follow-up, meaning there is incomplete data. If there is an effective placebo, this may not be differential (biased) loss but it reduces the sample left for analysis. The still-bigger problem is that some people do not adhere (comply) with the intervention. There is a temptation to restrict the analysis to those who adhere but the gold standard is compare the groups as originally constituted, this being an 'intention-to-treat' analysis.

So far we have considered trials of individuals but the unit of study may be larger, for example, families, neighbourhoods, workplaces, schools, hospitals, and even countries. These are called cluster trials. The principles are similar to those discussed. Specialized methods of analysis that take account of the clustering are often needed.

As with other designs there are many variants of trials, and for details you should consult advanced or specialist books. Other matters related to analysis are in section 9.11. We now turn to something similar—natural experiments.

9.7.3 Natural experiments and the special case of Mendelian randomization

The hallmark of the trial is that the intervention under evaluation has been imposed on the study participants by the investigator (or a collaborating individual or agency). Other kinds of studies, especially cohort studies, can also be thought of as also exploring interventions, for example, smoking cigarettes, getting immunized against small pox, brushing your teeth, etc. These interventions are self-imposed, while external people or environmental factors may impose others. The key difference is that the investigator has no control over the level of exposure, and there is no randomization. So, confounding remains a potential, serious problem.

There are some circumstances where the distribution of the exposure among subgroups of a population is, effectively, random. For example, some places have, naturally, a high fluoride level in the water, while others do not. People who settle in an area do not know what the fluoride content is. Imagine we compared the level of caries, the decay of teeth that is protected by fluoride, in a 100 similar towns across a nation, half of which had high fluoride and half of which did not. If the residents and those doing the measurement did not know what the fluoride level was, this study would be like a trial where different amounts of fluoride were put into the water by the investigators. This is what is called a natural experiment, because nature has determined the level of exposure.

The phrase *natural experiment* has been extended to similar circumstances, even when the intervention has arisen from human endeavour. The most famous example is from Dr John Snow's investigation of the causes of cholera in London. At that time, water was supplied by several private water companies taking water from the River Thames. The river in London was contaminated, so in 1844 the British parliament required water companies to draw their water upstream of London. One of the suppliers, Lambeth Water Company, complied with this, while another, namely the Southwark and Vauxhall Company, did not. Both companies supplied water to houses in the vicinity where cholera was present. Effectively, a grand experiment had taken place though in an unplanned way. There seems to have been no order in the distribution of water, so it was virtually at random. John Snow investigated the distribution of both cholera cases and the source of water. He calculated there were 315 deaths/10 000 households being supplied water by the Southwark and Vauxhall Company compared to 37/10 000 for those supplied by the Lambeth Company. He also showed how the rate of cholera infection declined after the Lambeth Water Company changed its supply. Strictly speaking, this is not a trial or an experiment (and not natural), but it is close to being one.

Taking advantage of these kinds of circumstances can provide compelling evidence quickly and at low cost. There is a resurgence of interest in these kinds of 'natural experiments', especially in the evaluation of policy implementation. The collective term natural experiments is appealing.

In Chapter 3.3 and especially the end of section 3.3.1, I introduced the genetic process of meiosis and said it underpins the concept of Mendelian randomization. Since the last edition of this book, Mendelian randomization studies have established themselves as important contributors to epidemiology, especially in the testing of causal hypotheses. Mendelian randomization is the grandest of natural experiments, and unlike most natural experiments, the exposure really is very close to randomized, so they could be described as randomized, natural experiments. There is a difference from real trials, however, as the kind and amount of the intervention is dictated by nature, not the investigator. In section 3.3.1, we took an example of a gene variant that leads to high serum cholesterol and another that leads to a lower serum cholesterol. For simplicity, let us imagine there is only one gene and one chromosome that affects serum cholesterol. Let us further imagine that a mutation has occurred such that people with it have a 10 per cent higher serum cholesterol than others and that if both alleles are affected 20% higher cholesterol. This mutation might be perpetuated and become common in the population. In the population, then, we will have people with these variants:

(a) Higher cholesterol variant on both of the pair of chromosomes (10% increased cholesterol each, 20% in total assuming the effects add up)

(b) Higher cholesterol variant on one of the pair of chromosomes (10% increased cholesterol)

(c) Higher cholesterol variant on neither of the pair of chromosomes (normal amount of cholesterol)

Scenario (a) requires that both parents have the gene variant. Let us assume only one parent had it and concentrate on groups (b) and (c) for simplicity. Which group you belong to is determined at conception and at random by the process of meiosis. It is quite hard to think of how these two groups might be subjected either to bias or be different from each other, so potentially leading to confounding. If so this allows a direct test of the hypothesis that a 10 per cent rise in cholesterol leads to an increased incidence of, say, coronary heart disease. This hypothesis helps us assess causality.

We need to undertake gene testing on people to find those with the variants so described and also a source of outcomes data. In fact, virtually any sample of the population where this variant exists will do because the exposure here must precede the effect.

There are some important assumptions behind the method. There needs to be a gene variant that actually leads to a sufficient change in the risk factor of interest for it to make a difference. In our example, a 10–20 per cent increase in serum cholesterol meets this requirement. Then, there needs to be an assumption that a genetically determined rise in the level of a risk factor has an effect of the same kind as those from non-genetic factors that also alter the cholesterol (e.g. dietary fat). So, the genetic variant is acting as a proxy (or instrumental) variable, that is, it is an indirect measure of it. We have to assume that the possession of this proxy variable is not associated with and hence does not influence other factors that might alter the risk of the outcome, for example, dietary behaviour, exercise, smoking, or even another biochemical factor, say another lipid or inflammatory factor relevant to CHD. This is generally true, with the exception that genes tend to influence other genes, but it needs to be demonstrated.

It might be thought that Mendelian randomization studies are suitable only for physiological and biochemical risk factors but their applications have been much wider. There are gene variants that influence behaviours; for example, milk consumption is affected by gene variants for the gene that makes lactase, the enzyme that allow digestion of the milk sugar lactose. Those who have a variant that fosters persistence of lactose in the gut drink more milk. They do not usually consciously know this, or behave this way because they know. There are similar mechanisms that relate to alcohol consumption and even smoking cigarettes.

The special value of Mendelian randomization is for checking potential causal hypotheses. If the high cholesterol variant is associated with raised CHD incidence, then that fits with a well-established hypothesis based mainly on cohort studies and gives us confidence that the association is

Box 9.9 Three major assumptions of Mendelian randomization studies

1. The genotype is associated with the exposure of interest
2. The genotype is associated with the disease only through its effect on the exposure under study
3. The genotype is not associated with other factors (whether other genes, or phenotypic traits) that also affect the disease

causal. If it does not raise CHD, it alerts us that other studies that show the association may be confounded. Of course, the Mendelian randomization study may be wrong too.

These are still early days for Mendelian randomization studies in epidemiology. There are many complications that are beyond this book's scope but the general principles of study design all apply. Extension of these methods is occurring rapidly. The exemplar panel for this study illustrates this method. Three major assumptions of the method are in Box 9.9.

Exemplar 9.1: A Mendelian randomization study of high-density lipoprotein cholesterol (HDL-C) in relation to myocardial infarction (heart attack) (Voight, B.F. *et al.* 2012)

Background comments

The causal relationship between LDL-C, so-called 'bad' cholesterol, and CHD, of which myocardial infarction (MI) is one manifestation, is established. There is much evidence that another lipid HDL-C, so-called 'good' cholesterol, is protective against CHD. The evidence for this is less clear. In particular, there are important behaviours, for example, exercise which raises HDL-C, and traits (e.g. female sex) where HDL-C is higher, that would be confounding factors in this relationship. Changing HDL, however, is difficult and drugs to raise it have important side effects. It is important to be absolutely sure that the HDL-C/CHD relationship is causal to make public health policy. Randomized controlled trials (RCTs) to establish this are problematic. Mendelian randomization approaches are promising and in this context a necessary step.

The study by Voight *et al.*

There were more than 120 authors of this study, which is indicative of the need to pool resources for Mendelian randomization research. Sample sizes need to be large as the strength of the association of genotypes and the risk factor, here HDL-C, tends to be small.

The method

The genetic markers

The authors used a genome-wide association study (GWAS) approach to identify single nucleotide polymorphisms (SNPs)—mutations, but think of them as risk factors—that were associated with blood lipid concentrations. They identified one SNP that was on a gene specifically associated with HDL-C (LIPG ASN 396 seer). They used the data to construct a genetic score based on both this one gene and 14 other SNPs associated with HDL-C.

The study design

The authors used both (a) case–control and (b) cohort designs. They combined them so this work includes meta-analysis.

(a) MI cases (19 139) and controls without MI (50 812) were pooled from 30 individual studies. The candidate SNPs were compared in cases and controls. A pooled odds ratio was obtained. They called the change in odds ratio the risk.

(b) Six cohort studies with 50 763 participants had 4228 MI outcomes. The SNP that was specifically associated with HDL was used to measure the association with HDL cholesterol in cohort participants who had not had a previous MI or stroke. The association between genotype and HDL-C was measured in people who had 0, 1, or 2 copies of the gene variant (allele) specifically associated with HDL-C. From this measure, the predicted association between the genotype and MI was calculated.

The use of this specific genotype as an instrumental (proxy, unmeasured) variable was assessed statistically.

Results

I have produced a summary of the complex results in Tables A9.1 and A9.2 in appendix 9.1. Of the identified LDL-C SNPs associated with LDL-C levels, 9/10 were statistically significantly associated with MI in the case–control analysis. Only six of 15 HDL-C associated SNPs were associated as expected, that is, negatively; one was positively associated and for the others, there was no statistically significant association.

In this analysis, the specific HDL-C genotype was not statistically significantly associated with the outcome in the case–control study. Nonetheless, the investigators focused on this genotype because the six statistically significant SNPs were also associated with either a lower LDL-C or triglycerides, so they were not suitable for Mendelian randomization.

The specific HDL-C related SNP is uncommon in the population (2.5%). It was known to be associated with a 0.14 mmol/l greater HDL-C concentration. This specific SNP was not associated with known MI risk factors (10 are listed in the paper), so it was suitable for Mendelian randomization.

The authors calculated that carriage of this SNP should lead to a 13 per cent reduction in MI. Using odds ratios, they predicted the OR in carriers of this SNP would be 0.87 with a 95% CI of 0.84–0.91.

The test of the prediction was in six cohort studies. In fact, the OR was 1.10 with a 95% CI of 0.89–1.37. This further corroborated the result from the case–control study. They compared the result using a standard increase in HDL-C of 0.03 mmol/l (and 0.39 mmol/l) using epidemiological methods and Mendelian randomization, with former the results in the table A9.1. The results contradicted each other.

They, finally, compared a genetic risk score for LDL-C and HDL-C and the results showed an increased risk of MI with LDL-C and a small, much less than expected, and statistically not significant, reduced risk with HDL-C.

Discussion

The authors start by discussing animal experiments. In mice one study indicated that the specific gene variant under study reduced atherosclerosis, but another did not. Animal evidence was inconclusive. They then noted that trials of hormone replacement therapy and of niacin raised HDL but did not reduce MI. They then discussed the limitations of Mendelian randomization and the statistical power of the study. They noted three other Mendelian randomization studies gave similar findings. They judged their approach was sound. They concluded that some approaches to raising HDL-C might not lead to reduced MI.

Concluding remarks

This work exemplifies how genetic epidemiology dovetails with traditional epidemiological methods. Here case–control and cohort study designs have incorporated genotypes as risk factors. If we accept that the assumptions underpinning Mendelian randomization have been met—and here they seem to have been—we have the added value of a grand experiment of nature.

Overall, this evidence is powerful in concluding that a causal relationship between HDL-C and MI (and by reasonable extrapolation, other atherosclerotic cardiovascular disorders) has not been established. Our main caveat may be that non-genetic factors which raise or lower HDL-C may have different effects from genetic factors that do the same. Is that plausible? Whether it is or not, it still needs to be borne in mind.

These methods are a powerful addition to the epidemiological toolbox. The method has burst into epidemiology in the last 15 or so years and exemplifies how dynamic and cross-disciplinary our discipline is.

Source: data from Voight *et al.* Plasma HDL cholesterol and risk of myocardial infarction: a mendelian randomisation study. *The Lancet*, Volume 380, Issue 9841, pp. 572–80, Copyright © 2012 Elsevier Ltd.

9.8 Overlap in the conceptual basis of study designs, designs mixing methods, choices, birth/age/period effects and strengths, and weaknesses

Unlike most textbooks I have not devoted a chapter, or even a separate sub-chapter, for each study design. Rather, I have emphasized the unity of purpose and of conceptual approach. This unity goes beyond the point that has been well emphasized in recent years that case–control and cohort studies can be unified by conceptualizing them both as samples of a defined population followed over time in a defined area. Rather, and in addition, I have emphasized that in practical terms one design can easily become another.

The cross-sectional study, for example, can be repeated using the same sampling methods to evaluate changes in time. The participants in the second study will be different from those studied in the first, although there may be, by the laws of chance, some overlap. This is simply a repeat cross-sectional study (and not a cohort as sometimes implied). If some public health intervention had been applied between these studies, say a no-smoking in public places ban, this second study would make a contribution to evaluating the intervention. This is not a trial but it is like one—perhaps a natural experiment. If, however, the same sample is studied for a second time (i.e. it is followed up), the original cross-sectional study now becomes a cohort study. If an intervention such as a no-smoking ban were introduced in between, this could be said to be a 'before and after' trial, but it is neither controlled, nor randomized. As we have already noted, such a study would have low credibility, but conceptually it belongs to the evaluation/trial family.

The cohort study can also be turned into a trial. The key difference between a cohort design and a trial is that the investigator observes the study subjects in the former but imposes an intervention in the latter. If, during a cohort study, possibly in a subgroup, the investigator imposes an intervention, a trial begins. For those in the intervention group, it is no longer a cohort study.

Indeed, there have been proposals that as trials are so hard to recruit into they should be embedded in very large cohort studies, where people have already been recruited. The cohort study can also give birth to case–control studies. When people with a particular disease are compared with a comparison group, the study is a case–control study. Ideally, the case–control study should be of new, or incident, cases. Cases that are newly discovered in a cohort study are ideal. These are called nested case–control studies and they add value to the cohort by making the research process efficient. The point is that the cohort study can also provide the controls. If the numbers are large, only a sample of potential controls in the cohort may be needed. This is a good strategy especially if costly tests need to be done. Case–control studies need much smaller sample sizes for estimating relative risks than cohort studies. Therefore, tests might only be done on cases and the selected controls.

Cases in a clinical or population case series may be the starting point of a case–control study or a trial. The case series for other conditions may provide controls too. Case series registers may also provide the data on outcomes for a cohort study or trial. In the PODOSA trial we looked at earlier, the participants are linked with their permission to the Scottish Diabetes Register, which is a centralized database of all diagnosed patients (hence a population case series) (Bhopal *et al.* 2014). We are informed when our trial participants develop diabetes. A cross-sectional study of people in a case series is also possible, where people on the list are surveyed at a point in time.

These kinds of similarities and interrelations, overlooked in classifications which emphasize the distinctions in study design, integrate study designs. The important thing is to understand the principles behind, and the defining features of, a particular study design and what it can do.

Not every epidemiological study fits neatly into one of the basic five designs in Box 9.1. However, such atypical studies are usually variants and amalgams of the basic designs, which can be grasped with an understanding of the key features and purposes of the five designs discussed. Table 9.5 develops this point by listing a range of epidemiological studies with their focus and main aims, and then indicating some possible design options.

Table 9.5 Focus of aim and design of some epidemiological studies

Focus of study	Main aims	Some possible design(s)
Produce disease counts and description based on cases and incidence rates	Establish size of case-load; define characteristics of disease; generate hypotheses based on factors in common (similarity of cases)	(a) Case series, preferably part of a large well-established clinical or population disease register that can be associated with a population denominator (b) You would only undertake other studies if there is no case series available. But, if necessary you could achieve these goals with a cohort study, albeit a large one (as is happening in India and China)
Produce incidence rates of disease or death, in relation to risk factors, particularly to further understanding of causality	(a) Establish disease rates; assess variation over time, place, and characteristics of cases; generate or test hypotheses (b) As above plus study natural history of disease; seek associations between risk factors and disease taking account of confounding and moderating factors	(a) Population case series with cases related to population usually defined by a census or other register but causal understanding is likely to be limited (b) Cohort studies with populations defined by exposure to risk factors. Sometimes retrospective cohort studies will suffice but mostly prospective cohort studies will be needed

Table 9.5 Continued

Focus of study	Main aims	Some possible design(s)
Produce international disease frequency comparisons	Explore across countries similarities and differences in disease proportions or rates, explore the relative importance of environmental and genetic factors in disease, and generate hypotheses	(a) Population case series, related to population census or other register, or, in absence of data, (b) Multicentre cross-sectional study or, (c) Multicentre cohort study
Produce prevalence of disease or risk factors data	Quantify disease and risk factor burden; seek associations between disease and risk factors; generate hypotheses	(a) Cross-sectional study but if this is not feasible consider, (b) Case series of living people in a disease or at risk registers related to a population census or population register. You may be able to link to a source of risk factor data, e.g. primary care records
You have access to cases of a disease and you need an answer quickly, especially for rare diseases, on possible causes	Generate or test causal hypotheses by producing estimates of the association between a disease and risk factors	Case–control study
Evaluation of interventions	Quantify the impact of an intervention on health status taking into account the placebo effect and the need for comparability of groups To assess effectiveness of interventions in decreasing disease, improving health or reducing risk factors	Randomized controlled trial, or if this is impossible, less vigorous variants of trials When trials are impossible case–control designs and repeated cross-sectional studies may help Observations of change over time in population case series data

Before reading on, complete the exercise in Box 9.10.

Some of the strengths and weaknesses of each study design are given in Table 9.6. This is not a complete list. Full discussion of each point is beyond the scope of this book, and will be found in books concentrating on methods. The important point is that each study has strengths. The 'hierarchy of evidence', whereby the trial and meta-analysis of trials reigns supreme only applies to evaluation, particularly of drugs. Other designs are stronger for measuring the burden of disease and in generating, testing, and further exploring causal ideas.

As the history of epidemiology has demonstrated, causal understanding comes from all types of study, and above all through deep reflection on disease patterns, however they are generated (see Chapter 5, e.g. Table 5.9). Understanding the concepts behind each study is essential in choosing, interpreting, and evaluating reports of studies in the context of the research questions being addressed.

Investigators usually have a choice and they will often adopt a mix of methods. In general, the simpler, cheaper, and more practical approaches are adopted first. Experience indicates that the difficulty and expense of these studies, say per person in them, rises in order as follows: case series,

Box 9.10 Strengths and weaknesses of the study designs

Based on the principles of study design and your knowledge of the purposes of epidemiology, consider the relative strengths and weaknesses of clinical and population case series, cross-sectional, case–control and cohort studies, and trials. Put these in a table. You may find the following key words and phrases helpful in your reflection: ease, timing, maintenance and continuity, costs, ethics, data utilization, main contributions, observer and selection bias, analytic outputs.

population case series, cross-sectional, case–control, cohort, and trial. As we move along this sequence, there are additional nuances; for example, the ethical and recruitment problems raised by trials add complexity to the challenge of follow-up, which is otherwise shared with cohort studies. The case–control adds the complexity of a control group to the one of establishing an unbiased case series. The cross-sectional study adds the complexity of recruitment, consent, and a community base in comparison to a case series.

Often understanding the problem at hand requires several perspectives and, in particular, both cross-sectional and cohort analyses. Table 9.7 shows a classic and early example of the birth cohort effect and is adapted from that of Frost. Typically, we examine age group effects, most commonly at a point in time (cross-sectional), and then compare across time periods. Before reading on, do the exercise in Box 9.11. For simplicity of interpretation, let us assume that the data are completely accurate.

In 1880 the death rate was very high in the age group 0–4, low in 5–19, and high in the others. In 1930 it was much lower in the youngest age groups than in those over 20. In every age group the rates dropped rapidly over time.

One conclusion we could reach is that the disease has changed—from one that was most common in infancy in the nineteenth century to one of older age groups by 1930. We could speculate that resistance to the infection had increased in children by 1930 as compared to 1880, and that resistance declines in older ages. This implies an ageing effect. If we follow those born around 1880 (0–4, 5–9) (underlined), we see that they are the same group (cohort) that had a high rate in 1920 and 1930. In fact, all the high rate groups in 1930 come from cohorts who had very high rates when in the 0–4 age group.

An alternative interpretation for the age effects in 1930 is provided by this birth cohort analysis. The high rates in the older age groups in 1930 might not be a result of ageing itself, but of the high exposure in these groups to the tubercle bacillus in infancy several decades back. This is known as the *generation* or *birth cohort effect*. The age patterns at a point in time (say 1930) may reflect exposures to the causes in earlier life that are changing over time, and not necessarily the effects of ageing itself.

If there are time trends in exposure to causal agents—and there usually are—this explanation for differences by age group at a point in time needs to be remembered both for infections and chronic, non-infectious diseases. The overall message is this: reaching the right conclusions may need data from more than one study design.

We now turn to so-called ecological studies in epidemiology.

Table 9.6 Some of the strengths and weaknesses of each study design

Attribute	Clinical case series	Population case series	Cross-sectional	Case–control	Cohort	Trial
1 Difficulty	Easy to compile by clinicians or through clinicians, especially if specialist clinical societies are involved	Difficult, as needs large number of data contributors and complex registration systems to ensure quality, comparable data	Difficulty depends on the study. Studies of natural living populations are hard compared with those at schools or other institutions	Usually difficult because of need for appropriate control group and problem of recall bias. Much easier if part of a cohort study	Difficult because of added complexity of follow-up. Exceptions include maternity cohorts with short term birth outcomes	Difficulty exceeds the cohort because of technical and ethical challenges of creating and imposing an intervention
2 Timing to set up and report	May be available very quickly especially if health administration systems record diagnosis that has an ICD or other recognized code	Needs much planning time. Merging of data from clinical or administrative databases, if possible, can speed up the process greatly	Usually set up and finished within a few years	Usually finished within a few years except those on incident cases of rare diseases	Usually long-term (decades) though sometimes (e.g. studies of birth outcomes) they can be quick. Retrospective cohorts can be quick	Usually designed to give an answer within a few years or a decade, i.e. usually shorter than cohort studies
3 Maintenance and continuity	Easy as along as clinical commitment remains	Demands continuing effort on part of clinicians and administrators, especially to maintain quality	Study is usually stopped. Rarely, these studies are turned into cohorts by data linked or re-survey	Study is usually stopped	Long-term continuity is essential and problematic, particularly as observations are usually on free-living people	Similar to cohort studies but when trials are in patients with diseases, the commitment to the trial may be high and follow-up is in health systems
4 Costs	Costs are low because data are at hand	Costs are in total high but usually hidden in the administration of the health service and in the time of staff employed for other reasons. Costs are low per person	Costs depend on study but lower than cohort or trial of same size	Costs are usually comparable with cross-sectional studies and, as study size is usually small, the overall costs may be low	Costs are high, both because numbers studied are large and because costs of retaining staff and systems to collect data over many years are high	Costs are high for the same reason as the cohort study and there are additional costs of the intervention, obtaining approvals, and trial management

(continued)

Table 9.6 Continued

Attribute	Clinical case series	Population case series	Cross-sectional	Case–control	Cohort	Trial
5 Ethics (informed consent, confidentiality, etc.)	Ethical issues such as confidentiality are not usually difficult if the investigator is the clinician. However, unless it is service audit or evaluation ethical permission is needed	Data collection and storage systems must meet ever-stricter legal and ethical standards on consent and confidentiality. Use of administrative records for research needs ethical approval	Standard ethical issues, and of obtaining access to a sampling frame	Standard ethical issues as in clinical case series but also those of cross-sectional studies if using community controls	Confidentiality issues are considerable. Potential intrusion if repeated contact and measurement	The ethics of trials are complex and evolving, and hinge on the issues of uncertainty, doing no harm and informed consent
6 Data utilization	Data are likely to be used for both clinical and research purposes	Data are usually under-utilized, but relevant to health-care planning and research	Usually for research but under-utilized, as more information is collected than needed	As analysis is straight forward, data are usually fully analysed for research	Data tend to be under-utilized for both research and service planning	Data concerning the central questions are utilized. Secondary analysis is tempting but should be minimized
7 Main contribution	Contributes to clinical knowledge, health needs assessment, disease burden and sparking causal hypotheses	Contributes to understanding burden of disease, and sparking and testing causal hypotheses	Major contribution to burden of disease, substantial contribution to analysis of associations and may confirm or spark hypotheses	Major contribution to clinical knowledge, and sparking/testing causal hypotheses. Control group may supply risk factor data if based on representative samples	Major contribution to both burden of disease (incidence) and causal analysis	Main contribution is to understanding of effectiveness of interventions, and indirectly to disease mechanisms and causes

8 Observer bias	May be compiled by single or few observers, minimizing observer bias	Multiplicity of contributors, so vast problem of observer bias	Small studies may be done by one observer, but for most studies inter-observer bias is a problem	Small studies may be done by one observer; large studies usually need a few people so bias may be present	Usually requires multiple observers, who change over time so this is a huge problem	Usually requires multiple observers It is essential that the randomization process removes this problem but difficult in multicentre trials
9 Selection bias	Major problem except in the rare case of one or a few clinicians seeing all the cases in a locality	Minor problem if all unselected cases are included	Selection bias arising from non-response is almost inevitable	Studies of prevalent cases have selection bias, those of incident cases minimize this although control group may have low response rates	Selection bias due to non-response at baseline is augmented by loss to follow-up	Selection biases are particularly severe because non-participation may be high and because intervention may only be suitable for some of the target population
10 Confounding	Not an issue as groups are seldom compared	Big problem as limited data on potential confounders	Not a major issue as group comparisons are not primary purpose and data on confounders can be collected	Major challenge as confounders must be identified and measured retrospectively	Major challenge but confounders can be measured prospectively and repeatedly	Not a problem if trial is successfully randomized and loss to follow-up is low and similar in both groups
11 Analytic output	Case numbers, percentages, proportional morbidity/mortality ratio	Main output is disease rates, in association with census or population register data	Main output is prevalence proportions	Proportions exposed and odds ratios	Incidence rate and relative risk or rate, and survival	Incidence rates, relative risks, survival and numbers needed to treat or prevent

Table 9.7 Analysing by time, age, and birth cohort, age-specific death rates per 100 000 per year from tuberculosis (all forms) among males, Massachusetts, 1880–1930

Age	Year					
	1880	**1890**	**1900**	**1910**	**1920**	**1930**
0–4	<u>760</u>	578	309	209	108	41
5–9	<u>43</u>	49	31	21	24	11
10–19	126	<u>115</u>	90	63	49	21
20–29	444	361	<u>288</u>	207	149	81
30–39	378	368	296	<u>253</u>	164	115
40–49	364	336	253	253	<u>175</u>	118
50–59	366	325	267	252	171	<u>127</u>
60–69	475	346	304	246	172	95
70+	672	396	343	163	127	95

Reproduced with permission from Frost WH. The age selection of mortality from tuberculosis in successive decades. *American Journal of Hygiene*, Volume 30, 91–96, Copyright © 1939 Oxford University Press.

9.9 Ecological studies: mostly mode of analysis?

9.9.1 Overview

Ecology is the scientific study of organisms in relation to their environment. As we discussed in Chapter 1 epidemiology is an ecological discipline, and generally all, or at least most epidemiological studies are ecological. The phrase 'ecological study', however, has come to mean 'In epidemiology a study in which the units of analysis are populations or groups of people, rather than individuals' (*A Dictionary of Epidemiology*). The unit of analysis in epidemiology is always the group, so on this definition, all epidemiology is ecological.

Box 9.11 Age trends, time trends, and cohort effects in tuberculosis in Table 9.7

- What is your assessment of death rates with increasing age in 1880 and 1930? Examine and describe each of these columns.

- What are the changes in rates across time in the age groups for example, look at 0–4, 30–39, and 60–69 years?

- What conclusion do you reach—for example, is tuberculosis more common in the older age groups in 1930? Is this because of ageing itself?

- What alternative explanation(s) is/are there for the rising rates by age group in 1930 other than an age effect?

- What impression is created by observing the death rates in those born in 1880 as the population grows older? This is illustrated by the line. (Note: 0–4 and 5–9 year olds become 10–19 year olds in 1890.)

Usually, though, epidemiological data analysis is on aggregate measures originally made on individuals. The *Dictionary of Epidemiology* gives as an example an ecological study of the association between median income and cancer mortality rates in states and countries. In such a study, the cancer mortality rates are likely to derive from individual data from a population case series held in a database (registry) of cancers and/or deaths, and median income from a census or other cross-sectional studies. In this example, the investigators have chosen to analyse their data by place (rather than, say, age, sex, or social class). This choice is not an inherent design feature but a mode of analysis. This type of analysis is also sometimes called correlational, demographic, or descriptive. For example, McMahon and Trichopoulos (1996) inform us that ecological studies are descriptive studies based on routinely collected information. In this book these studies are described as population case series or registry studies, because the label ecological is not necessary and is potentially misleading. If the label is to be used, then it should be reserved for studies where the variables measure a feature of the place (environment) and not of individuals then aggregated as populations. How, then, should we conceptualize the ecological study?

There are variables which are not based on individual data and that are useful in epidemiology. Such variables were discussed in Chapter 2 (section 2.5 in particular) and in section 9.3. Sometimes such variables are merely a substitute for individualized data, which would be better but may not exist. For example, information on the duties (taxes) collected by governments on products such as alcohol and tobacco exists over long periods of time. Such data may be a partial substitute for information on consumption patterns in individuals and populations. Such data also provide additional information, for example, on government policy, the state of the economy, and the legal status of these products. These data may be even better than individual data, for example, alcohol duties indicate far more alcohol is bought than that reported in surveys.

Other variables that relate to a place may have no equivalent individual level counterpart but have intrinsic importance in epidemiology (see also Chapter 2): the weather, expenditure on roads, the type of political structure, or amount of land devoted to growing fruit and vegetables. These variables are ecological, particularly those relating to the natural environment. Such variables can be studied on their own with descriptions of time trends, variation between places, and differences by the characteristics of the populations in these places. Variables can be correlated with each other, for example, the relationship between cars in the country and particulate air pollution. Assuming such a study helps us to study living organisms in relation to their environment, it is an ecological study, albeit a simple one, and if it sheds light on the population-level pattern of disease, it is also epidemiology.

There are other circumstances in which exposure data relating to a place and not to individuals (say hardness of the water supply) are correlated with health data collected on individuals but summarized by place rather than another variable (e.g. sex). In this circumstance, the boundaries are blurred especially as hardness of water is a proxy for the water drunk by individuals. Here the study could simply be described as a population case series (or registry) study. Conceptually, the ecological component is an issue of data analysis here and not of study design. Cross-sectional, case–control, and cohort studies and trials (and not just population case series) could also be analysed in this way. Indeed, in trials randomization is commonly at aggregate level (e.g. schools). These are cluster randomized trials. We don't call them ecological trials. This thinking leads us to modify our Box 9.1 as in Table 9.8.

In Table 9.8 ecological studies are considered to be those using aggregate data on places. Here the ecological design is not defined on using aggregate information on individuals, simply because all of epidemiology does that. Studies on individuals of any design, however, can be analysed geographically. In practice, such analyses take place on population case series and large cross-sectional studies such as censuses. For other studies, the numbers of people enrolled and

Table 9.8 Design by mode of analysis

	By aggregate data on individuals	By aggregate data on places (ecological)
Ecological	–	√
Case series		
– clinical	√	(√)
– population	√	√
Cross-sectional	√	(√)
Case–control	√	(√)
Cohort	√	(√)
Trial	√	(√)

the geographical spread, is usually too small. This is reflected by placing brackets around the tick in Table 9.8. There is a worldwide movement to create epidemiological cohort studies comprising millions, even tens of millions, of people. Those studies will be amenable to this kind of analysis. There is also a great deal of work on trials where randomization is not of individuals but places. These kinds of designs require analysis at two or more levels—known as multilevel (or mixed) modelling. This is a topic for advanced studies and beyond this book's scope.

9.9.2 Some fallacies: ecological, atomistic, and homogeneity

Ecological analyses are subject to the ecological fallacy (see Pearce 2000). This fallacy states that the association found with aggregate data may not apply to individuals; for example, in aggregate a population with a higher risk of disease may have a higher exposure to the risk factors, but this association may not apply to individuals. Imagine a study of the rate of coronary heart disease in the capital cities of the world relating to average income. Coronary heart disease probably will be higher in the richer cities than in the poorer ones. This finding would fit the general view that coronary heart disease is a disease of affluence. We might predict from such a finding that rich people in the individual cities have more risk of CHD than poor people. In fact, we would then have been trapped by the ecological fallacy as currently, in the industrialized world the opposite is the case: within cities such as London, Washington DC, and Stockholm, poor people have higher CHD rates than rich ones. The forces that cause high rates of disease at a population level are different from those at an individual level, as we discussed in Chapter 2.

The ecological fallacy is usually interpreted as a major weakness of ecological analyses (not of true ecological studies). The ecological analyses, however, inform us about forces which act on whole populations that may be in conflict with those that act on individuals (see also Chapter 2). Rather than a weakness, it is a strength, for it gives us an alternative and broader perspective. Before reading on, reconsider the exercise in Box 9.5.

Studies of individuals are prone to the opposite of the ecological fallacy, the so-called atomistic fallacy, which is by contrast to the ecological fallacy seldom discussed. Here, the fallacy is to wrongly assume from observations on the causes of disease in individuals that the same forces apply to whole populations. For example, at an individual level a high income or a marker of material success, such as employment or access to a car, is associated with a lower rate of suicide. This does not mean that populations or societies which are rich have a lower rate of suicide or better mental health. The opposite seems to be true. As in the previous example of CHD and wealth, the forces that cause or prevent disease at the individual level, for suicide factors such as family support and employment, are different from those that work at societal level (e.g. social cohesion and expectations).

A third fallacy, which I have named the fallacy of homogeneity, arises from the misinterpretation of population data from heterogeneous populations. This fallacy is most likely to arise in population case series analyses because of limitations in the detail available on the study populations. For example, studies of ethnic groups often use broad labels such as White, Black, Hispanic, or Asian etc. European-origin 'White' populations in England have a lower all-cause standardized mortality ratio (SMR) than those born in the Indian subcontinent (often called South Asians). While this is true, the highest mortality is actually within the Irish-born living in England, who are included in the White population, whose all-cause SMR is much higher than that of the Indian subcontinent-born population. To take a second example, the South Asian population is often described as having lower smoking prevalence than White populations. Again, while this is true, the highest recorded prevalence of smoking is actually within a subgroup of the South Asian population, in Bangladeshi men, as is the lowest prevalence, in the subgroups of Indian men and all women. These examples emphasize how extrapolating from one level to another (individuals to subgroups to whole populations) is not a straightforward matter. It is not the case that one kind of level of examination is better or worse than another. The perspectives are different but collectively give more insight than singly.

9.10 **Size of the study**

In planning a study, the size of the study population is a crucial matter. Studies that are larger than they need to be are inefficient and wasteful, not only of money but also scarce epidemiological expertise, public goodwill, and time. There is one exception to this rule; that is, studies based on data that have already been collected and computerized. The extra costs of analysing all the data available may be trivial. Studies that are too small may provide misleading answers, or at least, imprecise ones.

Estimation of a desired study size is a complex issue, and one that is core to most statistics courses (and beyond this book). The specific details vary for each study design. The principles, however, can be stated succinctly as follows:

♦ The sample size will be dictated by the research questions and stated study hypotheses.

♦ The study hypotheses need to be summarized and specified in a way that can be quantified; for example, 'That the predicted cumulative incidence rate of a disease is two per cent per year, and that exposure to a risk factor (say smoking) doubles the cumulative incidence'.

♦ The precision of the answer required needs to be stated. A study wishing to establish the relative risk precisely (narrow confidence intervals) will be larger than one accepting an imprecise estimate.

♦ In studies where the hypothesis is based on a difference between groups in the outcome, the size of the minimum difference that it is important to detect should be stated (alternatively, state the size of the difference expected). The smaller this difference, the larger the study will need to be.

♦ The sample size should be large enough to keep low the chances of two types of statistical error. Type 1 error is rejecting a null hypothesis when it is true. In most epidemiological studies a null hypothesis is one stating that there is no difference between comparison groups or there is no association between a risk factor and a disease. In making this error, one is claiming a difference when there is, in reality, none in the source (base) population, and apparent differences have occurred by chance. In most research, by tradition, we wish the probability of making such an error to be lower than five per cent. The smaller the type 1 error the larger the study.

♦ Type 2 error is failing to reject a null hypothesis when it is false. In epidemiology, this usually means declaring there is no difference between comparison groups or there is no association between a risk factor and a disease, when, in the source (base) population, there is. Most studies aim to have less than 10–20 per cent probability of such an error. The power of a study is the probability that a type 2 error will not occur (so most studies aim for a power of 80 % or more). The greater the power, the larger the study needs to be.

With this type of information, the stage is set to calculate sample size. Each study design, however, imposes its own specific requirements, and the reader will find guidance in books on statistical and epidemiological methods. Sample size calculation is not an exact discipline and requires scientific judgement. Furthermore, sample size calculations are usually based on simple outcomes and analyses, whereas most studies usually examine a range of outcomes using a range of complex multivariate methods. To specify sample size properly requires a great deal of pre-specification of data and an analysis strategy, and that may be impossible or very difficult to achieve in advance. This said, a pre-analysis written analysis plan is mandatory for trials and recommended for all other studies. It is advisable to take statistical advice on the size of the study. There are no general answers to how large a study should be but most studies are too small even for main analyses, and certainly so for subgroup analyses. That is one reason why meta-analysis is so often needed.

9.11 Data analysis and interpretation in epidemiological studies: underpinning questions

The principles outlined in all the earlier chapters will be required to interpret data properly, particularly taking into account error, bias, and frameworks for analysis of associations (Chapters 3, 4, and 5). There is a multitude of choice in data analysis—the reader will need to consult one of many suitable textbooks—but the principles behind, and the formulae for, the basic measurements are in Chapters 7 and 8.

The following simple account, nonetheless, provides a logical approach that will underpin the analysis plan, which should be prepared in advance of beginning the analysis. When new ideas emerge and changes are made the analysis plan should be revised with careful documentation of the change. Before reading on try the exercise in Box 9.12. You may wish to tackle one or a few of the questions at a time—some answers are given in sequential paragraphs.

9.11.1 Planning the analysis

Planning the analysis in advance requires, above all else, resolve to do it, steely discipline, and a great deal of foresight. Foresight comes with experience and from knowledge, particularly on the nature of the desired end point, whether in the style of a thesis, report, or scientific article. Every study design presents choices, but the principal outputs for each study design are given in Table 9.6 (row 11 analytic output). For calculating measures of association, the 2 × 2 table (Chapter 8, Table 8.8) provides the standard way to present data. While the details of the presentation differ by end product, the principles are identical. Sometimes, the analysis plan will be mandatory, and this is most likely in large-scale trials where the end points are preset. Then the analysis plan will be summarized in the research proposal, expanded in the protocol, and then set out in detail prior to data analysis. Ideally, the analysis plan should be published, for example, on a website, before the analysis begins. This does not, of course, prevent further analysis beyond that

Box 9.12 Questions underpinning the analysis

- ◆ How do I plan the analysis?
- ◆ What is my primary focus (or foci) for the analysis?
- ◆ How can I show that my data set is sufficiently error free for analysis?
- ◆ How can I show my data set contains valid data?
- ◆ How can I show the potential for generalization beyond the study population?
- ◆ How can I demonstrate the burden of disease and of the risk factors so others can use the data?
- ◆ How can I demonstrate the comparability (or otherwise) of my subpopulations that I wish to compare and contrast?
- ◆ How can I summarize these contrasts?
- ◆ How can I check whether effect modification/statistical interaction is present?
- ◆ How can I show these contrasts are not a result of error, bias, or confounding?
- ◆ How can I assess whether interesting my results, for example, apparent associations are just by chance?
- ◆ How can I assess the likelihood of causality?
- ◆ How do I write the findings up so they are both clear and sound?

specified, but this later analysis will be considered as secondary, and, therefore, not definitive. The objectives are:

1. to minimize bias, especially investigators' preferences on what analysis to present and publish
2. to minimize type 1 errors, which are increased with multiple comparisons (see section 9.10)
3. to retain focus and avoid what are called data dredging or fishing exercises for interesting findings
4. to test prior hypotheses.

This same approach is rare for other kinds of studies, partly because there is more scope and need for creativity in the analysis, and partly because there is seldom an external requirement for pre-specification. Prior written specification of the analysis strategy is, nonetheless, highly recommended for the reasons listed. This does not preclude creative exploration of the data but this should be identified as such.

One effective tool for aiding this step is the creation of 'dummy' tables, or analysis of a simulation (fake) data set, or a combination of these. In dummy tables the writer thinks out the sequence of the analysis and prepares a table legend and data layout for each required table, specifying the outcome variables in relation to exposure variables (cross tabulations). The statistical tests can be stated and columns/rows to accommodate the results of the tests can be inserted. Table 8.16 is a simple example of a dummy table, but the reader can easily imagine other tables without data. The approach can be extended to graphs and any other form of data output. Usually, at this stage, it is better to envisage the tabular output. Dummy tables are very hard to prepare but this approach is much preferred to diving into the analysis and hoping to turn up something interesting. The usual result of that approach, particularly for the novice, is a sense of drowning in data. This applies to primary research and systematic reviews alike. How are we to make the choices of which dummy tables to produce?

9.11.2 **Focus**

The analysis plan and dummy tables require you to focus on the research questions and/or aims and/or specific objectives of the work. These are the guide posts, while the proposal or protocol (including the literature review) provides the map. In doctoral and postdoctoral research we aim to fill the gaps in the map, or extend it, or less commonly, in cases of doubt, to confirm the map is correct. So, there is an onus for creativity and novelty. For health-service work and undergraduate/masters level work, it is often enough to follow the paths set out in previous publications.

Once you have a clear analysis plan (presumably agreed with study steering committees, collaborators, or supervisors as appropriate) you proceed to analysis. Mostly analysis is done by computer (except for very small data sets), so let us assume this. You will need to abide by data protection principles and laws and ethical committee (review board) rulings. As far as possible you should anonymize your data set and trim it so only those data required at this stage are in the analysis file. Identifying data (e.g. names), should be held securely and separately. You may need to enter ('punch') your data onto an appropriate database. Of course, if you are analysing someone else's computerized data, you will avoid this step. The best, though expensive, approach to data entry from paper is double entry (independently done). This minimizes the inevitable human errors that arise at entry. If the data were entered directly (i.e. not recorded on paper) into a computer, such errors will probably be impossible to rectify but you should look for them—they can be very subtle, but you should know the data entry rules in this case.

9.11.3 **Errors**

The investigator's first task is to check the data set for resolvable errors. Sometimes these will be obvious, for example, a male is said to have a diagnostic code for cervical cancer (either the sex code or diagnostic code is wrong), or a person is said to be 174 years of age (probably the correct age is 17 years or 74 years). Sometimes errors will not be obvious, for example, the code key for male is said to be 1, when it is 2. The entered data can sometimes be compared with those on original materials (e.g. questionnaires).

It is even more important for investigators to check secondary data sets, because their unfamiliarity with them will make errors hard to detect during the analysis. Unfortunately, too often researchers wrongly start with an assumption that such checks have already been done. That is unlikely.

This checking stage is often referred to as cleaning the data. Given the structure of the data set is sound we can turn to its content.

9.11.4 **Validity and qualities of variables**

Readers are probably familiar with the self-explanatory phrase 'garbage in, garbage out'. Unfortunately, garbage data are not easy to distinguish from quality data, particularly when summarized and tabulated. Epidemiologists who have collected their own data have a sense of their quality, but this is not true for data they have borrowed for analysis. In Chapter 7 we considered issues around data quality (e.g. the numerator), and in Chapter 6, we covered sensitivity and specificity as indicators of validity of the screening test compared to a gold standard. The principles and methods outlined there apply here.

There is no short-cut for the investigator—information is essential on the timeliness, completeness, repeatability, accuracy or validity (i.e. the truth) of data and precision of measurements. For secondary data sets, we need to get this information from those who collected the data. To take an example, the database says that a female of 49 years has an income between £30–40 000 per year and has diabetes. We want to know, for example, whether sex is self-reported or observed, age is self-reported or from medical records, whether income is self-reported or from an employer (or agency) database, and whether diabetes is self-reported, from medical records, or based on blood tests (if so which ones). We want to know which coding schemes were used and for diagnoses, what definitions were applied. For each of these we want to know the validity of the data. Self-report of sex and age is likely to be accurate, but self-report of income and diabetes will not be. The amount of inaccuracy needs to be estimated. To reiterate, it must not be assumed, as is often the case, that data obtained from external agencies, whether governmental or not, are accurate. It is especially important for investigators to rigorously assess the value of such data. The investigator retains the responsibility for the outcome of these secondary analyses, not the person or agency supplying the data.

We are now ready to choose an appropriate statistical analysis computer package. The choices of computer packages are many and the reader will need to consult statistical and computing colleagues and other books. The important thing is that the package meets the need. There is no merit in working with a complex package like SAS* or Stata* if Microsoft Excel* will do.

It is not essential but in practice epidemiological data are processed by computers as numbers. Many variables are not, however, numbers so they need to be recoded.

The simplest kind of categorical variable consists of two possibilities and is also the commonest and perhaps most important type, for example, dead or alive, diseased or not, male or female, adult or child, etc. These categorical variables are called binary (or dichotomous). We can easily and arbitrarily assign a number, for example, 1 for alive and 2 for dead (or vice versa). (Our computer could probably cope with L for alive and D for dead but numbers are easier than letters.)

The variable may have more than two categories, for example, socio-economic status, race or ethnicity, etc. Whenever possible we should not reduce such a variable to a binary one because in simplification there is always a loss of information.

In socio-economic status the variables will usually have a logical order (e.g. high, intermediate, or low socio-economic circumstances). If there is a logical order then numbers can also be assigned logically (e.g. 1, 2, 3). This kind of variable is called ordinal.

Ethnic or racial group, however, has no logical order so each category needs a code number. It would make sense, however, for the investigator to set out the categories in some logical way, for example, the ethnic groups associated with the Far East might be grouped together and so be assigned adjacent numbers. Categories without an order are called nominal variables. (Clearly, there is no natural standard numerical difference between the categories of the aforementioned variables.) Let us say we were studying the number of cigarettes bought by individuals for private consumption in a week. The number will range from zero to several hundred. There is a standard interval between the numbers and the quantity is whole numbers. This is an example of a numerical variable. These variables have no fractions, so are called discrete. If fractions are permitted, as in the weight of tobacco bought, this would be a continuous variable. In practice many continuous variables are measured to the nearest whole number (e.g. blood pressure). Others may be measured using a fraction and rounded to the nearest whole number.

In epidemiological measurements, we use the positive numbers from zero upwards. So, we should be careful when we see negative numbers in epidemiological data, including in confidence intervals.

These considerations have relevance to data analysis and interpretation. The numerical qualities of variables as discussed here can be summarized as:

Categorical variables can be nominal (no intrinsic quantitative order—numbers are assigned after measurement) and these can be

◆ Binary

◆ Non-binary

Categorical variables can also be ordinal (intrinsic quantitative order).

Numerical variables can be (intrinsic quantitative order and measurement is usually in numbers)

◆ Discrete (whole numbers)

◆ Continuous (whole numbers and fractions)

We have already discussed in Chapter 1 that the investigators have to assign functions to variables, for example, whether they are to be treated as exposures, intermediates, confounders, effect modifiers, or outcomes.

9.11.5 **Generalization**

Virtually all epidemiological studies are designed to be generalized beyond the study population to the source population, and perhaps even beyond that. The few exceptions are likely to be local, problem solving exercises, either for health-care planning or public health investigations, for example, to track down the food associated with an outbreak of diarrhoea and vomiting. This is epidemiology but it is service, not research. The goal of epidemiological research is to advance generalizable knowledge. This does not have to be causal. To discover that a disease or risk factor is commoner than it once was, or that we thought it was, is also a research advance. To discover a better method of doing epidemiology is a particularly important advance. Causal understanding is often generalizable. Epidemiology should be published in a way that permits assessment of its generalizability. It may well be that colleagues in Osaka, Japan will be hoping to generalize from work done in Buenos Aires, Argentina, or vice versa.

Future researchers in the same place will want to compare their results with yours. Having already stated the methods, date of fieldwork (often missing in publications), etc., you should now describe your study populations, compared with that in the source population as in the sampling frame, and if possible the target population, as in the census of that city, state, or nation, as appropriate. The description should include demographic (e.g. sex, age, ethnic group), socio-economic (e.g. income, class structure, etc.), behaviour (e.g. smoking), and health status (e.g. blood pressure, height, weight) data. This type of descriptive overview table is usually large. The investigator and reader can immediately see the kind of population recruited, and the potential selection biases that have arisen in the process. The Osakan reader in Japan then can assess whether the Buenos Aires study population's information is of value to Osaka.

Dementia is a serious problem that we need to understand better, and pooling knowledge internationally is desirable. It may well be that a study of the frequency of potential risk factors, dementia incidence, and associations between risk factors and dementia, will be of intense interest globally both for its methods and results. Indeed, a study that gives new insights in a locality may do the same internationally. It is for this reason that most epidemiological journals have adopted a vision, mission, and reach that is international rather than national.

9.11.6 **Burden of disease and needs assessment**

The kind of overview table considered in the previous section helps to assess the burden of disease or risk factors. If this is an important aim then proceed with analysis of variables like those in Table 8.14. The analysis may be done by sex, age group, social class group, ethnic group, etc. For burden of risk factors the key outputs will be prevalence proportions and for disease, either incidence rates or prevalence proportions. For data sets containing time of onset of the outcome, diurnal, weekly, seasonal, annual, and secular trends may be described. Where geographical variations are of interest, the data may be analysed by point pattern analysis, or by small area, region, nation, or even continent. This type of analysis is of time, place, and person—the epidemiological triad (Box 2.1 and Table 2.1). The prime outputs will be absolute measures (Table 7.1). This kind of descriptive work is vital and should not be omitted. Investigators are gaining an understanding of their population and their data, and generating new ideas that can be incorporated into the analysis strategy—potentially as secondary analysis.

While the relationship between risk factors and outcomes may be analysed at this stage for the whole population, this is unlikely to be very interesting. The principles, however, will be same as in comparing subgroups, as we shall discuss next.

9.11.7 **Comparability**

Mostly, epidemiological studies are designed to compare subpopulations, and to test one or more hypotheses about subgroup difference(s). The first step is to set out your overview table (see section 9.11.6) but for the comparison populations side-by-side. For simplicity we assume there are only two comparison populations, but there could be several—perhaps hundreds, as in international studies. (In the latter case the study groups will probably go in rows rather than columns.)

Our comparison overview table needs to include every variable that we believe is relevant to the question at hand and—here is the challenge—to make explicit those variables that we believe are relevant but we have no data on. Reflect on the exercise in Box 9.13 before reading on.

The key question is this: are there differences, other than fruit consumption, in factors that play a role in explaining the pathway between fruit consumption and cancer? If not, which is improbable, you may proceed to analysis. If so, as is likely, reflect on whether there may be, among the differences, some confounding.

We may find that low fruit consumers are more likely to be poor, to be male, to be older, to be smokers, and to drink more alcohol. Adjusting the results for age and sex may be appropriate at this stage. We may also find high fruit consumers also eat more vegetables, whole grain foods, fish, and white meat. Disentangling the effects of such factors is going to be a challenge—the challenge being to isolate the independent effects of fruit. At this stage the investigators may find so many differences, and discover that other data items of relevance (e.g. exercise habits, ethnic group) have not been collected, that a sound causal analysis is not feasible, at least with the study design at hand. They may even concede that further analysis should not be done. It is a wonder, however, that this course of action—rather inaction—is seldom taken, to the detriment of the science of epidemiology, through the genesis of spurious associations. At this stage of the analysis we are still using, mainly, absolute (actual) measures.

Box 9.13 **Fruit eating and cancer study: need for an overview table comparing groups**

There is a great deal of interest in lifestyle factors such as exercise, diet, alcohol, and illicit drug-taking on health. Imagine we are interested in fruit consumption and the occurrence of cancers. The comparison may be between high and low consumers of fruit. Why is an overview table of the kind recommended in section 9.11.6, by fruit-consuming category, critical?

These numerous differences are a major and important finding and need to be published, not least to inform others of the research challenges of pursuing this line of enquiry. It is poor epidemiology to fail to do this kind of analysis rigorously prior to presenting data on the strength of the association.

9.11.8 Summarizing the contrasts

Let us assume that the biases and mismeasurement errors in risk factors, outcomes and confounders have been estimated; and the number of confounders is relatively small and amenable to control. We can now proceed to contrast the risks in high and low fruit eaters using relative measures, preferably the relative risk (or prevalence proportion ratio in cross-sectional studies, and odds ratio in case–control studies). You could also do the contrast by using differences in absolute risks/rates but relative measures are more commonly used.

If there are demonstrably no confounding factors of note, there is no need for further control of confounders. This absence of confounding factors is unlikely except for trials.

If there are no confounding factors, you can calculate the relative risks (or other ratios) directly from incidence rates (or equivalent). If age and sex are the only confounders, you can adjust the incidence rates for age and sex before calculating the relative risks (and possibly stratify the data by sex and only adjust for age). If there are several confounding factors the data are then best analysed using one or more of the many multivariable methods (e.g. multiple regression, logistic regression, Cox regression, etc. depending on the kind of data). The adjusted results answer the question: what would the contrast have been if the study group and the control group were similar in relation to the variables entered in the model as confounders. Multivariable methods will calculate a relative risk with (and without) adjustment for confounding factors, both individually for each risk factor and collectively, for a group of risk factors. When exposures are graded relative risks can be calculated at varying levels (doses) of the risk to give the 'dose–response' relationship.

9.11.9 Interactions

Interactions were discussed in Chapter 5. An interaction will be detected by testing whether the relative risk in one group (say high fruit-eating men), differs to an important extent from that in another group (say high fruit-eating women). If so, the effect of fruit on cancer is interacting with the variable, sex. If there is interaction, the groups should not be combined but analysed separately. This is a complex area of data analysis. The analyst should state whether the study hypotheses a test of departure from addition or multiplication of risks. The model should follow the hypothesis.

9.11.10 Accounting for error, bias, and confounding

The interpretation is problematic when the data are of poor quality. Quantitative methods for handling confounding are well developed in epidemiology as discussed in Chapter 4 and briefly in section 9.11.8 in this chapter and elsewhere. Even with rigorous efforts, confounding may remain—this is residual confounding. This may be because some confounders are not measured and those that that are may be imprecise, and even be mismeasured such that there is a misclassification, for example, a person who takes exercise is misclassified as a non-exerciser. Commonly, publications mention residual confounders but usually proceed to interpret the results as if it did not actually occur. That is bad practice.

For mismeasurement and misclassification errors, techniques for quantitative adjustment of the relative risks or other summary measures are well developed. They need, however, a second set of measures, usually from a subsample. The relative risk can be corrected for measurement errors (regression dilution bias, e.g. see section 4.2.6). These corrections usually lead to a higher relative risk.

For most biases researchers provide a qualitative assessment, usually in the strengths and weaknesses part of the discussion of the publication. It is easy, however, to then proceed to interpret the results as if these biases did not actually occur. Methods are available, and are evolving, for quantifying the possible effects of a wide range of biases, including calculating bias-adjusted relative risks. The alternative scenarios following such analysis should be presented. Indeed, there is an argument for the primary output to be the fully bias-adjusted results, or, perhaps better for there to be a range of possible results to be shown.

9.11.11 How can I assess whether my results are the play of chance?

Once we have evaluated the role of errors in study design, execution, and measurement, confounding and bias we are, at last, ready to assess the role of chance in our results. Most studies are on subsamples of the population.

It may be that we obtained a result, let us say, 42 per cent of our study sample were smokers. Perhaps if we had a different sample the result would have been 32 per cent or 52 per cent. That is quite possible unless we had, originally, studied the whole population or virtually the whole population. How can we handle this problem of difference arising from chance in sampling?

We have three main strategies, two being rarely feasible, and the other almost universally applied, although often inappropriately.

The first strategy is to study everyone or almost everyone. This is sometimes possible even apart from censuses, for example, studying all newborn babies in a country, or all children as they enter school, or all people admitted to hospitals. In these special circumstances, the results you have are the most precise possible (but we will also see a third strategy being applied— read on for explanation). There is no sampling error and chance is not a factor.

The second strategy is to repeat the study, perhaps in simplified form, with several different samples. If the results are much the same, there will be confidence that the original estimate was about right. The problem is that this strategy is usually slow and costly, unless the data already exist for the second or third study; in which case, why not study the larger group in the first place?

The third strategy is to rely on statistical theory. If we can assume that our study subjects are a sample of the source (base) population, and if we know how the sample relates to that population, we can utilize statistical probability theories to answer important questions relating to our study's estimate.

If we had done our study repeatedly taking our samples in the same and known way, what would have been the range of values for the estimate of interest? If our sample is a random sample from a known population the result will follow a known statistical distribution—for example, for a variable such as smoking/non-smoking, it is the binary distribution. From this we can calculate confidence intervals around our point estimates. The confidence interval is just two numbers between which our estimate lies. Taking our example of 42 per cent smokers, the interval might be 35–49 per cent. The interval is dependent on the level of probability we wish to achieve. Typically, this probability is 95 per cent, that is, we want the interval to include our estimate and the 95 per cent of the closest estimates in this distribution. We could, equally, ask for 90 per cent of the closest estimates or 99 per cent of them. Conceptually, this is like taking 100 random samples and taking the mean value from the sample and 95 per cent of the values closest to the mean value.

It is of interest to note that the observed value sits in the middle of the distribution so is the modal (most likely), median, or mean value in the normal distribution. The values at the ends of the interval are less likely. We should, therefore, pay more attention to our result than the edges of the confidence interval.

We can and should calculate confidence intervals around key summary measures in our studies. Techniques are available for most such measures.

In comparing two groups, we could ask (i) are they different, and (ii) by how much are they different, and with a confidence interval around the difference. The second is preferred. Answering the first question has traditionally used the same concepts of sampling and probability but expressed as a P-value (P for probability). Here, instead of a confidence interval around the difference, a single number is calculated for example, $p = 0.04$ (the expression $p < 0.05$ is a poor alternative as it loses information, but is common). This means that the probability of getting a difference of the size seen, or larger than that, by chance alone is 0.04 or four per cent. This is often interpreted as being statistically significant. This approach to analysis and data interpretation is not recommended except, and then with careful interpretation, when alternatives are not available. Statistically significant should not be equated to significant, whether clinically, in public health terms, or epidemiologically.

The issues raised here so briefly are statistical and, except for a few central concepts, beyond this book. They rest on complex matters based on probability distributions. The availability of computer programmes means that these complexities are not sufficiently considered. For example, very often the study samples are not random samples at all and yet investigators calculate confidence intervals or P-values when these are not valid. In addition to training in statistics, most epidemiologists will need to work in partnership with statisticians, not least because advances are occurring rapidly and most epidemiologists will not be able to follow them themselves.

9.11.12 **Causality**

The investigator is now able to apply the frameworks for assessing the association for example, between fruit eating and cancer. If the association is real, and not artefact, and chance is considered an unlikely player, then the causal frameworks can be applied. The aforementioned analysis only contributes to strength of the association (and sometimes dose–response), and possibly specificity. The methods may clarify temporality. A systematic review will help assess consistency, a meta-analysis will help in quantifying the strength of the association, while a general review will guide us on biological plausibility (see section 5.6.2). We will look for experimental confirmation from human trials (if any), laboratory studies especially on mammalian cells or whole mammals, natural experiments, and genetic studies based on Mendelian randomization. Table 5.9 shows how different study designs contribute towards judgements of cause and effect. As discussed in Chapter 5, causality is not a product of data analysis—but the analysis makes a strong contribution. Table 9.9 lists causal and non-causal terms.

9.11.13 **Reviews, systematic reviews, and meta-analysis**

Examining the body of published work on a topic of research is known by the quaint term literature review, so a request to read the literature is not, in science, a direction to read Shakespeare. The time-honoured approach was to examine past work in chronological order. That is still to be recommended but, except for the most esoteric of topics, there will be so much to read that some selection will be necessary. In standard literature reviews, the selection is left to the discretion of the reviewer. The reviewers synthesize the scientific literature that they judge is necessary to answer the questions posed. In doing so, reviewers may focus on the work of well-known authorities in the field (particularly themselves!), more recent work, large-scale work, or other people's reviews. More pragmatically, they may choose work that is readily available, in a language they read, or that is published in the journals with high reputation. In modern times, work that can be found in electronic databases and can be downloaded for free on the internet is particularly popular. The problem with this traditional form of reviewing is bias, and the result is erroneous conclusions. This traditional approach is also inefficient, from society's perspective, even though it may conserve the time of the researcher. The researcher's selective approach may miss some important original research work. Since original research work usually costs hundreds of thousands, and even millions, of pounds it is wasteful to miss it.

This is not to say there is no role for such reviews. They are essential for the following:

◆ self-education and education of others, especially on the general principles of a subject;

◆ as a preliminary way of sketching out the need for research;

◆ as the prelude to a systematic review or meta-analysis;

◆ where there is sparse information—insufficient to justify a systematic review;

◆ as the basis of a commentary on published research;

◆ to support a viewpoint, where strict objectivity is not the aim (e.g. in a debate).

The traditional review was in narrative form with an emphasis on the conclusions generated by others' work. The traditional review did not, however, exclude the possibility of extracting the empirical findings of other research. Usually, however, these were presented in text format. The best traditional reviews were analytic and, if necessary, constructively critical but there was no formal way of assessing the quality of the studies.

The traditional review serves those disciplines where generalization is relatively easily or where strict objectivity is not the goal. For example, in describing the action of an enzyme or an eye muscle, a traditional review would probably be enough. Even one definitive article, or even one previous review, might suffice.

What about reviews of topics such as whether salt causes high blood pressure, or whether HIV causes AIDS? The production and marketing of salt is a multi-billion-pound endeavour. Every human being's quality of life will be affected by an erroneous review that concluded either that there is no causal link, or that there is one. The causal relation between the amount of salt taken and high blood pressure is unlikely to hold, alike, in South African miners, and Ford Motor Company executives. There have been strong, political views against the acceptance of HIV as the fundamental cause of AIDS, most obviously and recently in South Africa. A selective and biased review in the hands of politicians who do not believe in HIV could lead to many people dying unnecessarily.

The need for the best possible evidence, especially for making decisions on expensive health-service interventions, the need to make reviewing easier so more people can be involved, and the imperative to minimize error and bias have combined to lead to an explosion in the methods and outputs of systematic reviews. A systematic review has the following characteristics:

1. It is managed in the manner of a research project with a clear, written plan (protocol) stating the context (usually by a traditional review), goals, questions, methods, analysis, and outputs. This is a systematic approach.

2. It is aiming to review everything published that is relevant to the goals. If it does not review everything then it reviews a sample, with the selection of the sample being unbiased. Mostly, the sample is based on defining timeframes and places. The search for relevant data is systematic.

3. The information from original research is usually extracted (often into a form) and entered into a database or tables in a systematic way, and presented in some logical way.

4. The data extracted from point 3 are the focus of the review rather than the text of the original articles. The findings are the extracted results and are synthesized and discussed collectively.

The author of the systematic review has the dual challenge of pinpointing and dealing with the errors and biases in the original papers, and those that arise from compiling the results in this way. Many of the biases and errors occurring in primary research are mirrored in these synthesized data sets.

In our example of salt and high blood pressure, we are likely to find tens of thousands of articles on the subject. Thousands of others may be difficult to find. It may need a working lifetime to find and read them. Yet, the results may be required in a year, to assist in a forthcoming health policy.

The usual solution is to clarify and narrow the research questions, and hence the goals and scope of the review. We may, say, narrow it to—does salt cause high blood pressure in warm climate countries (or specify the countries), and specify a timescale for the fieldwork of the research (say, 1965 onwards). It is common but not usually good practice to restrict the review to English language publications. In this example, we may also restrict to case–control and cohort studies and trials in human populations. We would start our search of publications using electronic search engines and databases, before looking at reference lists in publications, and consulting experts. By this time, we should have a good idea of the resources needed to complete the review. If there are so many articles that it is still beyond the resources available, further inclusion and exclusion criteria will be needed, for example, restricting to cohort studies, or trials.

One logical solution, when there is a great deal of material, is to restrict studies to the best possible study design for that question. For a question such as how much type 2 diabetes there is in society, we may restrict to cross-sectional studies. For the question of what is the association between obesity and type 2 diabetes, we may restrict to cohort studies.

The evidence that is now at hand can be interpreted using the frameworks in Chapters 4 and 5. While we can search for evidence to support the guidelines for causality, it is clear that the systematic review is, in itself, the basis of a judgement on consistency. Consistency is particularly powerful when the evidence comes from a range of study designs, so there is a case for either including several designs within the one systematic review or doing a series of systematic reviews, for example, salt/blood pressure reviews of case–control and cohort studies separately. Other types of evidence (e.g. laboratory research) can be considered in the discussion.

Imagine now that we find 10 cohort studies all showing that people eating more salt, say X grams more, have about 50 per cent more hypertension than those who eat less salt, with the results of individual studies ranging from 35–65 per cent excess. Assume we have checked out these studies, there are no imperfections of note, and that everything points to a causal relation. What else can we do? What other additional analysis is possible?

Every estimate of risk has a random error and this can be estimated by calculating confidence intervals (CI) around it. The narrower the CI, the greater the precision. In one of the studies, one may find the excess is 40 per cent with a CI of 25–55 per cent. The range of the CI is narrower when the sample size is larger. A larger sample size can be mimicked by combining the 10 studies. Ideally, we would obtain the original data from the 10 studies and re-analyse them together. In practice, that is often not feasible. There are statistical techniques for combining the studies even without obtaining the original data. Either approach to combining data is known as meta-analysis.

In epidemiology it is unusual for studies either to be done in the same way, or to give the same results. The differences in the methods between the studies might give rise to different results. Alternatively, differences in the populations might do so. It is not easy to disentangle these possibilities. It is not at all improbable that of our 10 studies, two show that high salt is associated with lower blood pressure, three show no association, and five show higher blood pressure. What are we to do now? Is there some rigorous way of summarizing or synthesizing these results?

The epidemiologist foresees this need and adopts in the previously stated protocol an approach to extract value from this muddled picture:

1. Are some of these studies too unreliable to include in the meta-analysis? These will be sifted out early.
2. Are studies of different sizes (almost certainly)? If so, the larger studies will be given more weight (both judgementally and statistically)?
3. Are some studies of higher quality than others? These will be given more weight.
4. Is it reliable to combine data? This will be judged on: (a) methods being sufficiently similar and; (b) a statistical test (of heterogeneity) to see whether the effects are too different for them, reasonably, to be explained by random errors.
5. If the variation in findings is too great to explain by methodological or random variation, then, until shown otherwise, the best explanation is that the differences reflect the real population differences in the relation of salt to blood pressure. It would be misleading to combine all the studies, but it might be possible to aggregate some on the basis of some prior or coherent approach, for example, those in countries with warm climates separately from those in cold climates.

In adopting the meta-analytic method, we are getting better understanding of the strength and dose–response of the association.

So systematic reviews and meta-analyses provide direct input into two causal guidelines—consistency and strength of associations. In applied epidemiology, they provide more precise data on the burden of disease, and the effect of interventions.

This account is of the principles of systematic reviews, but there is a vast pool of technical knowledge and technical solutions. There are many websites and books for the interested reader—some of them, including the Cochrane and Campbell Collaboration websites, are listed in the bibliography.

9.11.14 **Write up**

After this costly and hard work, the failure to write up and present the findings for dissemination at conferences and, more importantly, in journal articles borders on the unethical. The omission will cause publication bias (section 4.2.8). The partial exception to this assertion is work done primarily for the education of the investigator (e.g. theses). (Doctoral theses' abstracts are, however, logged on electronic databases but students should aim to publish the new findings.)

The writing up of the work for publication is beyond the scope of this book. Your work will be assessed by editors and peer reviewers who are experienced in critical appraisal, so write with the questions in section 10.13 in mind. Alert readers will want these questions answered. The competition for publication is intense. Fortunately, in recent years open access journals have appeared and will publish all reliable work (albeit usually on payment of a fee).

Chapter 10 introduces the art of critical appraisal—a skill vital to data interpretation.

In your writing, take care to distinguish associations and causal associations. Table 9.9 sets out some causal and non-causal language for associations.

9.12 **Twenty questions on study design**

Consider which of the questions in Table 9.10 could be answered reasonably well with a clinical case series, population case series, cross-sectional study, a case–control study, cohort study, trial, or a truly ecological study.

Overall, make your choice for each question bearing in mind the strengths and weaknesses of each study design. Remember, most questions can be answered with a number of study designs

Table 9.9 Causal and non-causal terms for associations

Causal terms (should be used rarely*)	Association-related terms (should be used routinely)
Cause	Association
Effect	Link
Influence	Relation(ship)
Result	Correlation
Outcome	Prediction/predictor
Impact	Marker (risk)
	Risk factor
	Connection

*They will often be appropriate in trials and in authoritative statements on causality based on a thorough review of the evidence by objective scholars and researchers.

and there is seldom a single correct answer. Equally, sometimes more than one design, or a hybrid design is needed.

The exercise is designed to enable you to think about the questions and study designs.

You will find my answers in Appendix 9.2.

9.13 **Conclusion**

Study designs are best thought of as interlinked and mutually supporting methods. The various designs have similar purposes, are rooted in population concepts of health and disease, and are conceptually overlapping. They are also subject to similar errors, biases, and problems of sampling, and similar challenges in data collection, analysis, and interpretation. Epidemiologists may use several or a mix of designs to solve a problem, and it may be difficult to name them. Most studies can be distinguished by their focus on either disease or exposure, the relationship of the observation to calendar time and the natural history of disease, and whether there is an imposed intervention or not.

Epidemiological designs are based on the fundamental theories discussed earlier, particularly that differential exposure to the causes of disease leads to differential population patterns of disease. Only one design—the cohort study—tests this particular theory directly. The trial tests it indirectly by seeing whether drugs or preventive procedures that interfere with the putative causes will prevent or control diseases, thus leading to more favourable outcomes. Trials that deliberately exposed people to the causes of disease would be unethical. This is done on animals, especially where there are animal models of human diseases. Overall, human trials help evaluate hypotheses on control of disease rather than generate causal hypotheses. The other designs (case series, case–control, and cross-sectional) test the theory indirectly and retrospectively. The data from such studies help to develop and refine causal theories of disease. The process of designing studies and interpreting data, and especially the unanswered questions arising, drives advances in methods and techniques.

This chapter only skims the vast experience on study design and analysis; hopefully sufficiently to allow the reader to understand more advanced writings and to link earlier concepts to methods. To implement a study requires a knowledge of scientific writing, winning research grants, management of staff and resources, preparation of data collection forms, sampling methods, measurement and data collection, statistics, computing, and data interpretation (and other skills, all beyond the scope of this book). Many of these additional areas are general and are shared, at least, across many of the social and population sciences.

Table 9.10 Twenty questions: potential and preferred designs

Question	Potential study designs	Your preferred study design with reason
1 Is leukaemia increasing in its incidence?		
2 What factors are, potentially, causes of leukaemia?		
3 What proportion of the population is exposed to virus X?		
4 Does exposure to drugs to treat epilepsy in pregnant mothers lead to congenital malformations in their offspring?		
5 Does flying on long-distance aeroplane flights increase the risk of pulmonary embolism, i.e. blood clots in the lung?		
6 What proportion of those taking long-distance aeroplane flights develop deep venous thrombosis?		
7 What are the side effects of oral contraceptives?		
8 Are oral contraceptives more effective for the prevention of pregnancy than other methods, e.g. the condom?		
9 What are the risk factors for fatal pedestrian accidents?		
10 Does having a maximum speed limit of 30 miles per hour (about 48 kilometres per hour) reduce fatal pedestrian accidents, as compared to 40 miles per hour, in inhabited areas?		
11 Is the heart disease mortality rate on the rise or on the decline?		
12 Why is the incidence of heart disease mortality changing?		
13 Would doubling the amount of exercise in the population reduce the incidence of heart disease?		
14 What is the relationship between the wealth of the country as measured with the GNP and the consumption of illicit drugs, e.g. heroin, and legal drugs, e.g. alcohol?		
15 What proportion of school children are obese?		
16 Do farm subsidies to dairy farmers lead to increased consumption of dairy products in the population?		
17 What is the cause of a rare disease of your choice, e.g., phaechromocytoma, a tumour of the adrenal gland?		
18 How many cases of AIDS, or any other similar infectious disease of your choice, should the health service be planning for in 5, 10, and 20 years from now?		
19 Is the amount of fruit and vegetable consumption increasing or decreasing? What is likely to happen in 10 years from now?		
20 Would screening all adults for diabetes using blood tests improve the health of the population? Would this be cost-effective?		

Study design is constantly changing, as most recently witnessed in the rise of Mendelian rand-omization studies. We can already see the upcoming revolution will be in harnessing the power of data linkage to create mega-databases that will permit not only the study designs we know of, but also those awaiting invention.

The final chapter considers the art of reading and interpreting an epidemiological study, dis-cussed in the context of epidemiological theory, ethics, and practice. This skill, known as critical appraisal, is essential, and is best built on a sound foundation of understanding epidemiological concepts and their related methods.

Summary

Epidemiological studies have seemingly distinct designs but they are unified by their common goals to understand the frequency and causes of disease, by their strategy of seeking associations between exposures (potential causes) and outcomes (disease), by their utilization of survey meth-ods, and by their basis in defined populations. This explains why they complement each other, for example, in assessing the weight of evidence for cause and effect, and why apparently small changes can change the design.

The case series (or register-based study) lies at the core of the epidemiological method. It is usually based on a list or register of cases compiled by one or a group of clinicians. A case series is a coherent set of cases of a disease (or similar problem). A population case series is based on a register of such cases compiled for a defined population and time. Such registers include records of deaths, cancers, notifiable diseases, and hospitalizations. Cases can be analysed as rates over time, between places, and by population characteristics to generate understanding of the burden of disease and to generate associations. If such cases are compared with a control group, we have a case–control study. Case–control studies are analysed by comparing the exposure to risk factors in cases to those in controls—the analysis usually uses the odds ratio, which may provide a good estimate of the relative risk.

In a population studied at a specific time and place (a cross-section), measurements can be made of disease, the factors which may cause disease, or both simultaneously. This is a cross-sectional study and its primary output is prevalence data, though associations between risk factors and disease can be generated and hypotheses tested. Such a study might be used to identify cases of a particular disease in a population. If the characteristics of this group of cases are compared with a control group we have, again, a case–control study (of prevalent cases). If the population in a cross-sectional study is followed up to measure health outcomes, this study design becomes a cohort study.

Cohort studies produce data on disease incidence and are especially good on associations between risk factors and disease outcomes. Cases discovered in the course of follow-up in a cohort study may be compared with a comparison group and, once again, give rise to a (nested) case–control study.

If the population, perhaps but not necessarily so, of a cohort study, is divided into two groups, and the investigators impose a health intervention upon one of the groups, and follow up to meas-ure outcomes, the design is that of a trial. Trials produce data on incidence in treated populations in comparison with those untreated. They are used, primarily, to test rather than generate hypoth-eses, and their prime output is information on effectiveness of health interventions. Usually, due to ethical issues, trials are not actually embedded within cohort studies but done on populations selected specially for them. Natural experiments, including Mendelian randomization studies, may provide strong evidence.

Studies based on aggregated data, usually formed from geographically defined units of population, are commonly referred to as ecological studies but they usually are not as such. They usually represent a mode of analysis, rather than a design. All five epidemiological designs could, in theory, be analysed using geographically aggregated data. In practice, only population case series and very large cross-sectional studies such as the census lend themselves to such a form of analysis, because other designs usually have insufficient numbers. This is changing with the creation of massive population-based cross-sectional and cohort studies.

In all epidemiological studies, interpretation and application of data are easier when the relationship between the population being observed and the source and target populations is understood. For example, case series studies need a population base to construct rates; the cross-sectional study needs a case or population register to construct a sampling frame; the case–control study should, ideally, be on a defined, representative population of incident cases with a sample of controls from the same population source; the cohort study should inform about risk factor–disease outcome relations in the wider populations; and the results of most trials are only useful if they apply outside the study population actually recruited. For proof of concept, preliminary studies, a population base of this kind may be unnecessary.

The principles for the analysis of all studies are similar: prepare an analysis plan based on the study research questions and/or objectives; check the data for errors, mismeasurement, bias, and confounding; describe your study population's characteristics in relation to the source and target populations; describe your comparison groups with particular reference to potential confounding factors; undertake the analysis, producing summary measures appropriate to the study design that take into account the effects of confounding and interacting factors; interpret the data in the light of frameworks for discriminating real and artefactual associations; apply causal reasoning to associations if appropriate to the goals of the study; and write up your results for a critical audience answering the core questions underlying the appraisal of epidemiological research. In many of these steps, including moving to the next stage of research, the causal graph will be valuable. Your work may be set in the context of traditional, systematic, and meta-analytic reviews.

All designs can contribute, though unequally, to measuring disease burden for health policy and planning, and to testing causal hypotheses. The distinction between designs which serve one function or the other is not clear-cut.

Sample questions

Question 1 What population selection biases may arise in a cross-sectional study assessing the population burden of a disease?

Answer Population selection biases include the following:

- an incomplete sampling frame (list of people eligible)
- errors in the sampling frame
- failing to invite a sample representative of the population
- failure of the invitation to reach the person invited
- failure of the person invited to understand the invitation
- non-response/non-participation
- incomplete participation, for example, missing some questions and not giving blood tests.

Question 2 In a case–control study of diabetes mellitus (of type 2) in middle age and its possible link to obesity in childhood, the following data were obtained:

Of 950 people who had diabetes, 60 had demonstrable obesity in childhood. Of 900 people who did not have diabetes, 40 had had obesity in childhood.

(i) Put these data into a 2 × 2 table with all appropriate labels and numbers.

(ii) Calculate the odds ratio using the no diabetes group as the control population.

(iii) Do such data from case–control studies demonstrate cause and effect? In your answer, refer to the framework whereby associations are considered as causal or not causal (or real/artefact).

Answer (i)
See Table 9.11.

Table 9.11 Relationship between type 2 diabetes mellitus in middle age and obesity in childhood

		Diabetes Mellitus	**No Diabetes Mellitus**	**Totals**
Obesity in	+	60	40	100
Childhood	–	890	860	1750
		950	900	1850

Answer (ii)

$$OR = \frac{60 \times 860}{890 \times 40} = \frac{51\ 600}{35\ 600} = 1.45.$$

Answer (iii)
Case–control studies test a hypothesis and yield an association, usually measured by the odds ratio, which may be a good estimate of the equivalent relative risk from a cohort study. The association contributes to a cause and effect analysis but is not, in itself, enough.

The analysis of cause and effect should exclude data and study design artefacts (errors, biases, confounding) before applying a framework for causal analysis to what seems to be a real association, for example, that of Bradford Hill, or other guidelines for causal reasoning. Rarely do the data from case–control studies turn out to be causal and definitive on their own. More often, they make a small contribution to a larger body of work.

Question 3 (a) In a cross-sectional study of asthma in two cities (say city A and city B) the investigators studied children aged 10–15 years. They asked them to self-report on whether they had asthma. The study was in a classroom setting. A sample of schools was studied. They found that in city A, of 3300 children studied 300 reported a diagnosis of asthma while in city B, of 2700 children studied 400 reported asthma.

(i) Put these data into a 2 × 2 table.

(ii) Calculate the prevalence proportion ratio, first with city A as the study group and B as control, and then vice versa.

(iii) Set out, systematically, potential explanations for the higher prevalence of asthma in city B. (Note: clinical explanations are *not* required.)

Answer (i)

See Table 9.12.

Table 9.12 Results of the asthma study presented in a 2 × 2 table

Place	Asthma		
	Yes	**No**	**Totals**
City A	300	3000	3300
City B	400	2300	2700
Totals	700	5300	6000

Answer (ii)

Prevalence proportion in city A = 300/3300 = 0.091 = 9.1%

Prevalence proportion in city B = 400/2700 = 0.148 = 14.8%

Prevalence proportion ratio:

$$\frac{\text{City A proportion}}{\text{City B proportion}} = \frac{9.1\%}{14.8\%} = 0.61$$

or

$$\frac{\text{City B proportion}}{\text{City A proportion}} = \frac{14.8\%}{9.1\%} = 1.62.$$

Answer (iii) The two major explanations are that the results are an artefact or they are real. If artefact, then it could be chance, error in study design, or data collection methods that have led to bias or confounding. For example, we may not be comparing like-with-like. City B schools may have access to better health-care facilities that are giving the diagnosis of asthma. City A children might just think they are 'chesty' or even normal when they have the same symptoms. Or city B children and their parents may be more articulate and therefore self-report asthma more.

Alternatively, the difference may be real and can be analysed by the epidemiological triad of host, agent, and environment. City B children may be more susceptible to the disease, more exposed to agents that cause disease, or be living in environments where asthma-causing agents thrive, for example, modern housing where ventilation is low.

Question 4 In a randomized, double-blind controlled clinical trial of the value of dietary iron supplementation in preventing sickness absence from work in women, a university department of epidemiology did a study which compared two groups. The intervention group of 4300 women had the supplement. The trial outcome, sickness absence, was obtained from employment records one year later. Two-hundred-and-seventy (270) people were recorded as having at least one day off work.

The control group was 4150 women who had an inactive ingredient that looked similar to the dietary supplementation, that is, a placebo. Three-hundred-and-fifty (350) women were recorded as having at least one day off work in the same time period.

(i) Place these data in an appropriate 2 × 2 table.

(ii) Estimate the number of people who need to be given the supplement to prevent one or more days of sickness absence.

(iii) Do you believe this trial shows the effectiveness of dietary iron supplementation in preventing sickness absence? Write a short letter to the chief executive officer of a health authority or equivalent health-service funding body giving three reasons why you think the results show a benefit, and three reasons why the benefit might not be real.

Answer (i)

See Table 9.13.

Table 9.13 Results of the trial of the prevention of sickness absence from work in women through dietary iron supplementation presented in a 2 × 2 table

| | Sickness absence (one or more day/year) | | |
	Yes	No	Totals
Intervention group	270	4030	4300
Control group	350	2300	2700
Total	620	7830	8450

Answer (ii)

Number needed to prevent or treat (reciprocal of the difference in incidence rates):

$$= \frac{1}{(350/4150) - (270/4300)}$$

$$= \frac{1}{0.084 - 0.063}$$

$$= \frac{1}{0.021} = 47.6.$$

Answer (iii)

Dear Chief Executive,

Re: Iron supplementation to reduce sickness absence in women

I urge you to note the results of a recent iron supplementation trial carefully. First, because the trial was both randomized and double-blind, any bias in allocation to study groups and ascertainment of the outcome of interest is unlikely to explain the findings. Second, the use of randomization also ensured comparability of the two groups, and therefore, any confounding with respect to both known and unknown factors is unlikely. Third, the use of a placebo ensured that the outcome is likely to be due to the actual trial intervention rather than to any extra attention the intervention group received or their belief in the intervention.

Notwithstanding these strengths, potential errors still need to be considered. Although unlikely, benefits could have arisen by chance. Bias could have occurred if the study subjects or the researchers who collected the data correctly guessed whether they were on the actual treatment or a placebo. As iron has some specific effects, for example, constipation and dark stools, recipients may indeed have guessed the allocation. Third, there may be errors in the employment records of sickness absence. I also note that although the trial was randomized, there were more people in the intervention than control group. I have no explanation for this but it may matter so we need to learn more.

Yours sincerely,
A. N. Epidemiologist

Question 5 In a cohort study following up 7000 people for an average of five years, 3000 people took a vitamin supplement and 4000 did not. There were 57 cases of cancer in the vitamin supplement group, and 43 cases of cancer in the other group.

(i) Put these data into a 2 × 2 table.

(ii) Calculate the incidence rate in each group using the person–time denominator. For simplicity, first, as the disease is rare you may refrain from adjusting the denominator for those developing the outcome. Then, do adjust the denominator to account for a change in the population at risk as best as you can with this limited information.

(iii) What information do these findings offer for concluding that vitamin supplementation increases the risk of cancer?

Answer (i)

See Table 9.14.

Table 9.14 Results of a cohort study on the use of a vitamin supplement and cancer incidence presented in a 2 × 2 table

Risk factor	Disease outcome		Totals
	Cancer	No cancer	
Vitamin supplement	57	2943	3000
No vitamin supplement	43	3957	4000
Total	100	6900	7000

Answer (ii) Incidence rate (person-years) in the vitamin supplement group:

$$= \frac{57}{3000 \times 5} = \frac{57}{15\,000} = 0.0038 = 3.8/1000 \text{ person-years.}$$

Incidence rate in the no vitamin supplement group:

$$= \frac{43}{20\,000} = 0.0022 = 2.2/1000 \text{ person-years.}$$

More exact calculation would remove from the denominator 142.5 years (57 cases × 2.5 years) for the vitamin group and 107.5 years (43 cases × 2.5 years) for the no vitamin group, as people with the outcome contribute half of the time that non-cases do. This rests on the assumption that cases occur evenly over the time interval.

Answer (iii) The rate of cancer is about 70 per cent higher in the vitamin supplement group. The steps will be to consider the role of chance, bias, and confounding. Among the most important questions to answer is whether the two groups were alike, other than in relation to vitamin taking. Cancers are, for example, more common in older people and those who smoke. It may be that the two groups differ in these and other important ways. If the differences cannot be explained in these ways, then there is a case for applying the epidemiological guidelines for causal reasoning. If the evidence looks convincing a trial is the next step to gather more definitive evidence. In many of these steps, including moving to the next stage of research, the causal graph will be valuable.

Question 6 In a trial of the value of double glazing in preventing sickness absence from work, a housing department compared two groups. The first consisted of 3200 houses where the windows had been replaced. The head of household's sickness absence record was recorded by self-completion questionnaire—one year later. Two-hundred-and-seventy (270) people reported at least one day off work.

The control group was 20 750 homes awaiting double glazing; 2350 people reported at least one day off work in the same time period.

(i) Place these data in an appropriate 2 × 2 table.

(ii) Calculate the number of houses needed to be double glazed to prevent one or more sickness absences.

(iii) Do you believe the results of this trial? Write a short letter to the health authority giving *six* reasons why the results might be unreliable.

Answer (i)

Table 9.15 Results of the trial of double glazing preventing sickness from work presented in a 2 × 2 table

Exposure	Sickness absence		Totals
	Off work	Not off work	
Windows replaced	270	2930	3200
Windows not replaced	2350	18 400	20 750
Totals	**2620**	**21 330**	**23 950**

See Table 9.15.

Answer (ii)

Number needed to prevent

= Inverse of: difference in incidence in control group – incidence in study group

$$= \frac{1}{(2350 \div 20\ 750) - (270 \div 3200)}$$

$$= \frac{1}{0.113 - 0.084}$$

$$= \frac{1}{0.029}$$

$$= 34.5.$$

Answer (iii)

Dear Health Authority,

I urge you to evaluate the results of the double glazing trial with caution, as the results may be unreliable. First, the trial was not randomized. The people living in the two groups of houses may have been different to start with. Second, we may be seeing a placebo effect, that is, the benefits are non-specific. Third, there is the possibility of reporting bias, that is, the data on the sickness absence may be inaccurate. Fourth, it may be that those completing the questionnaire are more likely to report a benefit. Fifth, this might be a chance result. Finally, we have no data on the benefits in relation to the costs.

Yours sincerely,

A. N. Epidemiologist

References

Barbenel, J., Jordan, M., Nicol, S., and Clark, M.O. (1977) Incidence of pressure-sores in the Greater Glasgow Health Board area. *Lancet*, **2**, 548–50.

Bhopal, R.S., Moffatt, S., Pless-Mulloli, T., *et al.* (1998) Does living near a constellation of petrochemical, steel, and other industries impair health? *Occupational and Environmental Medicine*, **55**, 812–22.

Bhopal R.S., Douglas A., Wallia S., *et al.* (2014) Effect of a lifestyle intervention on weight change in south Asian individuals in the UK at high risk of type 2 diabetes: a family-cluster randomised controlled trial. *The Lancet Diabetes & Endocrinology*, **2**, 218–27.

Edwards, R., Pless-Mulloli, T., Howel, D., *et al.* (2006) Does living near heavy industry cause lung cancer in women? A case-control study using life grid interviews. *Thorax*, **61**, 1076–82.

Frost, W.H. (1998) The age of selection of mortality from tuberculosis in succesive decades. In: Buck, C., Llopis, A., Najera, E., and Terris, M. (eds). *The Challenge of Epidemiology: Issues and Selected Readings*. Washington, WA: Pan American Health Association, pp. 176–9.

Gregg, N.M. (1941) Congenital cataract following German measles in the mother. *Transactions of the Ophthalmological Society of Australia*, **3**, 35–46. Reprinted in Buch *et al.* 1988, pp. 426–34.

Harland, J., Unwin, N., Bhopal, R.S., *et al.* (1997) Low levels of cardiovascular risk factors and coronary heart disease in a UK Chinese population. *Journal of Epidemiology and Community Health*, **51**, 636–42.

Herbst, A.L., Ulfelder, H., and Poskanzer, D.C. (1971) Adenocarcinoma of the vagina. Association of maternal stilbestrol therapy with tumor appearance in young women. *New England Journal of Medicine*, **284**, 878–81.

McEachan, R.R., Santorelli, G., Bryant, M., *et al.* (2016) The HAPPY (Healthy and Active Parenting Programmme for early Years) feasibility randomised control trial: acceptability and feasibility of an intervention to reduce infant obesity. *BMC Public Health*, **16**, 211.

McMahon, B. and Trichopoulos, D. (1996) *Epidemiology*, 2nd edn. Boston, MA: Little, Brown.

Pearce, N. (2000) The ecological fallacy strikes back. *Journal of Epidemiology and Community Health*, **54**, 326–7.

Porta, M. (2014) *A Dictionary of Epidemiology*, 6th edn. New York, NY: Oxford University Press.

Voight, B.F., Peloso, G.M., Orho-Melander, M., *et al.* (2012) Plasma HDL cholesterol and risk of myocardial infarction: a mendelian randomisation study. *Lancet*, **380**, 572–580.

Appendix 9.1

Extra information for Mendelian randomization exemplar

Table A9.1 Summary table of results of Mendelian randomization study

1. Case–control study			
Risk factor	No. of SNPs	Range of increased risk (%) to	No. of SNPs statistically significantly associated with MI
LDL	10	3 to 16	9/10
HDL	15	−12 to 31	6/15
Specific HDL genotype (Ans 396 Ser)	1	−6% (95% CI–18 to 9)	0/1

Table A9.1 Continued

2. Cohort studies	No. of SNPs	Increased risk	No. of SNPs showing association
i. Standard analysis (4 cohorts) examining association with 0.03 mmol/l increase in plasma HDL-C			
Specific HDL genotype	1	−2 (95% CI −3 to −2)	4/4
ii. Mendelian randomization analysis (6 cohorts, including above 4)			
		+2 (95% CI −5 to 9)	0/1
iii. Genetic risk score for HDL-C			
	14	−7 (95% CI −32 to 26)	0/1
iv. Genetic risk score for LDL-C			
	13	+ 113 (95% CI 69 to 169)	1/1

Source: data from Voight BF, Peloso GM, Orho-Melander M, Frikke-Schmidt R, Barbalic M, Jensen MK et al. Plasma HDL cholesterol and risk of myocardial infarction: a mendelian randomisation study. *The Lancet*, Volume 380, Issue 9841, pp. 572–580, Copyright © 2012 Elsevier Ltd.

Table A9.2 Information provided for each SNP: example of the specific HDL associated polymorphism on the endothelial lipase gene (LIPG)

The alphanumeric identifier for the SNP	rs61755018
The chromosome and its location on the chromosome	18 or 21
Gene of interest	LIPG Asn396Ser
Major allele (variant) to minor allele (variant) frequency	Major allele A to Minor allele G (0.015 = 1.5%)
Allele modelled in analysis	G
Increase in plasma HDL-C (mmol/l) associated with allele of interest	0.14
Sample size – cases – controls	17 165 49 077
Observed change in MI risk (95% CI) for modelled allele	−6% (−18 to 9)
P-value for modelled allele and association with MI	0.41

Appendix 9.2

Answers to 20 epidemiological questions

Table A9.3 Twenty epidemiological questions—some possible answers

Question	Potential study designs	My preferred study design with reason
1 Is leukaemia increasing in its incidence?	Case series based on clinical or population disease registers (population case series)—particularly of cancer registrations	Cancer registration registers analysed as a population case series but ideally with a population register or census, so rates can be estimated
2 What factors are, potentially, causes of leukaemia?	Case–control studies Cohort studies/retrospective cohort studies Animal experiments Natural experiments of humans (note, if the question was on factors potentially protective from leukaemia, human trials would be possible)	Case–control studies because they give the answer efficiently and quickly These may well be nested within cohort studies
3 What proportion of the population is exposed to virus X?	Cross-sectional study Population registers recording people known to be infected with virus X, with the population denominator coming from the census or a population registration scheme	Cross-sectional study, as best method for prevalence data
4 Does exposure to drugs to treat epilepsy in pregnant mothers lead to congenital malformations in their offspring?	Case–control study Cohort study/retrospective cohort study Analysis of data from drug side effect registers Case series Trials comparing different drugs	Cohort study, which is quick and easy to assemble for pregnancy outcomes
5 Does flying on long-distance aeroplane flights increase the risk of pulmonary embolism, i.e. blood clots in the lung?	Case–control study Cohort studies/retrospective cohort study	Case–control study followed by cohort study if the initial study shows an association
6 What proportion of those taking long-distance aeroplane flights develop deep venous thrombosis?	Cohort study/retrospective cohort study	Cohort study (probably retrospective as it should be possible to construct a sample of long distance flyers)
7 What are the side effects of oral contraceptives?	Cohort studies/retrospective cohort studies Studies of reported side effects in drug surveillance schemes	Cohort study As the full range of side effects are unlikely to be in records, a prospective study is preferable

(*continued*)

Table A9.3 Continued

Question	Potential study designs	My preferred study design with reason
8 Are oral contraceptives more effective for the prevention of pregnancy than other methods, e.g. the condom?	Trials Cohort studies of people taking these forms of contraceptive	Trial, as best method of evaluation
9 What are the risk factors for fatal pedestrian accidents?	Case–control study Case series/population case series	Case–control study The challenge is getting controls—in one study these were pedestrians of the same age and sex passing by the spot at the time, day, and location of each accident
10 Does having a maximum speed limit of 30 miles per hour reduce fatal pedestrian accidents, as compared to 40 miles per hour?	Case–control studies National or international pragmatic evaluations based on case registers, i.e. population case series examining effect of changing speed limits Animal experiments Experiments using dummies simulating accidents Trials	Pragmatic before and after evaluations derived from population case series based on registers of accidents A trial, though theoretically correct, would be very difficult to do at reasonable cost
11 Is the heart disease mortality rate on the rise or on the decline?	Studies of population registers of disease, i.e. population case series Repeated cohort studies	Population case series, as most efficient, if data exist
12 Why is the incidence of heart disease mortality changing?	Modelling studies using information on risk factor–outcome relationships from cohort studies and, changing prevalence of risk factors from cross-sectional studies Repeated cohort studies	Modelling based on cohort studies and reported cross-sectional studies of risk factors The cohort studies establish the risk-factor-outcome relationship
13 Would doubling the amount of exercise in the population setting reduce the incidence of heart disease?	Trials, possibly examining intermediate outcomes Pragmatic, before and after evaluations International, regional, and local comparisons based on population case registers and information on exercise patterns based on cross-sectional studies	Trial, as the best method of evaluation
14 What is the relationship between the wealth of the country as measured with the GNP and the consumption of illicit drugs, e.g. heroin, and legal drugs, e.g. alcohol?	Ecological studies based on GNP and information on proxy indicators of consumption, e.g. excise duties on alcohol, or amount of heroin seized at ports	Ecological study

Table A9.3 Continued

Question	Potential study designs	My preferred study design with reason
15 What proportion of school children are obese?	Cross-sectional study Case series of a register of obese children	Cross-sectional study, as best method for prevalence data
16 Do farm subsidies to dairy farmers lead to increased consumption of dairy products in the population?	Ecological studies associating amount of subsidy to an indicator of consumption, e.g. milk produced. Cross-sectional studies measuring daily use over time, i.e. repeated studies timed appropriately Trials	Ecological studies as early and quick A trial of this kind of food policy would be extremely difficult
17 What is the cause of a rare disease of your choice, e.g. phaeochromocytoma, a tumour of the adrenal gland?	Case–control study Case series based on clinical or population registers	Case–control study (Prospective cohort studies would be nigh impossible as is true for most very rare outcomes and retrospective ones would be unlikely to be able to acquire the necessary risk factor data)
18 How many cases of AIDS, or any other similar infectious disease of your choice, should the health service be planning for 5, 10, and 20 years from now?	Modelling based on population case registers/surveillance systems of AIDS cases and trends in prevalence of HIV based on cross-sectional studies Expert consensus study, i.e. interview or questionnaire	Modelling based on a variety of data especially time trends in AIDS and (population case series) and cross-sectional studies of HIV prevalence
19 Is the amount of fruit and vegetable consumption increasing or decreasing? What is likely to happen in 10 years from now?	Repeat cross-sectional studies to ask people about their behaviour and intentions Ecological studies based on farming, marketing, and shopping practices	Repeat cross-sectional studies, as best method of gauging prevalence
20 Would screening all adults for diabetes using blood tests improve the health of the population? Would this be cost-effective?	Trials Pragmatic evaluations Modelling studies Health economics work on cost effectiveness, cost benefit, and cost utility	Trials with health economic study integrated

Chapter 10

Epidemiology in the past, present, and the future: Theory, ethics, context, and critical appraisal

Objectives

On completion of this chapter you should understand that:

◆ theory, method, and application are interrelated, therefore evolution in one leads to change in the others;

◆ epidemiology serves the community in a number of ways, but predominantly through its role as one of the underpinning sciences of public health and clinical care;

◆ ongoing vigorous debate on the future of epidemiology probably heralds a paradigm shift;

◆ epidemiology is both broadening and specializing;

◆ the context in which epidemiology is learned and practised is important in determining its nature;

◆ epidemiological codes of ethics and good conduct need to encompass both the scientific and the medical and public health applications;

◆ critical appraisal is an essential skill for epidemiologists and requires attention to fundamental issues including the social and geographical context and purposes of research;

◆ epidemiologists need to study their subject's history, classical studies, and contemporary research, and to join the debates that will shape the future of their discipline and the health status of global populations.

10.1 The interrelationship of theory, methods, and application: responding to criticisms of epidemiology

In about 50 years following the Second World War, epidemiology established its place at the heart of public health, clinical care, health policy, and service planning. This was achieved through astounding continuing advances in both infectious and environment related disorders and, especially, in understanding the causes of chronic disease related to behaviours. Of the latter the greatest triumph was, arguably, establishing tobacco as the cause of a large number of cancers, and cardiovascular and respiratory diseases. Notwithstanding these achievements, epidemiology entered the twenty-first century with both its exponents and critics questioning its foundations, record, and future.

Modern epidemiology has been accused of being atheoretical; divorced from its source of problems, theories, and applications (public health); the source of spurious, confusing, and misleading findings; and over-dependent on the 'black box' risk factor approach. Every day the media report hugely exaggerated claims and counter-claims about epidemiological studies. Some, but by no means all, of this questionable research is reported by people untrained in epidemiology but the discipline's reputation is still tarnished.

Almost invariably, investigators (and the media) are inferring or implying cause and effect relationships from mere statistical associations. As we have discussed, such associations are rarely causal. The fundamental axiom 'association is not causation' is violated constantly. Remarkably, it is commonplace for researchers to note this principle in passing and then to proceed to make causal claims unabashedly. The language of association and causation is entangled at least partly because of cross-disciplinary misinterpretation, often because disciplines use normal language in technical ways that are forgotten when translated across disciplines. Examples of this are the words significant, meaning a level of probability and not as most people understand (i.e. something that is important); and effect meaning the amount of change in a summary measure of association and not the impact of an intervention, as we would expect it to mean. In Table 9.9 I have provided some causal and non-causal terms. Causal terms should be used rarely, with the exception being randomized controlled trials, and major, consensual syntheses of data that are designed to summarize causal evidence from a body of literature.

Media publicity is, perhaps unfortunately, seen as a measure of success and is much coveted by researchers, their employers, and funders of research. Guarded conclusions that are so essential to good science do not make for exciting media reports. The result has been a profusion of unsound advice followed by the predictable and inevitable cynicism about epidemiological findings.

Science is, rightly, emphasizing engagement and knowledge sharing with the public. The need for education on core concepts that will enable the general public to absorb and appraise the information they are receiving is a topic for epidemiologists to consider. Alfredo Morabia, among others, has advocated teaching some epidemiology to school children.

Even more seriously, there have been questions about the relevance of epidemiology to resolving some major problems, such as the growing consumption of illegal drugs, the rising prevalence of smoking in developing countries, the obesity epidemic, climate change, and the omnipresent problem of health inequalities. To participate in the resolution of such problems, epidemiologists need to go beyond learning about, and advancing, methods and techniques. They also need to be aware of the changes in their environment and respond to them. Ideally, they would pick up coming changes early on. Some of the criticisms of epidemiology are old ones.

As early as 1978 Alwyn Smith criticized the atheoretical, empirical, methodological orientation of modern epidemiology and called for an integration of social, political, and biological frameworks of health and disease into epidemiology. In his 1985 review of the evolution of epidemiology in the United States of America, Mervyn Susser paid tribute to the methodological advances which had led to epidemiology reaching maturity as an academic discipline, but his words echoed some of Smith's concerns, and emphasized that epidemiology had originated as an applied public health discipline. Nancy Krieger (1992) concluded, based partly on an examination of textbooks, that attention has been diverted from theory and concepts of epidemiology to methods and technique. These and other more recent and equally influential observations, hopefully, will lead to a closer integration of theory, method, and application. Indeed, it was in response to such criticisms that I paid especial attention to theory in this book, and, more recently Krieger has responded to the challenge by publishing a textbook devoted to epidemiological theory (Krieger 2011).

The philosophy and theory underpinning epidemiology, as in most other scientific disciplines, is seldom made explicit, and is often taken for granted, and yet underpins all its work. It is a driver of change, and guides the paradigms within which epidemiology works.

Philosophically, epidemiology takes a positivist stance. The positivists' position is that problems can be solved and questions can be answered through the collection of data which are usually, but not always, quantitative. This stance has served epidemiology well. There are, however, limitations in the quantitative approach, which is excellent for description, but insufficient for generating understanding. This book has repeatedly emphasized that epidemiological advances may follow inspiration and insights that are not based on quantitative data—Semmelweis's inspiration being one (Chapter 5). In recent years we have seen greater incorporation of qualitative research into epidemiology, for example, to develop better measures, to gain understanding about how people think and behave, and to understanding why interventions offered in trials were, or were not, accepted.

Future epidemiology is likely to involve even closer ties between qualitative and quantitative approaches, and a greater attention to disease mechanisms, an approach that requires closer and work with social and biological scientists. Social scientists tend to be more theory orientated and want their work to be based on and contribute towards a pre-identified theoretical position. These collaborators will need to understand (and hopefully respect) the theories of epidemiology, so epidemiologists need to be able to know and communicate them.

The basic theory from which the causal contribution of epidemiology derives is that systematic variations in the pattern of health and disease exist in populations. These are a product of differences in either exposure or susceptibility to the causal factors. The fundamental epidemiological question is why these differences in exposure and susceptibility occur, and the challenge is to link explanations to the observed phenomena and to predict one from the other. Ultimately, such predictions could generate the 'laws' of health and disease in populations. These laws will not, however, be mathematical equations, as in physics, but could possibly be principles, as in the 10 Commandments. There is a great deal to do to achieve this goal, but we have already made great progress. The obvious example is the warning on cigarette packets 'Smoking kills'. That is, effectively, a law of health and disease based on epidemiology. We are probably able to say much the same for high blood pressure. The evidence base for adiposity, physical activity, nutrition, sleep, and many other factors needs to reach the same level of certainty.

Epidemiological theory attributes the causes of disease to an interaction within the causal triad of host, agent, and environment. This triad works particularly well for toxic and infectious diseases, but to make it more widely applicable it needs to be developed in more detail. Development will be derived from the expanding fields described by the labels of genetic, social, life-course, and chronic disease epidemiology. This way of causal thinking was discussed in Chapters 1, 2, 3, and 5.

Epidemiologists need to think deeply about the forces that generate health and disease in populations so their specific studies are based on, and contribute to, the broader context of changing health states.

Before reading section 10.2, do the exercise in Box 10.1.

10.2 Fundamental influences on health and disease in populations

Figure 10.1 provides a simplified diagrammatic representation of the thinking to be explained here.

The fundamental influences on health and disease at the population level include changes in the natural environment; environmental changes arising from human invention, discovery, and

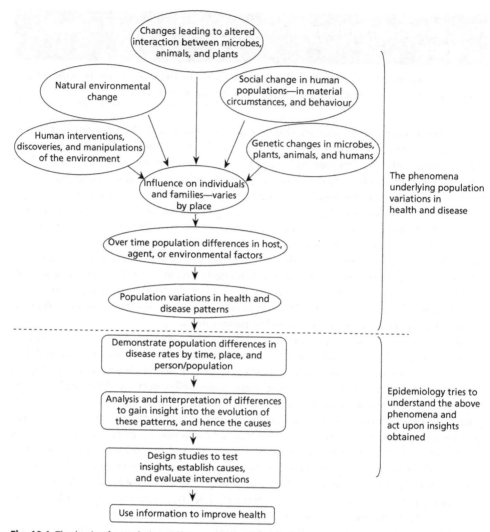

Fig. 10.1 The basis of population differences in health and disease pattern: towards an epidemiological theory and strategy.

intervention; changes in the interaction between humans, microbes, and animals, usually for cultural reasons; changes in human socio-economic circumstances, cultures, and behaviours; and the genetic evolution of plants, microbes, animals, and humans.

These complex and interacting influences, exerting their effect over long spans of time (for human genetic effects, likely to be measured in hundreds or thousands of years), are the underlying causes of population patterns in disease. Their initial impact may be small and on individuals and families or small groups. Over time, due to their varying circumstances and varying changes, populations begin to differ from each other, leading to the population patterns in disease and health that epidemiologists demonstrate. In Figure 10.1, all of these are shown above the dotted line. This is the raw material for epidemiology to study.

Epidemiological methods are designed to quantify variations in diseases and in their causes, to seek and quantify associations between them, and to generate and test resultant hypotheses, which are usually couched in more specific terms than those just mentioned. Nonetheless, they are embedded in this framework of influencing factors. The first step is to describe patterns over time, and by place and person.

Variations in disease frequency give rise to hypotheses which might help to explain the patterns observed, and give insight into the natural history and causes of disease. Classical epidemiological study designs (such as case–control and cohort) can be used to test such insights (Chapter 9) and, if supported, epidemiological guidelines can be applied to assess the likelihood of associations representing cause and effect (Chapter 5). Epidemiological models of cause (such as the triangle of causation) and directed acyclic graphs can help to conceptualize interventions for disease control (Chapter 5). Knowledge of cause and effect is essential to developing rational scientific interventions to prevent, control, and treat disease. To ensure these interventions work they need to be evaluated. Epidemiological study designs are also used for evaluating screening and diagnostic tests (Chapter 6), in evaluating preventive and other procedures in public health, in assessing the efficacy of drugs and other interventions in curative medicine, and in studies of prognosis. While all the study designs may contribute to evaluation, the most powerful one is the randomized controlled trial (Chapter 9).

The remaining challenge is to synthesize information from diverse epidemiological studies and other sciences, so that the evidence can be used to develop policy and services. The successful implementation of these policies takes epidemiology into partnership with the art and science of public health and clinical care. This takes us full circle because these interventions, in improving health, act as a fundamental influence on population patterns of health and disease. They will not be implemented evenly, or affect populations evenly, so new patterns will emerge to puzzle and challenge future epidemiology. We see here the enmeshing of epidemiological science with practice, a topic we consider next.

10.3 **Theory and practice: role of epidemiology**

As many, if not most, important advances derive from practical problems in public health and clinical care, epidemiological theory, research, and practice should intertwine. Gerry Morris, in his classic book *Uses of Epidemiology* (first published in 1957, and expanded in 1964) portrayed epidemiology as a discipline with multiple applications as reflected in his chapter headings: trends in disease; community diagnosis; working of health services; individual chances; completing the clinical picture; identification of syndromes; causal search, etc. In many contemporary textbooks, by comparison, the vision of epidemiology is narrower, and probably narrowing. In the 1980s we saw a major shift in epidemiology and this was described as 'modern epidemiology' (the title of Kenneth Rothman's influential textbook *Modern Epidemiology* may have echoed this movement, or perhaps gave rise to the use of the phrase (1986)). Textbooks placed an increasing emphasis on method, technique, and analysis implying that epidemiology is primarily about measuring disease in populations, and not how diseases develop, propagate, and are prevented in populations. Measuring disease, however, is merely the means to the end. This is not to deny the value of the advances in method in technique. Indeed, this book has benefited from these advances, which continue apace.

One vital question under current debate is whether epidemiology is primarily an applied discipline with population health goals, or a science where methods, technique, and theory are mainly aiming at the extension of knowledge (Rothman *et al.* 1998). Whatever the outcome of the debate the fact is that epidemiology has a huge impact on health and health care. It is worth noting that most definitions of epidemiology continue to place a premium on applications, including the sixth, 2014 edition of the *Dictionary of Epidemiology*.

In measuring the frequency (incidence and prevalence) of disease in defined populations (Chapter 7), epidemiological studies almost invariably uncover more than the expected morbidity, demonstrating unmet health care need thus leading to expanded or new services (Chapter 6). Comparisons of disease patterns over time, between geographical areas, and by the characteristics of people within populations (e.g. by sex and age) also permit an understanding of how disease patterns are likely to change (Chapters 3 and 9), so assessing future health needs and helping in health-care planning. Disease trends, combined with information on demographic change and risk factor patterns, can be used to predict the future, and develop health targets. For example, epidemiological observations in the United Kingdom in the 1980s and 1990s on the trend in measles cases, with the prediction of an epidemic, gave priority to a national measles campaign targeted at school children; predictions of the HIV and AIDS epidemic in the mid-1980s gave priority to these problems; and the observations of variations in disease experience by socio-economic status have placed inequalities in health as one of the top ranking international and national priorities.

Not all health problems are predictable and not all have been predicted correctly. Our collective crystal ball did not predict the imminence or the size of the obesity epidemic. Predictions of the demise of infectious diseases in wealthy nations were wildly optimistic. By contrast to this, predictions of how much mortality from coronary heart disease was preventable, and how quickly, were underestimates even though two major risk factors have risen sharply (obesity and diabetes).

The traditional values of epidemiology are that it is concerned with the nature of health and disease in populations; that there is population group variation in disease that is worthy of scientific study; that it is important to medical and public health policy and practice; and that is it vital to prevent, control, and treat disease. There is no clash between these traditional values and modern developments in epidemiology, which emphasize measurement technique, study design, and analysis. Rather, the former drives the latter, and the latter enhances the traditional goals of epidemiology. To illustrate how theory, method, and application are interdependent I have chosen two topics of personal interest: setting priorities in health care and assessing the impact on health of local polluting industries. These topics also show how epidemiological techniques continue to develop.

10.4 **From practice to theory to techniques and back**

10.4.1 **Setting priorities in health and health care: illustrative topic 1**

> Setting priorities is an issue for any organization. The process should be sensible; it should be founded on science; it should be based on experience and research.
>
> Virginia Bottomley (1993)

Priority setting within health and health care is a complex mix of science and politics. Epidemiological data on disease frequency, patterns, causes, risk factors, and effectiveness stimulates the political debate on priority setting. Epidemiological criteria for priority setting (e.g. frequency and severity of disease) need to be merged with clinical, economic, and political ones to make sense of past priorities and to help determine new ones. National health policy initiatives are nowadays, but not in the past, founded on epidemiology.

Priority setting cannot rest on scientific data alone. Judgements need to be made within a decision-making framework. Some of the characteristics of diseases, conditions, and problems which tend to receive high priority, in practice, are listed in Box 10.2, which is based on my judgement shaped by groups of postgraduate public health students who have discussed the topic.

Box 10.2 Some characteristics of problems given high priority

A. **Epidemiological and other scientific factors**

The problem is:

- ◆ common
- ◆ becoming commoner
- ◆ is commoner than expected, compared with other populations we compare ourselves to
- ◆ severe in its effects
- ◆ long-lasting
- ◆ communicable from person-to-person
- ◆ epidemic
- ◆ acquired externally, or iatrogenically, that is, from medical interventions
- ◆ one of the younger age groups
- ◆ preventable or treatable in a cost-effective way

B. **Social, economic, and political factors**

The problem is:

- ◆ of high media, public, and political interest
- ◆ economically important
- ◆ lobbied for by pressure groups or powerful individuals, especially politicians
- ◆ low in social stigma
- ◆ not seen as self-inflicted
- ◆ of interest to health professions including researchers

*Problems which do not have these characteristics, or have opposite characteristics, are given low priority.

Source: data from Bhopal RS. Setting priorities for health care in ethnic minority groups. In: Rawaf S, Bahl V, eds. *Health Needs Assessment in Ethnic Minority Groups*. London: Royal College of Physicians, Copyright © 1998 RCP.

Epidemiology, alone, provides quantitative information on how common problems are and how they are changing. In conjunction with other clinical sciences, epidemiology has a key role in studying the outcome of disease in terms of chronicity, severity, and case-fatality and in setting out the prospects for prevention, control, and treatment. With social, laboratory, and clinical sciences, epidemiology helps to define the relative importance of genetic, lifestyle, and external environmental factors in the causation of disease. The role of epidemiology is in providing background scientific information—part (a) of Box 10.2—that permits characterization of the importance of health problems at various geographical scales and in different population subgroups.

The epidemiological principle influenced by public health, which has limitations for individual patient care, is that the most important problems are those that cause the greatest loss of life and illness, and are most amenable to prevention or effective treatment. The degree of loss can be expressed as the loss of life and the loss of life free of illness or disability (DALY) and with the loss of quality of life (QALY) (as discussed in Chapter 8). It is, unfortunately, true that this perspective can undermine the prospects for people with rare conditions potentially requiring expensive policy interventions and even expensive individual level interventions. In the United Kingdom, for example, under the guidance of the National Institute for Clinical and Public Health Excellence (NICE) interventions that cost up to £30 000 (about $45 000 and €45 000) gain National Health Service support while more expensive ones do not. Very often the costly interventions are for rare problems. A call has been made by scientists and media alike in Scotland to supplement the vitamin D intake of the Scottish population to prevent, potentially, multiple sclerosis, a rare but lifelong, serious neurological disease. This call has not been supported, not least because doing a randomized controlled trial to demonstrate the postulated benefits would be problematic and extremely costly. By contrast, vitamin D trials for many other commoner conditions have been implemented.

To illustrate how epidemiology can contribute, Table 10.1 provides data on the number of deaths, the death rate, potential years of life lost (PYLL), and the standardized mortality ratios (SMR) for five health problems in an English health authority. In terms of providing diagnostic, advisory, and caring services, the data in Table 10.1, combined with basic clinical knowledge about the mode of presentation and severity of disease, show that cancers, ischaemic heart disease, and cerebrovascular disease potentially have high priority. These three problems would be high priorities on the basis of the frequency data alone, but their major contributions to PYLL and the high SMR for cancer and ischaemic heart disease add to their priority status. Accidents and suicide cause relatively few deaths but the PYLL data enhance their priority status. Accidents also show a high SMR.

The debate started by these data needs to be refined with information on numbers needed to treat for the efficacy of treatment and to prevent for preventive strategies (as discussed next in regard to risk factors), by adding the burden of disability and calculating disability-adjusted life years (DALYs), and by including economic factors, for example, by using quality-adjusted life years (QALYs) (Chapter 8).

Epidemiology also assesses the presence and impact of risk factors that influence mortality and morbidity. These data can be combined to estimate the risk of disease in a population that is attributable to one or more risk factors (Chapter 8). In conjunction with evaluation research these data, in turn, can be incorporated into health policy. For example, researchers have shown major variations in coronary heart disease (CHD) over time, between places, and within subgroups of populations, and have defined a number of important risk factors amenable to change of which smoking, hypertension, and high cholesterol are the best studied. Cross-sectional studies have defined the prevalence of risk factors in populations across the world, cohort and case–control

Table 10.1 The number of deaths, standardized mortality ratio (SMR) and potential years of life lost (PYLL) for selected causes of death, Newcastle upon Tyne, England, 1993

Cause of death	Number of deaths	Death rate per 10 000 population	PYLL	SMR
Cancer	943	335	6243	125
Ischaemic heart disease	884	314	3550	112
Cerebrovascular disease	348	124	1073	104
Accidents	72	26	1261	126
Suicide	26	9	870	94
All causes	3482	1236	19 264	116

SMR, standardized mortality ratio; PYLL, potential years of life lost.

Reproduced by kind permission of Dr Mike Lavender.

studies have linked risk factors to disease, and population-based trials have assessed the efficacy of preventive strategies. Health economics has been influential in helping to define the most cost-effective interventions that address the major issues highlighted by epidemiology. The sum of this knowledge contributes to judging the priority to be given to CHD prevention, in relation to the prevention of other diseases, and in relation to curative and palliative interventions. CHD has enjoyed top priority in many industrialized nations for several decades and is now rising in the priority list of many developing countries. Epidemiology is responsible for this.

Epidemiology provides information to use in the process of priority setting, which is ultimately, however, a political one. Some of the important political factors are given in Box 10.2 part (b). The scientific factors and social/economic/political factors are not independent. Clearly, problems that are common and severe are more likely to interest health professionals and also to be of economic and political interest. Problems that are of interest to pressure groups and politicians are more likely to be studied scientifically, and more data will become available to define the burden (and previously hidden burden) of disease and the scope for prevention or cure, thus raising its priority. The influence of politics and society on science, and vice versa, is an ethical matter (see section 10.10). Coronary heart disease, and especially heart attack (myocardial infarction) meets every one of the social, economic, and political characteristics of a high priority. It enjoys this status in industrialized, wealthy countries and efforts to raise it to a top ranking priority in developing countries are only slowly succeeding, because while the epidemiological data are clear enough the other factors are often not present. A recent United Nations summit has helped engineer change towards a higher political priority.

Few topics fall more clearly into the domain of applied epidemiology than priority setting. The role of epidemiology, though vast, is often not made explicit. Epidemiological theories, methods, and data combine with other disciplines to help form difficult judgements on priorities. When the causation of a disease is known, it is easy to overlook the role of epidemiology, both in macro and micro decision-making, but historical examples make it clear. In the case of cholera, the size of the problem gave it priority (macro), but which action should take priority: cleansing the streets of filth to reduce miasma or securing water supplies uncontaminated by sewage (micro)? In the case of pellagra (disease X in Chapter 1) its importance was clear because it was common and severe (macro) but should we prioritize quarantine measures, assuming it is an infection, or supplement the diet, assuming it is a nutritional deficiency (micro)? For coronary heart disease, do we prioritize cholesterol reduction or supplement the diet with antioxidants or fish oils or fish itself to reduce endothelial dysfunction (micro)? New variant CJD (Creutzfeldt–Jakob disease) in humans, arising from bovine spongiform encephalopathy (BSE) in cattle, was a priority on epidemiological grounds because it was increasing, externally acquired, severe, and potentially could result in an explosive epidemic (macro consideration). Time has shown that the feared epidemic did not occur, and the topic has quietly slipped as a priority. Theories on causation, and predictions of the size of the epidemic, were central to prioritizing this problem but there is great uncertainty on these at present. These examples illustrate the interdependence of theory, method, and data in applied epidemiology.

In conclusion, this topic illustrates how epidemiological understanding of causation is complementary to descriptive data on the burden of disease. Epidemiological theories of causation and data both help us to develop a sense of priority, and guide public health, health policy, and medical care services. The needs of policy and practice have provided the stimulus for modes of analysis (PYLL, attributable risk, NNT, DALYs, QALYs, etc.) that are not essential to causal epidemiology. In turn, these now classical measures are being further developed, for example, population impact numbers. The application of epidemiological knowledge spurs new questions and advancement of both method and theory; for example, the description of inequalities in health by epidemiologists is now giving way to understanding their causes and mechanisms especially with social scientists and with attention to co-factors; for example, sex, ethnicity and utilizing the concept of intersectionality.

10.4.2 Impact on health of local polluting industries: Teesside study of environment and health: illustrative topic 2

Research on industrial pollution and the health of nearby populations is usually done in the midst of media publicity and sometimes pending litigation. In our study of air pollution from petrochemical and steel industries and the health of people in Teesside (also see Chapter 4, Exemplar 4.1), my colleagues and I started with the testimony of general medical practitioners and with an analysis of mortality statistics. General practitioners feared, as had successive public health professionals for the previous hundred years, that the pollution caused premature death, cancer, asthma, and other chest problems. Routine statistics showed high mortality in the geographical areas close to industry. This type of problem typifies public health's dependence both on epidemiological theory, which is usually unspoken, and its method, which is explicit.

The first step in any investigation is to choose the theoretical framework within which to work. This was not done deliberatively or consciously, but automatically, by following the paths, traditions, and exemplars (paradigms) of environmental epidemiology. Only in retrospect is it clear to me that ours was a positivist approach, based on epidemiological, empirical, objectively collected data. It is also clear, in retrospect, that we gave less emphasis to alternatives, for example, qualitative studies of the public and industry employees, and toxicological approaches focusing on analysis of the chemicals produced by industry. These alternatives were secondary components. Other researchers from different disciplines may well have re-orientated the studies to prioritize such alternatives.

The second step was to propose hypotheses and study designs. We had several hypotheses of which the key one was that the risk of mortality and disease, particularly for respiratory health, would be higher than expected in populations living close to industry. We defined four populations in geographical areas at varying distances from the main industrial complexes. We wrote in the study protocol that an association would be worthy of serious consideration as causal if there was a gradient in the outcome with distance within the three areas in Teesside (called A, B, C), and if the three areas together had a higher outcome rate than a fourth area some 20 miles distant in the city of Sunderland (called S). We applied a mixture of designs, including modelling of historical land use, air pollution patterns currently and in the past (truly ecological studies), analysis of population case series of mortality from routine statistics, cross-sectional analysis of primary care use (by selected diagnosis), and cross-sectional studies of self-reported health in the community using questionnaires.

The third step was to agree on how the data were to be analysed and interpreted. Our framework of causal thinking was based, in essence, on the causal guidelines discussed in Chapter 5. We agreed that proximity of residence to industry was the key proxy measure for exposure to industrial pollution.

These decisions were based on important values, assumptions, and theories of health and disease. For example, the values and assumptions included that empirical data are more reliable than the testimony of local people; and that an epidemiological approach would be better than a toxicological one where we focused on measuring the air quality, or chemicals in blood or other human tissues, rather than health status. The underlying theory of health and disease was that long-term exposure to low levels of industrial air pollution does harm, rather than good. This alternative might seem absurd but it is not. Up until the 1950s many people proclaimed the health benefits of smoking tobacco (as indeed is still widely believed for chewing tobacco). This message was advertised in medical journals. The theory rests on data and is not secure until it does so. For the kind of pollutants we were concerned with, our theoretical stance was solid. Such factors are seldom made explicit but they play a vital role in guiding the research and its interpretation. Indeed, they were not made explicit in the Teesside study, but in retrospect and on reflection, their importance is clear.

We found that the death rates for lung cancer in women in area A, which was closest to industry, were exceptionally high and in line with the pattern predicted in our prior hypothesis. There was less clear-cut evidence for associations with proximity for some other respiratory health outcomes. For virtually every other cause of death and cancer, while health was poor, there was no such pattern. There was no evidence in favour of our prior hypothesis for birthweight, sex ratios at birth, and perinatal mortality in infants; for self-reported health; and for general practice consultation patterns.

We applied our real-artefact and causal frameworks to analyse these associations (see Chapters 4 and 5). We concluded that there was evidence that local industrial pollution had a potentially causal role in the high rates of lung cancer in women, but that for a wide range of other health concerns, alternative explanations were necessary. While there was no room for complacency, some reassurance was possible. How, then, were we to explain the many indicators of very poor health of people living in these areas closest to industry, if we were not willing to attribute them to industrial air pollution? We put particular emphasis on socio-economic deprivation and environmental degradation as causes of the general poor health in Teesside. We recommended a focus on poverty, new research on lung cancer in women and new studies of air quality around industry focusing on the public's concern. Our work provided data to resolve a public health problem that had been exercising medical officers of health since the beginning of the twentieth century.

The follow-up research included a case–control study of the association between proximity of residence to industry (as a proxy for long-term air pollution exposure) and lung cancer in women. Numerous studies of air pollution and lung cancer have been conducted and the pitfalls of tackling this topic are well documented. These pitfalls include the need to collect lifelong data retrospectively, using recall on both residential history (the key exposure variable) and on strong confounding factors including smoking and occupational history. The study used matched controls and an innovative 'life-grid' method for data collection. Here, a person's major life events are mapped on a time line, for example, going to primary school, secondary school, first job, moving house, marriage, having children, etc. Then, the enquiry about exposures is also mapped both generally, and specifically, in relation to these life events. This life-grid approach has been developed in the social sciences but is proving useful in epidemiology. The case–control study supported the earlier work, thus adding to the evidence in favour of a causal role for exposure to industrial air pollution in lung cancer in women (Edwards et al. 2006).

This work exemplifies how an outwardly atheoretical, pragmatic, public health-orientated project may be founded on important epidemiological theories and concepts. It also shows how epidemiology reaches out across disciplines to do the work—here toxicologists, geographers, statisticians, physicians, anthropologists, and epidemiologists worked together. When required, we went beyond epidemiology, for example, ecological studies of land use, and the use of the life-grid method for recall.

Those readers who do not share these epidemiological theories and concepts, and who are neither familiar with nor confident about the methods, will not be comfortable with the results. The public, for example, may give more credence to individual case histories of illness, and general observations on the quality of the environment, than to epidemiological data. Environmental scientists may remain unconvinced by the epidemiological findings unless the specific sources and nature of exposures can be directly linked to disease mechanisms. The crucial step, interpretation, is also dependent on theories and concepts. As epidemiologists need to communicate with both the public and other disciplines, it is important they understand how their theories and concepts compare with those of others including the theories of health and disease. Indeed, epidemiologists should know and make explicit the paradigms that their work falls into.

10.5 Paradigms: the evolution of sciences, including epidemiology

> In this essay, 'normal science' means research firmly based upon one or more past scientific achievements, achievements that some particular scientific community acknowledges for a time as supplying the foundation for its further practice.
>
> Thomas Kuhn (1996, p. 10)

Susser and Susser called for a fifth paradigm shift in epidemiology (Susser, 1996a,b). They identified four paradigm shifts (following the philosopher of science Kuhn) in epidemiology in the last three hundred years or so (Box 10.3) and advocated a new paradigm of multilevel eco-epidemiology, which ranges from molecule to macro environment. In doing this they struck a blow against the standard risk-factor–outcome analysis (adjusted for confounders) that characterized epidemiology in the late twentieth century. Understanding the significance of their call requires some knowledge of Kuhn's concept of scientific paradigms. Paradigms are 'shared ideas which account for relative fullness of their [i.e. scientists'] communications and their relative unanimity of judgement'. Kuhn's view is that sciences mostly work, at any one time, within a single paradigm driven by exemplars of successful work. Sciences that are maturing or changing do not have a dominant paradigm.

The idea of scientific paradigms is complex, with many nuances (Box 10.4). In the era of multiple, black box epidemiology, what might be the epidemiological equivalents of the four components? Symbolic generalizations could include the rise in relative risk associated with increasing exposure to a risk factor as strongly indicative of cause and effect. The model could be that chronic diseases arise from accumulated damage through exposure to risk factors over long timescales. The value that had pre-eminence was that causal understanding was achieved by studying these kinds of associations in populations. Exemplars were, above all else, cohort studies giving powerful insights on the effects of tobacco (e.g. Doll and Hill's British Doctors Study) and on a range of

---

Box 10.3 Four paradigms in epidemiology identified by the Sussers

Exploratory description of disease (e.g. Graunt's analysis of the London Bills of Mortality in 1662, and Ramazzini and occupational exposures, 1700). In this period there was a change to sickness being seen as a result of disease entities and not, as in the past, as humoral imbalance

- Miasma theory of disease: the idea that disease arose from foul emanations from pollution (eighteenth century)
- Germ theory of disease (nineteenth century)
- Multiple causes as captured in the black box metaphor (twentieth century)

Box 10.4 Four components of a paradigm, or a disciplinary matrix as identified by Kuhn

- Symbolic generalizations, for example, the laws of physics as given in mathematical formulae
- Beliefs in particular models, for example, heat as kinetic energy
- Values, for example, the key goal of science being accurate predictions
- Exemplars, that is, classic examples of problems and their solutions upon which Kuhn places special emphasis

---

cardiovascular risk factors (e.g. Framingham Study). Failure of the prevailing paradigm in solving current problems and explaining important observations inspires a search for a new paradigm that rapidly replaces the old one, which is then forgotten. This, he argues, is the foundation of scientific revolutions. Kuhn's ideas have been highly influential in the philosophy of science.

To call for a new paradigm as the Sussers did is, therefore, a severe provocation for it declares the current paradigm to be inadequate. There have, indeed, been a number of important and internationally published failures in recent years, especially in relationship to the potential benefits of hormone replacement therapy, a range of antioxidants, and many nutritional components. As I write in 2015, there is intense media and scientific discussion about the reversal of guidance warning against dairy fats, eggs, and other cholesterol-rich foods. In all these matters, cohort and/or case–control studies indicated benefits would accrue especially for cardiovascular diseases. Trials, sometimes done against fierce resistance, have not supported these observations.

Vigorous debate and resistance to change are identified by Kuhn as precursors to change. In the last 10 years, we have witnessed the much greater emphasis on trials and it is no coincidence that Mendelian randomization studies have gained in importance. The pendulum may have swung too far with many scholars and researchers proclaiming that causation cannot be concluded from observational studies (this is patently false). This debate also explains and justifies the rise of the directed acyclic graph as a tool for better causal analysis. New methods of statistical analysis are under development too. The vision of Susser and Susser is already in place, with epidemiology now orchestrating studies straddling variables from the gene mutation, molecules, biomarkers such as blood cholesterol, individuals, and many levels of spatial organization from home to region to country. Multilevel eco-epidemiology is here and, remarkably, has embedded itself in the short span of 20 years. We are in the middle of a shift almost without realizing it.

Current resistance to a broader role for academic epidemiology (e.g. in achieving tobacco control globally, especially in the developing world, or reducing health inequalities) might be explained as an intuition among epidemiologists that some of the dominant problems being identified lie outside the solution of current epidemiological concepts and methods. Kuhn's view strikes a chord:

> . . . one of the things a scientific community acquires with a paradigm is a criterion for choosing problems that, while the paradigm is taken for granted, can be assumed to have solutions. To a great extent these are the only problems that the community will admit as scientific or encourage its members to undertake.
>
> Kuhn (1966, p. 37)

Once exemplars for these kinds of mega problems are in place, no doubt views will change. This current debate in favour of new paradigms is fuelled by a combination of new patterns of disease (section 10.6), challenging new applications, a perception that the current risk factor-disease-out-come-based approach has not yielded the anticipated and solidly based advances, and the availability of new techniques of data acquisition and analysis.

10.6 Epidemiology: forces for change

Diseases wax and wane—mostly we do not know why and may never find out. This has a profound effect on medical practice. The pattern of diseases that doctors saw a hundred years ago is not today's. The pattern now is likely to be very different from that in 50–100 years. Some but not most changes are simply reflecting new diagnostic labels. Before reading on do the exercise in Box 10.5.

Examples of diseases never or rarely seen in contemporary medical practice in industrialized countries include smallpox (extinct), scurvy, beriberi, rickets, and erroneous diagnoses such as those previously attributed to masturbation, race, hysteria, or anatomical variants (the floating kidney) and so on. The Lancet ran a special column on discarded diagnoses that included sthenia, autointoxication, focal infection, typhomalaria, synochus, and many others.

Many other massive changes, some anticipated (e.g. those due to climate change) but most not (the impact of robots on health), will occur within our lifetimes. The shape of the average human body is transforming with ample nutrition causing substantial enlargement in height and, especially, bulk.

Diseases that physicians in a hundred years' time may not see include mesothelioma (a cancer resulting from asbestos), tuberculosis, polio, measles, and Guinea worm infestation. With luck, even conditions such as stroke and heart disease, at least in the currently industrialized countries, may be rare. AIDS may be conquered and a historical quirk by then.

Epidemiology, and epidemiologists, need to follow and adapt to these changes, and ideally predict them, preventing adverse outcomes if possible. It is difficult to predict, even in general terms, and impossible to specifically identify what new diseases, especially infections, are on their way. Even generalizations such as a rise in dementias given the increase in the number of very old people may well be wrong, especially if we can understand the causes and develop interventions. One adaptation that has already occurred is specialization within an expansion of the scope of epidemiology.

10.7 Scope of epidemiology and specialization

The scope of epidemiology has broadened with the discovery or invention of new applications and methods. This, and the changing pattern of diseases, has encouraged subdivisions of epidemiology, though sometimes these are artificial. There is, for example, infectious disease epidemiology, chronic disease epidemiology, health-care epidemiology, public health epidemiology, life-course epidemiology, social epidemiology, clinical epidemiology, and genetic epidemiology. In the *Dictionary of Epidemiology* (p. 96) there are 27 categories of epidemiology under the heading 'Epidemiology, Demarcation of'. This list could be longer, and new forms of epidemiology could

Box 10.5 Waning and waxing of diseases

Reflect on the diseases that contemporary doctors either do not, or extremely rarely, see. Now, reflect on diseases that may not be seen by doctors in a hundred years' time. Finally, what new diseases (or risk factors) can you foresee in the twenty-second century?

be proposed or created. Indeed, I possess a list of 56 titles used by epidemiologists. The important question is whether such divisions confer benefits, and whether these benefits exceed the costs.

The benefits are those of all forms of specialization, that is, narrowing the scope of work permits the researcher or practitioner to deepen the field, particularly by working closely with colleagues from other disciplines in the specialized field rather than with other general epidemiologists. Concepts and methods can be refined or developed to suit a specific application. Specific applications give rise to innovations that are often transferable.

The costs of specialization include: fragmentation of the discipline; a loss of breadth by the specialist individual or group; and a reduction in communication and cross-fertilization between epidemiologists working in the subdisciplines. These factors can impede cross-subdiscipline learning.

The fundamental concepts used in most subdivisions of epidemiology are similar. The same is true of the main measures of health and disease and study designs. The value of broad subdivisions such as chronic disease epidemiology is not clear, for the subdivision captures a vast territory, beyond the scope of even a specialist. The similarities between infectious disease and chronic disease epidemiology far outweigh the differences. In contrast, clinical epidemiology, in the sense of epidemiology applied to patients in the clinical setting, retains a relevant distinction, and its specific needs have driven the use of new techniques of data analysis and interpretation (e.g. numbers needed to treat). The term clinical epidemiology is sometimes used wrongly to distinguish medically qualified epidemiologists from others. The term clinical applies to the subject matter. Subspecialization is heavily influenced by the context in which epidemiology is practised.

10.8 The context of epidemiological work: academic and service in the USA and UK

Academic epidemiology in the United States is anchored in schools of public health which are mostly independent of medical schools. In large schools, departments of epidemiology may house hundreds of professional epidemiologists and this is where the next generation is trained (Bhopal 1998b). While there are also academic departments with epidemiologists in many medical schools, their influence is much smaller. In recent decades, partly driven by the imperative to do and teach research, fewer people with a service public health background have been appointed to these schools, the posts being filled with research scientists. The presence of clinically qualified staff (physicians and nurses) is also diminishing.

In such schools of public health, since the 1950s the vision of public health has become more scientific. The culture of science is hypothesis driven and centres on research grants and publication of scientific papers in journals. The prize is new knowledge. Issues of theory, measurement, analysis, and study design receive close attention, rather than their application in disease control or prevention, so their academic and service public health goals have diverged (Committee for the study of the future of Public Health 1988). Applied epidemiology is strong in Federal and State organizations, especially CDC (Centers for Disease Control and Prevention). In this environment, epidemiology is focused on identifying and resolving public health problems, including their evaluation.

In contrast to the United States, academic epidemiology in the United Kingdom is mostly associated with medical schools and the public health service within the NHS (National Health Service). These medical school epidemiology and public health departments tend to be multidisciplinary and have close links to like-minded clinicians, especially in primary care, and medical specialties where prevention is important, for example, respiratory and cardiovascular medicine, and infectious diseases. These circumstances promote comparatively close links between public health and medicine, and academia and service, and generate a focus on applied work. Despite much discussion to create more, only one major university-based school of public health on the USA model exists in the United Kingdom—the London School of Hygiene and Tropical Medicine. This is a large postgraduate institution.

The US School of Public Health type of environment is large enough to offer a career path for professional researchers. There, the epidemiologists see themselves, by and large, as professional epidemiologists. There are sufficient of them to form a professionalized, self-contained group and set up and sustain specialist organizations such as the Society for Epidemiological Research and the American College of Epidemiology. These are an addition to multidisciplinary societies such as the American Public Health Association. Many epidemiologists work in specialist departments of epidemiology.

In contrast to the United States, many epidemiologists in the United Kingdom perceive themselves first as statisticians, physicians, public health specialists, or social scientists. Medically qualified staff usually have a formal contract with the NHS and non-medical ones require one for research with the NHS. They mostly work in multidisciplinary departments where epidemiologists are usually a minority. Epidemiologists participate in multidisciplinary societies (Society for Social Medicine) or international, epidemiological ones (IEA—the International Epidemiological Association). There are no national epidemiology societies in the United Kingdom. Rigorous training in the science of epidemiology is harder to achieve than in the United States and most epidemiologists are trained through the public health disciplines.

The circumstances embed British epidemiologists within multidisciplinary and applied settings. The circumstances allow US epidemiologists the option of specializing and standing apart from applied public health.

In mainland Europe there is a mix of systems, with most countries having major national institutes that promote epidemiological research, perhaps closer to the USA model. Service for epidemiologists within the health-care system is less common in mainland Europe than in the United Kingdom, though this is changing.

Whatever the context, epidemiology is important in public health, as reflected in its definition.

10.9 The practice of epidemiology in public health

There is agreement that epidemiology is a key science that underpins public health and increasingly clinical practice. Yet, the gap between academic epidemiology and public health practice may be widening. Public health, according to the definition by the Committee of Inquiry (1988) chaired by Sir Donald Acheson, is: 'The science and art of preventing disease, prolonging life and promoting health through the organized efforts of society.' (A complete definition is in the *Dictionary of Epidemiology*.) Public health applies science in the social and political context, inevitably creating tensions between the scientific goal of gaining knowledge and the public health goal of improving health. These tensions are being partly resolved through an increasing emphasis internationally on evidence-based policy, clinical practice, and public health, with a special emphasis on evidence from clinical trials and systematic reviews/meta-analyses. This has created a common platform for academics and practitioners of medical sciences that are based on both individuals and populations.

Epidemiology can be put into practice in many ways, including: understanding the relative impact of biology, environment, and health care on disease (e.g. explaining the decline of tuberculosis); making the case for legislative change as was done following the London smog in 1953; setting up preventive programmes to tackle disease as done so vigorously in Finland to prevent CHD; predicting the future need for services using disease and HIV prevalence trends as in the field of AIDS; evaluating interventions; developing policy and clinical priorities; making clinical diagnosis in an individual patient; and providing the inspiration and methods for seeking new causal hypotheses as required for so many diseases (e.g. pancreatic cancer). So, there is no doubt about the role of epidemiology in public health practice. This role is, however, not usually the focus, but a by-product, of epidemiology.

Epidemiological textbooks usually proclaim the applications of epidemiology as the foundation science of public health, but most focus on design and methods for causal research, rather than demonstrating clearly how epidemiology helps public health practice. The exemplars and classic studies used are mainly causal investigations, yet much (maybe most) epidemiological effort in the public health field is on disease description and burden, prediction of trends, and evaluation of public health and clinical activity. (This book has sought a balanced perspective with equal weight to these domains.)

In a major review of epidemiology in 1985 Susser picked two studies that established the reputation of epidemiology in the modern era: the Framingham cohort study, and the case–control studies on smoking as a cause of lung cancer. Susser's choices, as opposed to other triumphs such as the poliomyelitis trial of 1954 (which he discusses in detail), illustrate the dilemma. While epidemiologists may spend much of their time working on applied public health work, they still respect causal contributions most, and this is reflected in their teaching even though several consensual reports concur that students need the broader perspectives rather than methods of study design.

As an applied science, epidemiology needs a code of ethics and good conduct that serves both its scientific and public health purposes.

10.10 **Ethical basis and proper conduct of epidemiology: the need for a code**

While written ethical codes for medical practice date back to Hippocrates, some 2000 years ago, the idea that science in general (not just medical science, or social science) should be governed by ethical codes is recent. To illustrate why epidemiology needs an ethical code I have chosen to discuss three issues of interest to me: manipulation of scientists by the tobacco industry; manipulation of authorship by researchers; and the purpose and direction of research on ethnicity and race (considered in depth because of its exceptional importance to epidemiology and public health in a millennium where all societies are becoming multiethnic ones).

10.10.1 **The tobacco industry manipulates researchers including epidemiologists**

The pervasive and often covert influence of the tobacco industry on scientific research and publication has posed mighty ethical challenges for research institutions, researchers, and journal editors. The tobacco industry has put its commercial interests before the health of society. Tobacco industry archives now on the web show how the industry has manipulated research to deflect attention from tobacco's impact on health, for example, by fostering controversy about the effects of passive smoking on health; countering authoritative review articles through an international network of paid scientific 'consultants' whose activities included writing critical letters to academic journals; publishing biased 'review' articles; establishing a 'learned society' on indoor air quality; and performing research into non-tobacco causes of lung cancer (see Barnes and Bero 1998).

The tobacco industry concealed or distorted evidence from its own research showing the addictive and harmful nature of smoking. Sadly, some epidemiologists were manipulated by the industry. Epidemiologists working on topics such as tobacco need to be armed with an ethical code to protect them against such manipulation, and to guide them in making the right decisions in difficult circumstances, particularly when they are offered resources to pursue what are, apparently, good works. These experiences also justify policies such as declaration of conflicts of interest, sources of funding, and external influences on the research process. Many reputable journals have stopped publishing work funded by tobacco companies. The lessons are relevant to other powerful industries because it is clear they are using similar strategies.

10.10.2 Authorship: manipulation by researchers

The authorship of scientific papers is hugely important for the status of universities and for the reputations of researchers (Bhopal *et al.* 1998b). There is a view that only work that has passed the scrutiny of peers is reliable and trustworthy (a view worthy of scrutiny, particularly as there is sparse evidence on the value, never mind cost-effectiveness of the hallowed tradition of peer review). The main way for peer scrutiny is through publication in peer-reviewed journals. Publication is a key factor in academic promotion, success in competing for an academic appointment (and sometimes in service appointments too), in winning research grants, and, in the United Kingdom, determining the finances coming into universities from the government grant. Not surprisingly, the pressure to publish is great, tempting individuals to accept authorship on papers to which they have not contributed sufficiently or even at all, a practice called 'gift authorship'. Richard Horton, editor of *The Lancet*, said, 'The mantle of authorship has become a heavy robe of fake majesty that conceals those who seek credit unworthily, priority unjustly and reward improperly' (Horton 1998).

The pressure to publish exciting groundbreaking papers in the 'top' journals has led to malpractice ranging from only reporting exciting results (publication bias) to publishing fraudulent, even manufactured, data.

The criteria for authorship prepared by the International Committee of Medical Journal Editors are commonly flouted (Box 10.6). Scientists, including epidemiologists, recognize that allocation

---

Box 10.6 The International Committee of Medical Journal Editors' criteria for authorship (2015)

The International Committee of Medical Journal Editors (ICMJE) recommends that authorship be based on the following four criteria:

- Substantial contributions to the conception or design of the work; or the acquisition, analysis, or interpretation of data for the work; AND

- Drafting the work or revising it critically for important intellectual content; AND

- Final approval of the version to be published; AND

- Agreement to be accountable for all aspects of the work in ensuring that questions related to the accuracy or integrity of any part of the work are appropriately investigated and resolved.

In addition to being accountable for the parts of the work he or she has done, an author should be able to identify which co-authors are responsible for specific other parts of the work. In addition, authors should have confidence in the integrity of the contributions of their co-authors.

Reproduced with permission from International Committee for Medical Journal Editors, *Defining the Role of Authors and Contributors*, http://www.icmje.org/recommendations/browse/roles-and-responsibilities/defining-the-role-of-authors-and-contributors.html, accessed 14 Sep. 2015. Copyright © 2015 ICMJE.

of authorship is complex and raises ethical issues central to scientific integrity. (See also section 10.12 for error in scientific papers.)

Epidemiologists should follow these criteria.

10.10.3 Ethnicity and race: purpose and direction in epidemiology

Ethnicity and race are among the top five or so variables in epidemiology. Their utilization, however, has put many researchers in peril of being judged as racist. Knowledge of the ample and awful history of racism in science and medicine provides the essential insight into how societies may abuse data on racial differences. Some two thousand years ago, Hippocrates contrasted the feebleness of the Asiatic races to the hardiness of the Europeans (see Chadwick and Mann 1950). Hippocrates' concept of race was of human groups shaped by their ancestry in different environments (especially climate). Nonetheless, this is a kind of stereotyping surely based on ignorance that has cascaded down the ages.

In the nineteenth century racial differences in anatomy, physiology, behaviour, and health status were avidly sought. The idea of races as distinct human species, which was long and seriously debated, gave way to races as biological subspecies. On this basis race is the group a person belongs to on the basis of physique (a concept that has been hotly contested). Before reading on, do the exercise in Box 10.7.

Racism results from the belief that some races are superior to others, which is used to devise and justify actions that create inequality among racial groups. In the nineteenth century, differences among races were usually assumed to be biological, interpreted to show superiority of White races, and used to justify policies which subordinated 'coloured' people.

Research focusing on problems more common in non-White groups, combined with data presentation techniques designed to highlight differences in comparison with the White population, so easily portrays the non-White groups as weaker. When research implies genetic factors, rather than environmental ones, as the cause of racial differences in health, racial minorities may be perceived as biologically (innately), and permanently weaker. (Such research tends to ignore findings of no difference and those showing non-White groups to be in better health.)

Science that indicated such weakness was used to help to justify slavery, social inequality, eugenics, immigration control, and the racist practice of medicine. Race-specific 'diseases' such as drapetomania (irrational and pathological desire of slaves to run away) were invented. The Tuskegee Syphilis Study in Alabama (discussed in Chapter 4 on bias) by the US Public Health Service, which lasted from 1932 to 1972, deceived and effectively bribed 600 Black subjects into cooperating with research which examined the progression of syphilis without treatment, even once penicillin (a cure) was available (see Jones 1993). In May 1997 President Clinton apologized on behalf of the United States of America to the survivors. Osborne and Feit (1992) concluded that much American health research on race and ethnicity contributes to the idea that some human groups are inferior.

Box 10.7 Ethnicity and race as artificial constructs

Reflect on whether there is some truth to the view that races and ethnic groups are socially constructed, artificial ways of categorizing human beings. Can you think of examples of times and places when the idea of race has been used to overtly political or social ends, particularly the suppression of some groups?

Modern genetics undermined the biological concept of race, and extreme Nazi racism indirectly discredited both race-based science and eugenics. Race classifications are now considered to be based on a few physical features (such as colour and facial features) of small direct importance to health, but which serve important social rather than biological purposes. Nonetheless, the idea of the biological basis of health differences by race (and somewhat less so for ethnicity) remains strong. Biology remains the defining feature of the twentieth-century race concept, supported by many contemporary dictionaries and encyclopaedias, and permeating biomedical thinking.

The view that race is primarily a social, not primarily biological, reality is, however, emergent and slowly strengthening in the new century, despite an upsurge of interest in race in genetics. With the new genetic technologies, we can map the genome and find how markers cluster differently in populations. Using these markers alone, the ancestral origins of a person can be deduced. At the level of continent, the markers correspond well to self-reported or assigned racial classification and so there is correlation between self-reported race and gene-marker defined race. This is hardly surprising as race is based on physical features, which are a result of ancestry in different continents. The paradoxical, and somewhat contradictory, result of this work has been reinforcement of the idea of the genetic unity of the human species and support for a biological basis for current racial classifications. The story is unfolding and its ultimate implications are unclear. In the meantime, ethnicity is overtaking race as the preferred variable for subgrouping humans.

The concept of ethnicity is that human beings identify themselves, or are identified by others, as belonging to a group because they differ culturally in fundamental ways including language, food, religion, lifestyle and, of course, their geographical origins, which have shaped their genetics and physique. Without question, ethnic group classifications are socially constructed. There is discrimination and prejudice targeted at groups defined by ethnicity, religion, country of birth, migration status, etc. The concept of racism has been extended to cover these areas. In epidemiological practice, perhaps unfortunately but understandably, race and ethnicity are often used as synonyms for overlapping underlying concepts.

Studies of ethnic and racial variations in disease pose a challenge to the maintenance of high ethical standards in epidemiology. The concepts of race and ethnicity are commonly applied in epidemiology in the hope of advancing causal understanding of disease. Contemporary race, ethnicity, and health research is mostly 'black box' epidemiology, concentrating on so-called ethnic health issues, and generating a multiplicity of interesting hypotheses. As Kiple and King (1981) discuss, the idea of a package of specific 'racial' or 'ethnic' diseases that deserve special attention and research has unfortunate echoes in history. 'Negro' susceptibility to particular diseases, such as leprosy, tetanus, pneumonia, scurvy, and sore eyes, was instrumental in 'branding blacks as an exotic breed', and the differences were explained by hypotheses on causation that can now be seen as nonsense. It may be that future generations will see current epidemiological work in the same light.

One of the most important observations in this field is that ethnic minority populations comprising of recent migrants and their offspring may have better health status than the majority population the country of settlement. This healthy immigrant effect (or paradox) diminishes with time. By contrast, long-settled minorities and colonized indigenous minorities tend to have worse health than the majority. There are important epidemiological challenges here that need careful, sensitive, and ethical research using the concepts of race and ethnicity.

Racial prejudice is fuelled by research portraying ethnic minorities as different, usually inferior to the majority. Infectious diseases, population growth, and culture are common foci for publicity. Epidemiologists must be aware of the attractions of their work to the media and of the potential impact of their work on race relations. This is not to argue that they should not do it, but that they should do it well and thoughtfully.

Race and ethnicity are epidemiological variables that show, dramatically and unequivocally, the importance of historical, political, social, and ethical awareness among epidemiologists.

10.11 Ethical guidelines for epidemiology and the clash of informed consent, data privacy, and the pursuit of epidemiology

Ethical guidelines for epidemiology include broad statements about the duties of epidemiologists to be honest and impartial, not to distort the truth, and to uphold the public interest rather than narrow sectional interests. Other guidelines have given more specific guidance, including that epidemiologists should not accept contractual obligations influencing conclusions from research; or accept grants or contracts in which the funder retains the right to edit or suppress results.

In 1998, the International Epidemiology Association's European Group published a code of practice for epidemiologists that has proven durable. This stated that, among other principles, some of which we have already explored, epidemiologists should:

- seek the truth in good faith without doing harm or jeopardizing personal integrity;
- judge their own work and ideas and those of colleagues in an impartial manner;
- disclose conflicts of interest to ethical review committees;
- publicly acknowledge all research sponsorship;
- publish all research with scientific merit;
- refuse requests to withhold findings, change or tone down the content of reports, or delay publication unreasonably;
- ensure sponsors agree in writing that results will be published regardless of outcome and agree to the independence of the investigators;
- declare sources of funding and possible conflicts of interests in publications.

In January 2007 an updated document was approved by the IEA Council and published by the IEA in 2010. In this revision, a plea is made for a balanced approach to ethical approval with a warning that ethical rules are becoming so strict that they are undermining observational epidemiology. The point is that individual informed consent is not taken for data in important databases, for example, cancer registers, and mortality registers. Despite this warning, from IEA and subsequently other organizations there is little doubt that increasing public and governmental concerns on data privacy are making access to health data for research more difficult. While exemptions for research exist and will continue, accessing such exemptions is not easy. Epidemiologists may find that a partial solution is working with staff within the health services or agencies responsible for data. Technical solutions are available so data does not physically leave the agency holding the data but is accessed remotely. These solutions can link data sets across the world remotely in a secure manner without data transfer.

The classical medical ethics framework of autonomy (respect for individual rights), beneficence (doing good), non-maleficence (doing no harm), and justice is adopted in this IEA document. Under autonomy the key issue for epidemiology is identified as informed consent, which is an ideal that often cannot be achieved, especially in the use of national, routinely collected databases. Linkage of databases is an especially tricky issue in relation to consent and data confidentiality (see exemplars in Chapters 7 and 8 for such studies). Studies show the public strongly supports database studies, but only by health researchers and professionals rather than commercial companies or government. Involving the public in such studies may help in gaining necessary approvals.

The commonest potential harm is disclosure of confidential data. Practical advice on how to avoid this is given by the IEA but the key is separating personal identifying data from the data set used for analysis. In judging whether the data set holds personal information readers might ask this: would a skilled investigative journalist be able to obtain private information about an individual given the data on that individual in your data set? (A full postcode/zip code and a diagnosis might be enough.) Since 2007 whole genome scanning has become common in epidemiology. DNA cannot be anonymized as we know from 'DNA fingerprinting' evidence used in criminal trials and paternity law suits. There is no solution. Theoretically individuals could be identified, for example, by the police from genetic data held in epidemiological databases.

The document supports the guidance on authorship now updated in Box 10.6. Numerous other issues are considered. This guidance from the IEA is core reading for the practising epidemiologist. The reader is encouraged to study these IEA guidelines in more detail (http://ieaweb.org/good-epidemiological-practice-gep/). To seek the truth and judge with impartiality (first and second bullet points above) requires, above all, a sound understanding of critical appraisal.

10.12 Critical appraisal in epidemiology: separating fact from error and fallacy

> Scepticism is the scalpel which frees accessible truth from the dead
> tissue of unfounded belief and wishful thinking.
>
> Skrabanek and McCormick (1992, p. 144)

In an era emphasizing scientific evidence as the foundation of medicine and public health, the scalpel of critical appraisal is as important to the twenty-first century doctor as the surgical scalpel was to the nineteenth century one. Epidemiologists have a prime role in keeping the scalpel sharp. Critical appraisal is important because much of what we believe as the truth is wrong, sometimes dangerously so. Before reading on do the exercise in Box 10.8.

Historical examples of harmful medical activities include the treatment of fevers and other common problems by cautery, bloodletting, purging, vomiting, and enemas. Many public health actions were equally wrong; for example, fumigation of towns to control epidemics of cholera, typhus, and yellow fever. At the time, however, these actions must have made sense to those who put them into practice. Furthermore, these kinds of actions fitted with the theories of the time, that is, humoral theory of disease in individuals and the miasma theory of disease in public health. These actions were neither arbitrary nor unscientific. As we already discussed some of these actions worked, for example, cleaning up the environment, but not for the stated reasons.

Examples of follies from the twentieth century include surgery for the floating kidney; ECT (electroconvulsive therapy) for a wide range of psychological and psychiatric disorders (it does

---

Box 10.8 Reflection on medical and public health activities shown to be wrong

Reflect on some medical and public health activities which were widely practised but are now known to be wrong, some dangerously so. Your reflection should include both historical activities, say, before the turn of the twentieth century, and ones that are more recent. Now, reflect on some current policies and practices that may meet the same fate.

work for severe depression); prolonged enforced bed rest after a heart attack when we now know that patients need to be mobilized within hours or days; and treatment of heart rhythm disorders during a heart attack with the drug lignocaine. These actions were, in retrospect, dangerous but at the time were state of the art.

Only with the 'retrospectoscope' can we identify follies and fallacies. Life and death decisions are being made on uncertain knowledge about the causes, prevention, diagnosis, and management of disease. For example, is hospital birth safer than home birth for a healthy mother? Is screening for cardiovascular risk factors including diabetes and cervical and breast cancer saving lives or causing unnecessary costs and anxiety? Are drugs for moderate/mild high blood pressure, obesity, depression, and anxiety effective and safe? Why are so many antibiotics prescribed for non-bacterial illnesses? Is folate supplementation of the diet, or as a vitamin supplement, good for heart disease? Do vitamin D or probiotics prevent diseases? Does health education about drugs and safer sex prevent or augment problems? Is butter good or bad for you? We often don't have clear-cut answers about the effectiveness or cost-effectiveness of the activities we undertake. Before reading on, do the exercise in Box 10.9.

The reasons why clear-cut answers to critically important questions do not exist include the following:

- the tendency and preference to base clinical and public health practice on personal experience and considered, collective peer judgement;
- the tendency to act on good, common-sense ideas, often based on general scientific principles, in the absence of firm research evidence of effectiveness and cost-effectiveness;
- the tendency to follow the ideas of distinguished colleagues and charismatic leaders, including politicians;
- the difficulty and expense of doing research that gives clear-cut answers;
- the inconsistency of findings—some action works in one place or time but not in another;
- the difficulty of reaching the correct interpretation of data;
- limitations of and error in research.

Error in science is common, as the regular notification of errors in every journal shows. The favoured image of the scientific process is of steady accumulation of sound knowledge. The fault with science, if any, is usually said to lie in the abuse of knowledge, rather than in its accumulation and interpretation. The scientific paper, the carrier of scientific knowledge, has the authority of its authors, the elaborate peer review system, and the editorial processes of the publishing journal, and is expected to be accurate.

Accuracy is a characteristic cherished and demanded by scientists. Both lay and expert readers may, however, easily overlook errors in published work, precisely because they are unexpected. Errors can then be perpetuated by quotation in secondary sources. The editorial and peer review processes are not foolproof against error. The publication and continued citation of fraudulent research provides the most extreme example of the limitations of current means of detecting and excluding error in scientific literature. Fraud, however, represents an important but small proportion of errors in the scientific literature. Several studies of the use of statistics in medical journals

Box 10.9 Reasons for the lack of clear answers

Reflect on and list reasons why, historically, medical and public health practice has not sought, or has not achieved, clear research-based answers to important questions.

have shown that error is a massive problem. Most errors are subtle and are made unwittingly by researchers who try hard to avoid them. Error is intrinsic to the research process.

Critical appraisal is the use of the 'scalpel of scepticism' to extract truth from error in research. In evaluating research, particularly epidemiological, researchers need to consider both technical excellence and its value in historical, political, social, and geographical context. This book has provided the background concepts to guide the reader in critical appraisal (particularly Chapters 3, 4, and 5). In preparation for application of these concepts, the reader will need to consult other books and papers (see references). Petr Skrabanek and James McCormick's (1992) book *Follies and Fallacies in Medicine* is a gold mine of examples, and the brief exposition in sections 10.12.1 to 10.12.2 is heavily based on their discussion of fallacies. (The book is available free on the internet—see references.)

10.12.1 **Some fallacies**

The fallacy of association being causation

Humankind needs explanations, and this need leads us to confuse association, which is easily demonstrated, with causation, which is problematic. This matter has been discussed throughout this book (Chapters 3–5). The axiom, 'association is not causation, but it may be', is a safeguard, as is remembering that an association between factor A and disease B may be a result of:

- Coincidence or chance;
- Confounding (A and B share a common cause D);
- B causes A (consequence or reverse causality);
- A causes B (cause).

This can be easily remembered as the four Cs (Chance, Confounding, Consequence, Cause).

The weight of evidence fallacy

The idea that pooling weak evidence can turn it into better evidence is tempting but sometimes wrong. (This principle has huge implications for the burgeoning field of systematic reviews and meta-analysis, which were rare when this folly was described.) It is wrong to discard discordant evidence, even if it is scanty. The Popperian view of science is that progress is made by rejecting or refining hypotheses and the example of the hypothesis 'Swans are white' is memorable. More is learned about this false hypothesis by observing a single black swan (common in New Zealand) than 1000 white ones. Pooling evidence is, of course, the goal of systematic reviews and meta-analyses and is important for the causal contribution of consistency (see Chapter 5). The lesson is that critical appraisal must underpin the review process. In addition, we should remember that the heterogeneity in the data we are pooling may be real, and in the process of gaining precision by summarizing data in a single summary, we are losing knowledge.

The fallacy of repeated citation

Is spinach a particularly good source of iron as claimed by the cartoon of Popeye the sailor man, and now widely known? The answer, according to Skrabanek and McCormick, is no. In the original paper reporting these data on the iron content of spinach, the decimal point was misplaced, giving a tenfold overestimate. (As I have not checked the original paper, this is an example of repeated citation.) The lesson is that you should examine data with a critical eye. It does seem implausible that spinach has more iron than similar leafy vegetables. The scientific method requires replication and that is good epidemiological practice.

The fallacy of authority

Simply because an article or book is published does not make it right. Equally, the fact that a paper or book is not published because it is rejected by peer review does not make it wrong. Rejection by peers is the fate of much innovative, groundbreaking research. The lesson is that all work, irrespective of author, needs objective examination. Two recent innovations in online publication could help with these problems. First, some online journals make space for readers' comments at any time after publication, for example, the rapid response system in the *British Medical Journal* (BMJ). Second, some of the journals are committed to publication of all research that is sound, irrespective of other subjective factors, for example, novelty value or human interest.

The fallacy of simple explanation

Scientists and the public alike have a preference for simple explanations (usually referred to in science as elegant or parsimonious hypotheses). The emphasis in epidemiology on searching for single risk factors as causes, as opposed to ways of summarizing and studying the complex interaction of multiple risk factors, is a reflection of this preference. A quotation from H. L. Mencken summarizes Skrabanek and McCormick's view (cited on p. 37 of their book) on this matter: 'for every complex problem there is a solution that is simple, direct and wrong' (see Chapter 5). Of course, sometimes there are simple explanations that are correct but these are exceptions.

The fallacy of risk

Skrabanek and McCormick discuss a World Health Organization (WHO) study showing that women who had used oral contraceptives for 2.5 years had a relative risk of 1.5 for cervical cancer, that is, 50 per cent more than those who did not. Is this association reflecting a causal relationship, they asked? Second, does it matter, and is it something for women to worry about? In terms of life expectancy, women aged 20–24 reduced, on average, their lifespan by 11 days. The principle here is: presented with a relative risk, ask yourself, what does it matter in terms of absolute risk? (See Chapters 7 and 8.) In recent years the emphasis on absolute risks has increased greatly, although more needs to be done.

The fallacy of inappropriate extrapolation

Just because something is unhealthy in excess (salt, milk, zinc, alcohol, weight, serum cholesterol, radiation, or water) does not mean it is unhealthy in moderation. Beware of investigators who extrapolate beyond their data, warn Skrabanek and McCormick. Equally, factors that are healthy in moderation may be unhealthy in excess (e.g. vitamins).

The fallacy of significance tests

Any difference between two groups, no matter how small or unimportant, can be shown to be statistically significant if the sample size is large enough. Skrabanek and McCormick ask us to (a) beware of statistically significant differences in big studies, and to (b) remember that the validity of the probability that a particular set of results has occurred by chance, shown by the significance tests (and illustrated by the *P*-value), depends on a prior hypothesis. They also remind us that statistically significant results are more likely to be published and that there may be unpublished studies showing no difference or the opposite (publication bias—see Chapter 4). In recent years these points have been taken on board in epidemiology, though less so in clinical research settings.

The fallacy of obfuscation

Beware of the use of complex language to obfuscate (to bewilder). The use of words such as 'essential', 'multifactorial', or 'functional', when describing diseases really means we don't know the causes. They are general labels to distinguish forms of disease where the causes are known, for example, renal hypertension means kidney problems are raising the blood pressure, while essential hypertension means no specific cause is known. Such words hide ignorance yet they give authority to the user. In epidemiology, we also have much jargon and possibly unnecessary complexity.

The fallacy of covert bias

Use of language, particularly adjectives, may reflect the bias of the investigator. One writer may see a difference as important, another as unimportant. The reader needs to avoid being misled by the bias of the writer. Generally, adjectives should be minimized in scientific writing.

This is a sample of the fascinating collection of fallacies so well described by these authors. So how are we to avoid them?

10.12.2 **The nature of critical appraisal**

Despite its name, critical appraisal is not just criticism with a kinship to a book, film, or theatre review that aims to assess how good the work is in relation to expectations and what has gone before. *Citizen Kane* is an acclaimed film, but one wouldn't judge it in relation to the state of knowledge or technology of today. Similarly, in appraising a scientific paper, we must give credit for ideas. Do not criticize a cross-sectional study because it is not a trial (but do so if it is interpreted as if it were one!). Give a balanced view. The starting point is a mindset that is determined to examine the research painstakingly to form an independent judgement and to extract the valid message.

The next step is for the reader to attempt critical appraisal. To make this meaningful the reader is advised to work on contemporary journal papers and prepare the appraisal as a letter (or rapid response electronically, if feasible) to the editor and, if it is good enough, to submit it for publication. The educational benefits of preparing a concise, critical evaluation of a scientific paper are considerable.

Researchers reviewing a field should routinely search for, summarize, and cite relevant journal correspondence and other comments. An original scientific paper is incomplete without the accompanying published comment. Online journals now offer the ideal of electronic linkage of corrections, retractions, and correspondence to original articles. Ideally, inter-library loan requests for a paper should be for the paper together with its related commentary, whether correspondence or editorial (sadly, this is not done). The next section outlines some questions of particular relevance in epidemiological appraisal.

10.13 **Some questions relevant to the appraisal of epidemiological research**

Austin Bradford Hill posed four simple questions to guide the thoughtful reading of scientific papers:

1 Why did the authors start?

2 What did they do?

3 What did they find?

4 What does it mean?

These four questions are an excellent starting point. Additional general questions include these:

- What is the importance of the research this paper describes?
- Is the research ethical and approved?
- Have the authors declared conflicts of interest and source of funding?
- Have the authors made explicit the concepts guiding their work and defined their terms?
- What are the objectives, hypotheses, and research questions under investigation?
- Were the methods appropriate to meeting the objectives, testing the hypotheses, and answering the research questions?
- Is the study sample of the right kind and size to meet the study objectives?
- What biases are inherent in the methods and what steps have been taken to minimize these?
- Do the results relate to the objectives, hypotheses, and research questions addressed?
- Do the discussion and conclusions provide an objective assessment of the findings and place them correctly in relation to other scientific literature?
- Does the discussion outline the limitations of the study?
- What is the next step in terms of policy, practice, and research?

Such general questions can be combined with those in Box 10.10 to produce a critical appraisal specific to epidemiological research.

Box 10.10 Some questions for appraisal of epidemiological studies

- Is an epidemiological approach appropriate to the problem under study?
- What is the study design and is it suitable for the problem addressed?
- Are the dates on which the sampling frame was compiled given?
- Is the date or time period over which data were collected (fieldwork) given?
- For conditions which have a cyclical pattern, has the timing of measurements been stated? For example, for blood pressure this would be time of day, time of week, month, and season.
- Has the target population, that is, the one to which the findings are to be applied, been defined?
- Have the precise geographical boundaries of the study been given? If this is not a geographically defined population, can the study population be related more generally to a place?
- Have the target and study populations been defined and described in terms of their social and economic standing, and geographical and cultural origins?
- Have the terms/labels used to describe populations or subpopulations been defined and justified?
- Is the study sample representative of the source and target population (particularly important for studies of prevalence and incidence of disease, but less so for studies of cause and effect relationships)?

- Are the results likely to be more widely generalizable?
- Are the sampling and measurement methods equivalent in the groups to be compared?
- Are the measurement errors estimated and if so do the results take these into account?
- Are compared populations or subgroups similar on key variables (confounding and interacting factors)?
- Where there are differences have the authors done adjustment using a weighting technique such as age standardization, or other statistical techniques such as logistic regression (see Chapters 4 and 8)?
- Do the statistical adjustments resolve any potential problems of confounding or might there be residual problems?
- Do the analyses provide information on both absolute and relative risks?
- Is there any analysis adjusting for estimated biases, for example, for non-response or loss to follow-up?
- If odds ratios are given, and used as an estimate of relative risk, are the required assumptions met? If not have appropriate adjustment formulae been applied?
- If the study is one exploring causality, is the causal framework and causal model given? Have the results been interpreted using that framework and model?
- Have the results been set in the context of a systematic review and/or meta-analysis?

The subject of critical appraisal is a large one, and the interested reader will be able to find guidance on how to critically appraise studies both in different fields of epidemiology and with different designs. A great deal of guidance on how to report research has been created recently and many journals now require authors to follow it (this is collected on the EQUATOR website—see websites section).

Some guidance adopts a checklist-type approach, with an attempt to assign numerical scores to the quality of the paper. The aim of some such checklists is to exclude papers from the review. I favour the mindset that we need to extract the value from each publication, excluding mainly on irrelevance to the question at hand, but otherwise only if the research is in error or is repetition. Exclusion is usually for practical reasons, purportedly saving a small amount of time or money. Currently, it is common practice for researchers to restrict their literature review to studies in English. This is a problem justified by lack of resources but will not be sustainable given access to cheap automated translation. It is also common and poor practice to restrict literature reviewing to certain dates, perhaps when electronic databases were started. Without a scientific reason this is not advised. The research excluded may have cost millions of pounds and may have the answers you wanted.

We now turn to the need to reflect on both the past and the future, as a means of continuing one's education in epidemiology.

10.14 Historical landmarks and the emergence of modern epidemiology

One path to a solid epidemiological education is to study the classics, or in Kuhn's terminology, exemplars. Exemplars provide inspiration as well as instruction. I have chosen three examples—see exemplar panel 10—to illustrate the value of historical studies to contemporary work, including lessons that are pertinent today.

Based on these kinds of early achievements, epidemiology and public health advanced rapidly with triumphant insights into the causes and control of diseases including puerperal fever, pellagra, typhus, beriberi, congenital rubella, adenocarcinoma of the vagina, lung cancer, coronary heart disease and, more recently, gastric ulcer and cancer, AIDS, cervical cancer, and sudden infant death syndrome. Many of these achievements were in partnership with other scientific disciplines but it would be a reasonable claim that epidemiology spurred, even initiated, the line of enquiry. These landmarks showed how society could conquer disease.

These are the kind of examples that provide inspiration and, rightly, take pride of place in our textbooks. Kuhn identified textbooks as vehicles for perpetuating scientific paradigms and as necessary for rapid progress by the novice, including through the study of exemplars (classics). The further reading lists at the end of the book offer choices on reading exemplars. Mistakes have also been made but its legacy has established epidemiology as having a vitally important role in medical science, though perhaps too ready to infer causality from data on associations. That is a challenge for the future.

Exemplar 10.1: Historical landmarks in the development of modern epidemiology

James Lind and scurvy

James Lind investigated scurvy and reported his findings in 1753 (see Lind 1753). He wrote 'Scurvy alone, during the last war, proved a more destructive enemy, and cut off more valuable lives, than the united efforts of the French and Spanish wars.' He also noted that scurvy 'raged with great violence in some journeys, not at all in others'. The first observation identified the immense size of the problem, the second told him that scurvy was preventable. To prevent it he needed to create the conditions where scurvy did not 'rage with great violence'.

He generated many causal hypotheses including the role of sea climate and particularly the moist air. He chose to investigate diet and conducted his historic experiment on the ship *Salisbury* in 1747 where he 'ordered' 12 patients, divided in pairs, to take cider, elixir vitriol, vinegar, sea water, an electuary (consisting of garlic, mustard seed, radishes, balsam of Peru, gum myrrh), and oranges and lemons. He found that 'the most sudden and visible good effects were perceived from the use of the oranges and lemons'.

Sadly, many lives were to be lost before his remedy was accepted and adopted about 90 years later. The British Navy then started providing limes as part of the rations, giving rise to the name 'limeys' for British sailors. A deficiency of vitamin C, found in fruit and vegetables, was shown in 1928 to be the cause of scurvy. Vitamin C was the first vitamin to be synthesized in 1932, nearly two hundred years after Lind's work.

This story illustrates the importance of reflecting on the differing patterns of disease— here, scurvy in some journeys and not in others—and then generating a number of plausible hypotheses and testing the most likely ones. It shows that putting research into policy and practice is a long-term endeavour. Finally, this story shows that precise mechanistic understanding, though valuable, is not crucial to put epidemiology into public health practice. The work is usually considered one of the first scientific trials (Chapter 9). The James Lind history, hosted on a website by the Royal College of Physicians of Edinburgh, commemorates this work by collecting historically important documents on evidence-based medicine and public health.

Edward Jenner and smallpox

Smallpox is one of history's most important diseases. The story of how Edward Jenner, a country-based medical practitioner in Gloucester, investigated the role of vaccination with cowpox virus is well known, but where did he get the idea? What was the observation that inspired him to take the cowpox virus from the hands of the milkmaid Sarah Nelmes and insert it into the arm of 'a lad of the name of Phipps' on 14 May 1796? The observation on which he reflected was this: that milkmaids have clear complexions and are generally free of pockmarks (a disease pattern) and that it is hard to inoculate them using smallpox virus; an observation that we could disparagingly call an 'old wives tale'. Jenner did not observe this himself, and he was not the first person to follow the path of vaccination. However, he did test, evaluate, and establish the practice. It is important to note that variolation, where a small amount of smallpox material was inoculated into healthy people to protect them from serious smallpox, was already established in Europe (it came from China). It worked but could be dangerous.

Jenner investigated this observation and the local practice of exposing people to cowpox as a means of protecting against smallpox. The farmer Benjamin Jesty, for example, had previously inoculated his family with cowpox.

Jenner inferred that milkmaids' exposure to the cowpox protected them from smallpox. If so, he thought, why not inoculate with cowpox, rather than with smallpox, a practice that was then widespread but risky. His gamble was to vaccinate Phipps, and then expose him to inoculation with the smallpox virus six weeks later. Phipps had no reaction to the later smallpox inoculation.

This kind of experiment could not be envisaged in modern times. Jenner studied 23 other people to convince himself the method worked. Jenner was certain he had demonstrated a new technique for the prevention of smallpox and, perhaps unusually, his contemporaries agreed (Jenner 1798). Jenner correctly forecast the elimination of smallpox, and expended much time and energy to promoting his work. In 1840 the British Government banned variolation and replaced it with the new technique—vaccination, the word derived from the Latin for cow (i.e. vacca).

The WHO declared smallpox to be eradicated in 1980, again nearly 200 years later. I believe this is history's supreme medical advance. Smallpox is the only disease to be completely eradicated through deliberate public health endeavour.

This story illustrates the need for scientists and health professionals to listen to the public with an open mind, and to test a hypothesis with an experiment (though do follow the ethical procedures of the times). Finally, it shows that those making a discovery need to be champions of its dissemination and implementation. It also reinforces the long timescales between discovery, and achievement of public health goals.

John Snow and cholera

The classic investigation of cholera by John Snow, one of the founders of epidemiology as we know it, also illustrates important principles. The pandemics of cholera in the nineteenth century sweeping from the east into Europe were causing terror, as thousands died. The description by Roy Porter gives a feel for the terror that an outbreak involving hundreds or thousands of people might cause.

> Internal disturbances, nausea and dizziness led to violent vomiting and diarrhea, with stools turning to a gray liquid (often described as 'rice water') until nothing emerged but water and fragments of intestinal membrane. Extreme muscular cramps followed, with an insatiable desire for water,

followed by a 'sinking stage' during which the pulse dropped and lethargy set in. Dehydrated and nearing death, the patient displayed the classic cholera physiognomy: puckered blue lips in a cadaverous face. There was no agreement about its cause; many treatments were tried; nothing worked.

Roy Porter (1997, p. 403)

At the time, the miasma theory was favoured. Miasma was atmospheric pollution arising from decaying organic matter. Miasma theory was not a sideline idea but the prevailing, dominant view of the time, underpinning much of public health. John Snow investigated this disease for 20 years, culminating in his study of what he described as 'the most terrible outbreak of cholera which ever occurred in this kingdom', the epidemic of cholera in Broad Street, Soho, London (Snow 1949). On reaching the scene, he immediately suspected some contamination of the water in the Broad Street pump, a conclusion he supported by his observations:

♦ that the dead lived or worked near the pump;

♦ a nearby workhouse and brewery had their own water supply and little cholera;

♦ people living far away but drinking Broad Street pump water were afflicted;

♦ the homes of people dying from cholera were clustered around the pump.

In further outbreaks in 1953, Snow undertook studies to establish that people living in the area of the outbreak whose drinking water came from the River Thames upstream of the City of London (supplied by the Lambeth Water Company) had much less cholera than those supplied from the Thames at the City of London (by the Southwark and Vauxhall Company). The former water was less likely to be contaminated by sewage.

Water, not miasma in the air, he concluded, is the source of the morbid matter that causes cholera. He published in 1849 and 1855, and gave evidence to many learned committees, including one in the House of Commons. He was unable to convince those in power and died in 1858 long before his ideas were accepted.

John Snow's now-classic book on cholera cost him two hundred pounds to publish and he sold 56 copies in three years, making 3 pounds, 12 shillings. The bacterium *Vibrio cholera* was identified by Robert Koch as the cause of the disease, but controversy continued thereafter. Only in the late 19th century did Snow's view prevail.

The lessons here are numerous. How much emphasis can we place on either the judgement of peers or committees in assessing the importance of research? It is also worth reflecting on the fact that John Snow was, primarily, an anaesthetist for whom epidemiology was a passion. All doctors, perhaps all health professionals, should see themselves as potential contributors to epidemiology. Perhaps the key lesson is that confronting an established theory (miasma) is a formidable challenge. Snow's development of concepts and methods, and his overall achievement is recognized as foundational for epidemiology.

10.15 **A reflection on the future of epidemiology**

In wealthy industrialized countries where the economy is stable or growing, the challenges for epidemiology will, increasingly, lie in the prevention and control of the diseases of older people—particularly the diseases of degeneration, especially of the brain, cardiovascular system, and bones/joints. The populations of many such countries have low death rates and low fertility rates, so the number of newborns is insufficient. A sustainable population structure is maintained by immigration. Paradoxically, the solutions to these problems of old age may lie in improving maternal, fetal, and infant health.

According to the fetal origins (or developmental origins) hypothesis, the environmental conditions that the fetus (or newborn) experiences programme metabolic adaptation, and lay the foundations for diseases of middle and later life. Relative poverty in early life, and wealth in later life, may be the basis of metabolic maladaptation, triggering diseases such as coronary heart disease and diabetes (the adaptation–dysadaptation hypothesis). These ideas seem important, even though the influences may have been exaggerated. The new field of epigenetics (see glossary and Chapter 3) promises to elucidate the mechanisms underlying the phenomenon. The study of risk factors and disease across the life course, indeed across generations, confronts epidemiology with immense conceptual and technical challenges.

The threats to health in wealthy countries include the fear and actuality of economic and environmental collapse, and the side effects of wealth, for example, obesity, physical inactivity, and even excessive time indoors.

The impact of environmental degradation and climate change is becoming a high priority for epidemiology. This is leading epidemiology to macro-level research and scholarship, away from individuals to ecologies, governmental systems, and industrial policy. In recent years we have seen a rise in studies of health from a global perspective. There is an emerging 'one health' movement which aims to integrate animal and human health. These ideas are combining with expansion of access to digitized health and risk factor data to create a new era where epidemiology works from the micro (e.g. gene products) to the macro (e.g. global burden of disease and risk factors).

In many relatively poor developing countries, the traditional public health problems of poverty (inadequate sanitation, inadequate nutrition, and the communicable diseases) are combining with those of the post-industrial era including cancer, heart disease, stroke, obesity, diabetes, road traffic accidents, environmental damage and climate change, to create a public health nightmare. Nonetheless, health status in most such countries is improving fast, with reduced death rates leading to population expansion even as fertility rates decline. These nations have relatively young populations so maternal and child health and the diseases of middle age are still commanding priorities.

Disentangling the interacting effects of changing circumstances of poverty and wealth in the causation of disease (the topic of health in populations in economic transition) is a vast challenge for epidemiology. In developing countries public health information systems and infrastructures are being put in place and we can see an explosion of epidemiological research. Much of this work is, unsurprisingly, basic epidemiology, based on simple information systems. As research can be done comparatively cheaply in these environments, however, we may well see a rapid expansion of advanced research, for example, clinical trials and biobanks, in developing countries. This work will produce more reliable data on burden of disease, for example, causes of death on a national scale, and help judge whether risk-factor–disease-outcomes, and interventional effects, follow the pattern already demonstrated in the wealthy industrialized countries. We can expect this will be the case, as already demonstrated for some diseases (e.g. lung cancer and CHD).

Economic and health inequalities will surely hold centre stage in public health epidemiology as they have done for two hundred years. Modern communications increasingly expose the injustice of gross waste in some countries, and horrendous poverty in others. The traditional 'solution' based on the moral regeneration of the poor through schooling on sobriety, frugality, and industry has proven insufficient. Poverty is now seen as a potent and direct cause of ill health, and vice versa. Good health, therefore, will be prioritized as a drive to economic prosperity too. Epidemiology has made a vast contribution both in describing such inequalities, and in helping to understand them, given the limitations of studying a matter of such complexity.

The future holds many ethical and technical challenges for epidemiology and health inequalities. In relation to inequalities related to socio-economic status, ethnic group or race, and sexual orientation, we have a tension between a societal structure based on economic inequality and a desire for health equality. Even the internationally renowned Social Determinants of Health mission of the WHO has not been able to find practical solutions in a time when economic inequality is generally rising (Marmot *et al.* 2012).

An interesting question is whether epidemiology should be an advocate for eradication of health inequalities (i.e. participate in the policy debate) or a dispassionate observer (i.e. seek the neutral stance theoretically associated with sciences). The technical challenge is whether epidemiology can provide insights on the mechanisms by which wealth and health interact, and whether it can design and implement efficient and solid trials of interventions that nations will adopt. This work falls into the growing realm of social epidemiology.

The human genome mapping project has reignited the question of the relative importance of genetic and environmental factors as the underlying causes of disease. A long-standing stance that in relation to public health and hence its ally, epidemiology, the environment is predominant, is being questioned and challenged. In assessing disease causation and prevention, even though the environment–gene interaction is all-important, the categorization of disease into 'genetic' or 'environmental' is often the first step. In future, we will see these interactions being pinpointed with new approaches to intervention. A few important principles will help to guide epidemiologists in the current tidal wave of genetic research which is also engulfing epidemiology.

Within populations, the genetic pool changes slowly and genetic variations between populations are small; in contrast, the environment changes rapidly, and differs greatly from place to place. The frequency of occurrence of most common diseases shows massive geographical and rapid time period variation. For instance, heart disease rates in Japan are a fraction of those in Europe. Even more strikingly, rates of many diseases, including heart disease, have been shown to vary as much as threefold between neighbouring areas within cities; areas distinguished by little more than their affluence. Variations in the incidence of cancer are also particularly striking, sometimes 20-fold differences, or even more. Geographical variations between populations appearing over short periods of time are not genetic (unless they reflect microbial genetic changes). Changes in the incidence of disease over brief timespans, say between single generations, point to the dominance of environmental causes. The causes of the current epidemic of obesity and of alcoholic liver disease, both doubling or more in about 10 years in Scotland, are not genetic as newspaper headlines sometimes claim, but environmental. This said, all biological phenomena must involve the genome to confer susceptibility. The new science of epigenetics offers the conceptual route to explaining how this occurs.

The incidence of many diseases has changed dramatically in recent decades. In the United Kingdom, for example, stroke, gastric cancer, chronic bronchitis and, most striking of all, infections including tuberculosis, have been in decline for over 100 years. At the same time, however, asthma, AIDS, skin cancers, and hip fractures are among problems that have increased. The epidemiological pattern of CHD exemplifies the oscillating nature of disease. While rare at the beginning of this century, CHD reached a peak in many industrialized countries in the 1960s, 1970s, or 1980s. However, the cause of this great epidemic has never been fully understood and now that it is in rapid decline the reasons are again much debated (epidemiology points to risk factor changes and medical advances both making major contributions).

The genetic contribution to disease causation is being clarified and there is a revolution in diagnostic and therapeutic medical techniques. However, the genetic revolution is unlikely to match the revolution in public health based on environmental change that has within a few generations added decades to the average human lifespan, which continues to rise fast. Genetic factors provide the stage in the great drama of disease causation, but the environment is still the leading player.

Epidemiology will need to embrace and benefit from the advances in genetics. While it is difficult to predict the changes that the advances in genetics will make to epidemiology, two are clear. First, advances in genetics will undoubtedly have an impact on the management of disease in the future, and ultimately on population disease patterns. As a minimum, genetic methods of diagnosis will raise the number of people known to be at risk, and probably the numbers actually diagnosed. This will not only apply to genetic diseases, but to most (if not all) diseases. The ultimate vision is for a whole genome scan at birth that provides a disease risk profile for everyone at low cost. Technically, this is possible but at present we do not have the understanding to use the information to advance public health. Secondly, epidemiologists will need to be trained in genetics to a much greater depth than at present. One beneficial side effect of genetic epidemiology is that studying small, interacting effects requires large studies. We now have biobanks containing demographic, anthropometric, social, lifestyle, biochemical, and genetic data on millions of people and shortly that will extend to perhaps tens of millions of people. This gold mine for epidemiological research will have benefits beyond genetics. For example, the UK Biobank Study of 500 000 people designed to study gene–environment interactions has given rise to a major paper on the prediction of death using traditional risk factors, a topic distant to its goals. Epidemiology will be able to capitalize on such data sets, especially as these kinds of studies promote easy access to researchers internationally.

Genetic epidemiology will deepen understanding of the interaction between the environment, lifestyle, and the gene, for example, demonstrating why some people have high serum cholesterol and how this causes atherosclerotic diseases. The public health dividend from such knowledge will come from altering the pattern of risk factors in the population. Reducing total serum cholesterol from the currently pathological level of 6 mmol/L and more in some populations, to a physiologically normal value of 4 mmol/L or even less, without mass medication, requires an understanding of how people and societies change. It is remarkable that in the 37 years since my medical graduation I have seen professional perceptions on the level of total cholesterol requiring clinical action drop from about 7 mmol/L, to about 6 mmol/L and now to 5 mmol/L. My figure of a healthy population average of 4 mmol/L still looks radical but it will probably soon be standard. It is not simply genetics and biochemistry that determines an individual and population's serum cholesterol level, but among other factors what and how food is grown, processed, purchased, cooked, and eaten. These factors are determined by more than personal taste. Trade agreements, agricultural policy, land use, farming and fishing, marketing, and economic subsidy are crucial determinants of costs, availability, and consumption. Epidemiologists who wish to study the causes of raised cholesterol in individuals and populations need to study these wider forces.

One of the challenges for epidemiology will be to avoid being deflected from its crucial purpose, which is understanding the causes and consequences of diseases in populations, and acquiring and presenting the evidence advocating appropriate actions to improve health. In addition to maintaining the solid ground of today's epidemiology, we will need to make much clearer and better observations on how diseases are generated through the interactions that people make when living in groups, in other words, the social and population determinants of disease.

I am writing in September 2015 as a refugee crisis engulfs the Middle East, spilling into Europe, and one that may change Europe fundamentally. Vast migrations are taking place, some within countries, for example, the urbanization of the world. The creation of multiethnic, multiracial societies is a fast-moving, probably irreversible trend. The movement and mixing of people from global trade, international travel for work and education, climate change, war and urbanization and intermarriage across ethnic and racial groups heralds exciting opportunities and momentous challenges for epidemiology. Epidemiologists will need to work ever more closely with social scientists who have a sounder understanding of how societies work and can be changed to promote health.

There has been a massive increase in knowledge of methods, which has not been matched with development of theoretical frameworks of health and disease in populations. Development of theory and concepts is a pressing need. Among the priorities are the design and analysis of mixed method studies to examine causality in its true, multilevel, ecological context. The development of graphic methods for outlining causal pathways as the basis for causal work is promising. Large-scale data sets with information at various levels, powerful computer technology, and new forms of analysis are required, and are all in development. Data mining techniques using powerful computers are also available. These may be applied on linked data sets on tens of millions, perhaps hundreds of millions, or even billions, of people. This is the era of 'big data', that is, large, complex data sets that cannot be easily analysed by traditional means. They may require hypothesis-free computer driven analysis. Who knows, such analysis algorithms for epidemiology may become superior to humans, just as those for chess are far superior to the world champion.

Epidemiologists will need political and public support to navigate through ethical and legal constraints on the acquisition and analysis of such data. The impact of such approaches on epidemiology is hard to predict but we should be fearful of being overwhelmed by the discovery of thousands of non-causal associations. An even closer collaboration between epidemiologists and researchers in other fields, including informatics, will be a stimulus to such advances.

Epidemiology as a discipline will continue to grow and will remain a vital area of knowledge for all clinical and public health researchers. Epidemiology will help them to envision the causes of ill health and diseases and the health needs of their populations. From this vision will flow the coherent global, national and local policies, laws, and health-care systems to generate health from the pattern of disease. Perhaps in due course, epidemiology will also lead in generating from all this work, a coherent theory of population health.

Summary

The philosophy and theory underpinning epidemiology is seldom made explicit, and yet it underpins our work, drives change, and guides our paradigms. Epidemiology takes a positivist, philosophical stance grounded in empirical data. The basic theory is that systematic variations in the pattern of health and disease exist in populations and these are a product of differences in the prevalence of, or susceptibility to, the causal factors. Most epidemiology works within the multifactorial risk factor paradigm, though we are progressing towards a multilevel, eco-epidemiology, paradigm.

Epidemiological methods are designed to quantify variations in disease patterns and their potential causes, to establish associations, and to test resultant hypotheses. Diseases arise from complex interactions of causal forces. This knowledge is applied to prevent, control, and treat disease. Influential exemplars, especially on the causes of smoking and heart disease, have established the multifactorial paradigm and epidemiology's place in the modern world. Philosophy, theory, method, exemplars, and application are interdependent.

A vigorous ongoing debate on the future of epidemiology, and the paradigms within which it works, is being fuelled by a combination of the changing pattern of disease; advances in partner disciplines—for example, genetics and informatics; new challenging applications; a perception that the current risk-factor–disease–outcome-based approach is no longer yielding the anticipated advances; and availability of new techniques of data acquisition and analysis. Major changes are anticipated. Already, epidemiology is both broadening and specializing. We can see the further rise of genetic epidemiology and, at the opposite spectrum, of social epidemiology. Life-course epidemiology will encompass both. Epidemiology using data on whole populations, comprising tens of millions, if not hundreds of millions of people, is on the horizon. Studies on billions of people may occur within this century.

While epidemiology is applied in several health domains, it is a prime force in public health, whether influencing policy, strategy and planning decisions, or in disease prevention and control. It is an underpinning (but not sole) science of public health. It also has a big role in clinical medicine, especially in providing evidence. This imposes on epidemiology the need for a code of ethics and good conduct that serves both its scientific and its applied purposes.

Errors in study design, data collection, and interpretation may impair human health. Critical evaluation of research is, therefore, a crucial skill, and essential in the ethical conduct of epidemiology. In evaluating research, epidemiologists need to attend both to its technical excellence, and to its value in the historical, political, social, and geographical context. Epidemiology is rooted in the populations it studies, and in place and time, but it seeks generalization of findings, to improve health more widely.

These obligations require epidemiologists to have an understanding of the wide determinants of health and disease. This can only be achieved by broad studies of our own and related key disciplines combined with following contemporary debates on the future of epidemiology.

Sample question

Question 1 Why is an ethical code important in epidemiology?

Answer Epidemiology studies human (and animal) populations, and deals with matters of life and death. The findings influence both the public directly as they are popular with the media, and indirectly via public health and clinical professional practice and policy. Erroneous information, and erroneous hypotheses and theories, may lead to a great deal of harm. Where information is of value, there is an obligation to bring it to the attention of those who can apply it to benefit human health.

The research process that leads to such information raises all the ethical issues of human research, for example, informed consent by participants, confidentiality of data, autonomy of participants, respect for participants, and equity. Equity means fairness and is an undeveloped issue needing attention, though there have been attempts; for example, the US National Institute of Health requires studies to include men and women and racial/ethnic minority groups.

For these and other related reasons, an ethical code is important in epidemiology.

Acknowledgement

I acknowledge the work of Dr Mike Lavender in helping me think through the text that describes Table 10.1.

References

Barnes, D.E. and Bero, L.A. (1998) Why review articles on the health effects of passive smoking reach different conclusions. *Journal of the American Medical Association*, **279**, 1566–70.

Bhopal, R.S. (1998a) Setting priorities for health care in ethnic minority groups. In: Rawaf, S. and Bahl, V. (eds) *Health Needs Assessment in Ethnic Minority Groups*, pp. 57–64. London, UK: Royal College of Physicians.

Bhopal, R.S. (1998b) The context and role of the American School of Public Health: Implications for the UK. *Journal of Public Health Medicine*, **20**, 144–48.

Bhopal, R.S., Rankin, J., McColl, E., *et al.* (1997) The vexed question of authorship: views of researchers in a British medical faculty. *British Medical Journal*, **314**, 1009–12.

Bottomley, V. (1993) Priority setting in the NHS. Ch 3 in *Rationing in Action*, pp. 25–32. London, UK: BMJ Publishing Group.

Chadwick, J. and Mann, W.N. (1950) *The Medical works of Hippocrates*. Oxford, UK: Blackwell Scientific.

Committee for the Study of the Future of Public Health (Institute of Medicine) (1988) *The Future of Public Health*. Washington, DC: National Academy Press.

Committee of Inquiry (1988) *Public Health in England*. London, UK: HMSO.

Edwards, R., Pless-Mulloli, T., Howel, D., *et al.* (2006) Does living near heavy industry cause lung cancer in women? A case control study using life grid interviews. *Thorax* **62**, 1076–82.

Horton, R. (1998) The unmasked carnival of science. *Lancet*, **351**, 688–9.

Jenner, E. (1798) *An inquiry in to the causes and effects of the variolae vaccine.* Excerpt in Buck *et al.* 1988, pp. 31–32.

Jones, J.H. (1993) *Bad Blood: The Tuskegee Syphilis Experiment*, 2nd edn. New York, NY: Free Press.

Kiple, K.F. and King, V.H. (1981) *Another Dimension to the Black Diaspora.* London, UK: Cambridge University Press.

Krieger, N. (1992) The making of public health data: paradigms, politics, and policy. *Journal of Public Health Policy*, **65**, 412–27.

Krieger, N. (2011) *Epidemiology and the People's Health: Theory and Context.* New York, NY: Oxford University Press.

Kuhn, T.S. (1996) *The Structure of Scientific Revolutions*, 3rd edn. Chicago, IL: The University of Chicago Press.

Lind, J. (1753) *A Treatise of the Scurvy in three parts, containing an inquiry into the nature, causes, and cure of the scurvy.* Excerpted from James Lind, *A Treatise of the Scurvy in Three Parts, Containing an enquiry into the nature, causes and cure of that disease, together with a critical and chronological view of what has been published on the subject.* Edinburgh, UK: Sands Murray and Cochran, and reprinted in Buck *et al.* 1988, pp. 20–3.

Marmot, M., Allen, J., Bell, R., Bloomer, E., Goldblatt, P. (2012) WHO European review of social determinants of health and the health divide. *Lancet*, **380**, 1011–29.

Morris, J.N. (1964) *Uses of Epidemiology*, 2nd edn. Baltimore, MD: The Williams and Wilkins Company.

Osborne, N.G. and Feit, M.D. (1992) The use of race in medical research. *Journal of the American Medical Association*, **267**, 275–9.

Porta, M. (2014) *A Dictionary of Epidemiology*, 6th edn. New York, NY: Oxford University Press.

Porter, R. (1997) *The Greatest Benefit to Mankind: A Medical Hhistory of Humanity from Antiquity to the Present.* London, UK: Harper Collins.

Rothman, K.J. (1986) *Modern Epidemiology*, 1st edn. Boston, MA: Little, Brown.

Rothman, K., Adami, H. and Trichopoulos, D. (1998) Should the mission of epidemiology include the eradication of poverty? *Lancet*, **352**, 810–13.

Skrabanek, P. and McCormick, J. (1992) *Follies and Fallacies in Medicine*, 2nd edn. Chippenham, UK: Tarragon Press. (Available at: http://chagall.med.cornell.edu/Skrabanek/Follies-and-Fallacies-in-Medicine.pdf),

Smith, A. (1978) The epidemiological basis of community medicine. In: Bennett, A.E. (ed.) *Recent Advances in Community Medicine*, pp. 1–10. Edinburgh, UK: Longman.

Snow, J. (1949) The cholera near Golden Square (extracted from *Snow on Cholera*, Cambridge, UK: Hybrid University Press.) Reprinted in Buck *et al.* 1988, pp. 415–18. *The Challenge of Epidemiology: Issues and Selected Readings*, pp. 415–18. Washington DC, WA: Pan American Health Organization.

Susser, M. (1985) Epidemiology in the United States after World War II: the evolution of technique. *Epidemiologic Reviews*, **7**, 147–77.

Susser, M. and Susser, E. (1996a) Choosing a future for epidemiology: II from black box to Chinese boxes and eco-epidemiology. *American Journal of Public Health*, **86**, 674–7.

Susser, M. and Susser, E. (1996b) Choosing a future of epidemiology: I eras and paradigms. *American Journal of Public Health*, **86**, 668–73.

Appendix 1

Possible curriculum for taught courses for undergraduate and postgraduate students and in continuing education

This book assumes literacy and numeracy at the level expected in a 16–17-year-old person who studies maths, English and science. No exposure to medicine, related professions, or medical sciences is necessary, though it is helpful. The book is designed for postgraduate and continuing professional education but has proven itself useful in a wider arena.

This book is primarily aimed at the Masters level student needing a broad grasp of the subject, and especially from a public health perspective.

There is no agreed standard curriculum or order of teaching in epidemiology. Skilful and experienced teachers will be able to match learners' needs to the time and resources available. In the second edition of this book, I included a table relating chapter and section headings to possible course content for postgraduate or continuing education level (25 contact hours and also for 20 contact hours), for undergraduates (10 contact hours) and for policy-makers and health service managers (four contact hours). This table has been removed in this edition but some readers might still find it useful (e-mail me for a copy at raj.bhopal@ed.ac.uk).

I have instead expanded my general observations on teaching epidemiology, in the light of several recent curriculum reviews especially targeted at Master of Public Health (MPH) level courses. These observations are personal and teachers will tailor courses to follow their own judgements.

The key objective for postgraduate students starting their studies is a thorough but broad grasp of the strengths and weaknesses of the epidemiological approach and the principles of sound data interpretation. Recent curricular reviews of MPH level courses have endorsed the approach taken by me, e.g. study design is not the dominant requirement at this level. Indeed, some recent reviews give little or no prominence to this at all. This book includes all the material required at this level and more.

I make the reasonable assumption that MPH students will undertake other relevant course,s e.g. on medical statistics and social sciences and these studies will dovetail with epidemiology. I have introduced many of the necessary principles and background required here.

Undergraduate students need to see the scope of the subject and its potential relevance to their own studies and subjects. Above all, the undergraduate's interest must be captured and held. Techniques are unlikely to be important for most such students (until they are doing their own projects, when they need to know a limited range of methods and techniques). The achievements of epidemiology—many of which are highlighted here—can inspire undergraduates. These however need to be balanced by the limitations and errors.

Policy-makers and managers need to see the grand scope of the subject and its potential relevance to the solution of their health and health service challenges. The route to this will usually lie with examples of the application of epidemiology in health services contexts and in health and health care policy. In addition, they need to grasp the core concepts and definitions to allow them to read reports and general papers. These concepts will include topics like error, rates, standardization, association, confounding (as not comparing like-with-like), and judging causality.

It is unlikely any teacher will need or want to teach everything in the book. After all, we teachers need to inculcate habits of self-learning among students. To teach on most of the content of the book is feasible (in my experience in both Masters and continuing education courses) in about 12 lectures (50 minutes each) with 12 practical sessions of the same length. This suits courses based on 15-week semesters as these usually have 12 or 13 teaching weeks. Teachers running shorter courses will need to make choices on material to be left out, or to be identified as for private study.

What about the order of teaching and learning? I have ensured that every chapter is independent. I have also introduced in Chapter 1 enough of the core ideas and methods to permit an understanding of later chapters. Teachers can follow their preferences. I have started with general principles and approaches (Chapters 1–5), applications, techniques and methods (Chapters 6–9) and then back to general principles (Chapter 10). This said, there is no chapter that is devoid of methods, and equally, none without principles. This order has worked for me both for Masters' students studying over 15 weeks and professionals learning epidemiology in one week. If you don't have a preference, you can follow the order of the book.

Many courses are taught online. The scope for student–teacher interaction is more limited than in classroom teaching. I have written the book to be an interactive experience so that online students may feel they are communicating directly with their teacher.